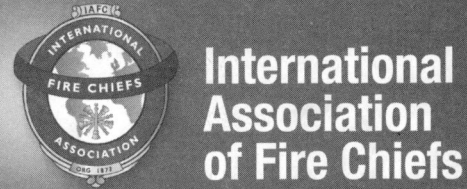
International Association of Fire Chiefs

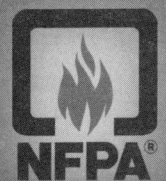
National Fire Protection Association

Fundamentals of Fire Fighter Skills

FOURTH EDITION

Student Workbook

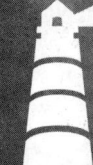

JONES & BARTLETT LEARNING

Jones & Bartlett Learning
World Headquarters
5 Wall Street
Burlington, MA 01803
978-443-5000
info@jblearning.com
www.jblearning.com
www.psglearning.com

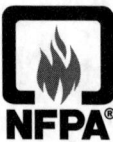

National Fire Protection Association
1 Batterymarch Park
Quincy, MA 02169
www.NFPA.org

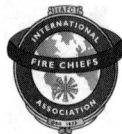

International Association of Fire Chiefs
4025 Fair Ridge Drive
Fairfax, VA 22033
www.IAFC.org

Jones & Bartlett Learning books and products are available through most bookstores and online booksellers. To contact the Jones & Bartlett Learning Public Safety Group directly, call 800-832-0034, fax 978-443-8000, or visit our website, www.psglearning.com.

> Substantial discounts on bulk quantities of Jones & Bartlett Learning publications are available to corporations, professional associations, and other qualified organizations. For details and specific discount information, contact the special sales department at Jones & Bartlett Learning via the above contact information or send an email to specialsales@jblearning.com.

Copyright © 2020 by Jones & Bartlett Learning, LLC, an Ascend Learning Company and the National Fire Protection Association (NFPA).

All rights reserved. No part of the material protected by this copyright may be reproduced or utilized in any form, electronic or mechanical, including photocopying, recording, or by any information storage and retrieval system, without written permission from the copyright owner.

The content, statements, views, and opinions herein are the sole expression of the respective authors and not that of Jones & Bartlett Learning, LLC. Reference herein to any specific commercial product, process, or service by trade name, trademark, manufacturer, or otherwise does not constitute or imply its endorsement or recommendation by Jones & Bartlett Learning, LLC and such reference shall not be used for advertising or product endorsement purposes. All trademarks displayed are the trademarks of the parties noted herein. *Fundamentals of Fire Fighter Skills, Fourth Edition Student Workbook* is an independent publication and has not been authorized, sponsored, or otherwise approved by the owners of the trademarks or service marks referenced in this product.

There may be images in this book that feature models; these models do not necessarily endorse, represent, or participate in the activities represented in the images. Any screenshots in this product are for educational and instructive purposes only. Any individuals and scenarios featured in the case studies throughout this product may be real or fictitious, but are used for instructional purposes only.

The NFPA, IAFC, and the publisher have made every effort to ensure that contributors to *Fundamentals of Fire Fighter Skills, Fourth Edition Student Workbook* materials are knowledgeable authorities in their fields. Readers are nevertheless advised that the statements and opinions are provided as guidelines and should not be construed as official NFPA and IAFC policy. The recommendations in this publication or the accompanying resource manual do not indicate an exclusive course of action. Variations taking into account the individual circumstances, and local protocols may be appropriate. The NFPA, IAFC, and the publisher disclaim any liability or responsibility for the consequences of any action taken in reliance on these statements or opinions.

Production Credits

General Manager and Executive Publisher: Kimberly Brophy
VP, Product Development: Christine Emerton
Executive Editor: Bill Larkin
Director, Relationship Management: Carolyn Pershouse
Director of Marketing Operations: Brian Rooney
VP, Manufacturing and Inventory Control: Therese Connell
Composition: S4Carlisle Publishing Services
Project Management: S4Carlisle Publishing Services
Cover Design: Kristin E. Parker
Text Design: Kristin E. Parker
Rights & Media Manager: Shannon Sheehan
Rights & Media Specialist: Thais Miller

Editorial Credits
Authors: Rudy Horist and Matt Muldoon

Cover Image (Title Page, Part Opener, Chapter Opener): © Glen E. Ellman
Printing and Binding: Sheridan Saline
Cover Printing: Sheridan Saline

ISBN: 978-1-284-14699-8

6048

Printed in the United States of America
26 25 24   10 9 8 7 6 5 4

Contents

> Note to the student: Consult your instructor for access to the Student Workbook Answer Key.

Section I Fire Fighter I.. 2
Chapter 1 The Fire Service 2
Chapter 2 Fire Fighter Health and Safety.. 8
Chapter 3 Personal Protective Equipment 16
Chapter 4 Fire Service Communications 40
Chapter 5 Fire Behavior 48
Chapter 6 Building Construction 56
Chapter 7 Portable Fire Extinguishers.. 64
Chapter 8 Fire Fighter Tools and Equipment 78
Chapter 9 Ropes and Knots.. 86
Chapter 10 Forcible Entry 102
Chapter 11 Ladders.. 116
Chapter 12 Search and Rescue 134
Chapter 13 Ventilation... 152
Chapter 14 Water Supply Systems.. 170
Chapter 15 Fire Hose, Appliances, and Nozzles 184
Chapter 16 Supply Line and Attack Line Evolutions 198
Chapter 17 Fire Suppression.. 218
Chapter 18 Fire Fighter Survival 238
Chapter 19 Salvage and Overhaul 256
Chapter 20 Fire Fighter Rehabilitation 272
Chapter 21 Wildland and Ground Cover Fires........................... 278

Section II Fire Fighter II 286
Chapter 22 Establishing and Transferring Command................. 286
Chapter 23 Advanced Fire Suppression 298
Chapter 24 Vehicle Rescue and Extrication 312
Chapter 25 Assisting Special Rescue Teams 326
Chapter 26 Fire Detection, Suppression, and Smoke Control Systems 334
Chapter 27 Fire and Life Safety Initiatives 342
Chapter 28 Fire Origin and Cause 350

Workbook Activities

The following activities have been designed to help you. Your instructor may require you to complete some or all of these activities as a regular part of your fire fighter training program. You are encouraged to complete any activity your instructor does not assign to you, as a way to enhance your learning in the classroom.

Chapter Review

The following exercises provide an opportunity to refresh your knowledge of this chapter.

Matching

Match each of the terms in the left column to the appropriate definition in the right column.

_____ 1. Fireplug   **A.** The position responsible for a fire company and for coordinating activities of that company among the shifts

_____ 2. Doff   **B.** A valve installed to control water accessed from wooden pipes

_____ 3. SCBA   **C.** Guiding and directing fire fighters to do what their fire department expects of them

_____ 4. Battalion chief   **D.** To take off

_____ 5. Fire hook   **E.** The position responsible for operating the fire apparatus

_____ 6. Don   **F.** A tool used to pull down burning structures

_____ 7. Safety officer   **G.** To put on

_____ 8. Captain   **H.** The position often in charge of running calls and supervising multiple stations or districts within a city

_____ 9. Driver/operator   **I.** The position with the authority to stop any firefighting activity until it can be done safely and correctly

_____ 10. Discipline   **J.** Air packs used by fire fighters to enter a hazardous atmosphere

Multiple Choice

Read each item carefully, and then select the best response.

_____ 1. To provide a uniform way to deal with emergency situations, departments develop and follow
  A. laws.
  B. regulations.
  C. standard operating procedures (SOPs).
  D. policies.

CHAPTER 1

_____ 2. In some fire departments, the preferred terminology for standard operating procedures is
   A. policies.
   B. regulations.
   C. rules.
   D. suggested operating guidelines.

_____ 3. The majority of fire departments consist of
   A. all career fire fighters.
   B. mostly career fire fighters.
   C. mostly volunteer fire fighters.
   D. all volunteer fire fighters.

_____ 4. The organizational structure of a fire department consists of a(n)
   A. chain of custody.
   B. incident management system.
   C. chain of command.
   D. division of labor.

_____ 5. New fire fighters usually report to a
   A. lieutenant.
   B. captain.
   C. battalion chief.
   D. division chief.

_____ 6. A comprehensive all-hazard approach of programs, activities, and services to reduce the loss of life and property is known as
   A. Learn Not to Burn.
   B. All Hazard Planning.
   C. Community Risk Reduction.
   D. Risk and Hazard Assessment.

_____ 7. In the 1700s, a fire mark indicated
   A. the homeowner had fire insurance.
   B. the homeowner was a career fire fighter.
   C. the homeowner was a volunteer fire fighter.
   D. the home had a previous fire.

_____ 8. The overall responsibility for the administration and operations of the department belongs to the
   A. battalion chief.
   B. chief of the department.
   C. incident commander.
   D. government.

_____ 9. The first water system valves or fire hydrants used by fire fighters were called
   A. fire taps.
   B. water valves.
   C. water boxes.
   D. fireplugs.

____ 10. The theory that each fire fighter answers to only one supervisor is referred to as
   A. unity of command.
   B. span of control.
   C. division of labor.
   D. discipline.

____ 11. Which of the following is not a form of discipline?
   A. SOPs
   B. Policies
   C. Span of control
   D. Training

____ 12. Augustus Caesar created what was probably the first fire department, called the Familia Publica, in
   A. 100 B.C.
   B. 24 B.C.
   C. 1 B.C.
   D. 10 A.D.

____ 13. The type of smoke detector that is activated by smaller, invisible products of combustion is a(n)
   A. combination alarm.
   B. photoelectric alarm.
   C. ionization alarm.
   D. combustion alarm.

____ 14. The first fire insurance company in the United States was established in 1736
   A. by George Washington.
   B. by Benjamin Franklin.
   C. in Charleston, South Carolina.
   D. by the Alexandria Fire Department.

____ 15. Colonial fire fighters had limited equipment. Most departments then had only buckets, ladders, and
   A. hand-powered pumpers.
   B. horse-drawn water carriages.
   C. fire hooks.
   D. hoses.

____ 16. The company responsible for securing a water source, deploying handlines, and putting water on the fire is the
   A. truck company.
   B. brush company.
   C. water company.
   D. engine company.

____ 17. The type of smoke detector that is activated by larger, visible products of combustion is a(n)
   A. photoelectric alarm.
   B. combination alarm.
   C. remote alarm.
   D. combination alarm.

____ 18. The company that specializes in forcible entry, ventilation, roof operations, search and rescue, and ground ladders is the
   A. truck company.
   B. brush company.
   C. water company.
   D. engine company.

____ 19. In 1871, a historic fire, which was believed to have been started by a cow, burned for three days, destroyed more than 2000 acres and 17,000 homes, and killed 300 people. This was the
   A. Great Chicago Fire.
   B. Peshtigo Fire.
   C. Green Bay Burn.
   D. Alexandria Fire.

_____ 20. The fire service draws its authority from the governing entity, and the head of the department is accountable to the
   A. fire chief.
   B. insurance companies.
   C. leaders of the governing body.
   D. civil servants.

Vocabulary
Define the following terms using the space provided.

1. Safety officer:

   _____
   _____
   _____

2. Paramedic:

   _____
   _____
   _____

3. Incident commander (IC):

   _____
   _____
   _____

4. Company officer:

   _____
   _____
   _____

5. Training officer:

   _____
   _____
   _____

Fill-In
Read each item carefully and then complete the statement by filling in the missing word(s).

1. _____ is a national strategic planning process for fire loss prevention.

2. When multiple agencies work together, a unified command system must be established. This system is referred to as the _____.

3. _____ provide specific information on the actions that should be taken to accomplish a certain task.

4. The first fire regulations in North America were established in Boston, Massachusetts, when the city banned _____ and _____.

5. _____ personnel administer prehospital care to people who are sick and injured.

6. The first volunteer fire company began in Philadelphia in 1735, under the leadership of _____.

7. Frederick Graff, sr., a fire fighter in New York City, developed the first _____ _____ in 1817.

8. The _____ developed the first municipal water systems.

9. In Washington, D.C., _____ _____ _____ were introduced as the first communication tool used to send coded telegraph signals to the fire departments.

10. Today, U.S. building codes are developed by the _____ and the ICC, the same organizations that develop U.S. fire codes and standards.

True/False

If you believe the statement to be more true than false, write the letter "T" in the space provided. If you believe the statement to be more false than true, write the letter "F."

1. _____ Captains report directly to chiefs.
2. _____ Covering a fire to ensure a low burn is called "banking."
3. _____ George Washington established one of the first fire departments in Alexandria, Virginia, in 1765.
4. _____ The fire fighter is responsible for dispatching units to an incident.
5. _____ The Peshtigo fire storm jumped the 60-mile-wide Green Bay and continued to burn on Wisconsin's northeast peninsula.
6. _____ The organizational structure of a fire department consists of a division of labor.
7. _____ The battalion chief is the second rank of promotion, responsible for managing a fire company.
8. _____ "Info techs" serve as liaisons between the IC and the news media.
9. _____ Today, almost all fire protection in the United States is funded directly or indirectly through tax dollars.
10. _____ Photoelectric smoke alarms react more quickly to fast-burning fires than ionization smoke alarms.

Short Answer

Complete this section with short written answers using the space provided.

1. Identify and describe the role of five companies common to most fire departments.

   _____
   _____
   _____
   _____

2. Identify the five E's of fire prevention.

   _____
   _____
   _____
   _____

3. Identify the four basic management principles utilized in most fire departments.

_____
_____
_____
_____

4. List the six basic steps of the Community Risk Reduction (CRR) process.

_____
_____
_____
_____
_____

5. Outline the roles and responsibilities of Fire Fighter II.

_____
_____
_____
_____

Fire Alarms

The following real case scenarios will give you an opportunity to explore the concerns associated with the history and orientation of the fire service. Read each scenario, then answer each question in detail.

1. You have chosen the fire services as a career and have worked hard to get to this point. You successfully completed the entry requirement and have been issued your bunker gear and uniform. Given that you need to keep yourself on target to become a proud and accomplished fire fighter, what must you do to succeed?

_____
_____
_____
_____
_____

2. You are outside the fire station washing the fire truck when you are approached by three children on bicycles. None of the children is wearing a helmet. They ask you if you will show them the truck and the station. How should you proceed?

_____
_____
_____
_____
_____

Fire Fighter Health and Safety

Workbook Activities

The following activities have been designed to help you. Your instructor may require you to complete some or all of these activities as a regular part of your fire fighter training program. You are encouraged to complete any activity your instructor does not assign to you, as a way to enhance your learning in the classroom.

Chapter Review

The following exercises provide an opportunity to refresh your knowledge of this chapter.

Matching

Match each of the terms in the left column to the appropriate definition in the right column.

_____ 1. Portable radio

_____ 2. Critical incident stress debriefing (CISD)

_____ 3. Employee assistance program (EAP)

_____ 4. Rapid intervention crew

_____ 5. Freelancing

_____ 6. Occupational Safety and Health Administration (OSHA)

_____ 7. Personnel accountability system

_____ 8. Rehabilitation

A. The dangerous practice of acting independently of command instructions

B. A minimum of two fully equipped personnel who are on-site, in a ready state, for immediate rescue of injured or trapped fire fighters

C. Readily identifies the locations and functions of all fire fighters at an incident

D. The federal agency that regulates worker safety and, in some cases, responder safety

E. Fire service programs that provide confidential help to fire fighters with personal issues

F. A portable communication device used by fire fighters

G. A process to provide periods of rest and recovery for emergency workers during an incident

H. Postincident meeting designed to assist rescue personnel in dealing with psychological trauma

Multiple Choice

Read each item carefully, and then select the best response.

_____ 1. A process to provide periods of rest and recovery for emergency workers during an incident is called
   A. recon.
   B. rehabilitation.
   C. RIC.
   D. relegate.

CHAPTER 2

_____ 2. Team members operating within a structure should maintain _____ contact with one another at all times.
   A. voice
   B. vision
   C. physical
   D. All of the above

_____ 3. According to the NFPA, approximately what percentage of fire fighter deaths occurs during training?
   A. 5 percent
   B. 14 percent
   C. 20 percent
   D. 25 percent

_____ 4. What is the second most common cause of fire fighter deaths?
   A. Explosions
   B. Exposure to diseases
   C. Motor vehicle crashes
   D. Roof collapses

_____ 5. The system in which two fire fighters work as a team for safety purposes is referred to as the
   A. incident management system.
   B. buddy system.
   C. personnel accountability system.
   D. personal alert system.

_____ 6. What is considered the leading cause of death among fire fighters?
   A. Vehicle accidents
   B. Smoke inhalation
   C. Heart attack
   D. Cancer

_____ 7. The written rules and procedures that outline how to perform various functions and operations are the
   A. general operating guidelines.
   B. Code of Federal Regulations.
   C. incident management system (IMS).
   D. standard operating procedures (SOPs).

_____ 8. The National Fire Protection Association (NFPA) standard regarding fire department occupational safety, health, and wellness is standard
   A. 1001.
   B. 1403.
   C. 1500.
   D. 1582.

_____ 9. According to the Firefighter Cancer Support Network, fire fighters have a _____ percent higher risk of being diagnosed with cancer than the general U.S. population.
   A. 5
   B. 9
   C. 15
   D. 33

_____ 10. Most fire fighter injuries and deaths are the result of
   A. equipment failure.
   B. preventable situations.
   C. burns and explosions.
   D. hazardous materials.

_____ 11. The National Fallen Firefighters Foundation has developed a fire fighter safety initiative designed to raise awareness of life safety issues. This program is known as
   A. Everyone Goes Home.
   B. NFA Safety.
   C. NFPA Safety.
   D. OSHA and Safety.

_____ 12. A good guideline is to consume _____ ounces of water for every 5 to 10 minutes of physical exertion.
   A. 1 to 2
   B. 5 to 8
   C. 8 to 10
   D. 10 to 12

_____ 13. In recent years, there have been _____ fire fighter suicides compared to line-of-duty deaths.
   A. more
   B. less
   C. just as many
   D. almost as many

_____ 14. When working at the scene of a highway incident, fire fighters should wear their normal PPE and
   A. helmets.
   B. high-visibility safety vests.
   C. roadway extrication gloves.
   D. SCBA.

_____ 15. When the speed of a vehicle doubles, the force exerted increases by a factor of _____.
   A. 2.
   B. 3.
   C. 4.
   D. 10.

Vocabulary

Define the following terms using the space provided.

1. Personnel accountability system:

   _____

   _____

   _____

2. Standard operating procedures (SOPs):

_____
_____
_____

3. Employee assistance program (EAP):

_____
_____
_____

4. The 16 Firefighter Life Safety Initiatives:

_____
_____
_____

5. Safety Officer:

_____
_____
_____

Fill-In

Read each item carefully, and then complete the statement by filling in the missing word(s).

1. _____ collisions are a major cause of fire fighter fatalities.

2. The _____ has developed programs with the goal of reducing line-of-duty deaths.

3. Some cancers do not present for _____ years or more after exposure to a carcinogen.

4. The _____ officer has the authority to stop any activity that is judged to be unsafe.

5. The patterns that develop during training continue during actual emergency incidents. Thus, developing _____, _____, _____ during training helps ensure safety later.

6. The National Fire Fighter _____-_____ provides a method for reporting situations that could have resulted in injuries or deaths.

7. All fire fighters—whether career or volunteer—should spend at least _____ _____ each day in physical fitness training.

8. _____ is the leading cause of death in the United States and a leading cause among fire fighters.

9. When fire fighters make independent decisions or do not follow command instructions, they are taking part in the dangerous practice of _____.

10. Emergency vehicle operators are subject to all _____ _____, unless a specific exemption is made.

True/False

If you believe the statement to be more true than false, write the letter "T" in the space provided. If you believe the statement to be more false than true, write the letter "F."

1. _____ A prompt response is just as high a priority as a safe response.
2. _____ Most fire departments have employee assistance programs to provide counseling services to support fire fighters.
3. _____ Freelancing is a good method of discovering new firefighting techniques.
4. _____ Most fire fighter injuries and deaths are the result of preventable situations.
5. _____ Every fire department must have a personnel accountability system.
6. _____ Members of rapid intervention teams are the first fire fighters to enter a structure in an emergency operation.
7. _____ Even with an emergency driving exemption, the operator can be found criminally or civilly liable if involved in a crash.
8. _____ Emergency vehicle operators are subject to all traffic regulations unless a specific exemption is made.
9. _____ On the fire ground, the company officer must always know where his or her teams are and what they are doing.
10. _____ Fire fighters need not be aware of their surroundings when performing their assigned tasks at an emergency scene.

Short Answer

Complete this section with short written answers using the space provided.

1. Identify five of the nine Guidelines for Safe Emergency Vehicle Response.

_____
_____
_____
_____

2. Describe the purpose of a critical incident stress debriefing (CISD).

_____
_____
_____
_____

3. Identify four guidelines to stay safe, both on and off the job.

___

4. Identify the four major components of a successful safety program.

___

5. Identify three groups that fire fighters must always consider when ensuring safety at the scene.

___

Fire Alarms
The following real case scenario will give you an opportunity to explore the concerns associated with fire fighter qualifications and safety. Read the scenario, and then answer the question in detail.

1. Your company officer has requested you to give a morning training lecture on the common causes of fire fighter deaths. Identify the common causes of fire fighter death, and outline some of the information you can use to support your lecture. What can you do to reduce the chance of death or injury?

___

2. You are asked to talk with a recruit fire fighter class on the topic of cancer in the fire service. What are the main points you will discuss with these new fire fighters?

_____
_____
_____
_____
_____
_____

Skill Drills

Skill Drill 2-1: Mounting Apparatus Fire Fighter I, NFPA 1001:4.3.2
Test your knowledge of the skill drill by filling in the correct words in the photo captions.

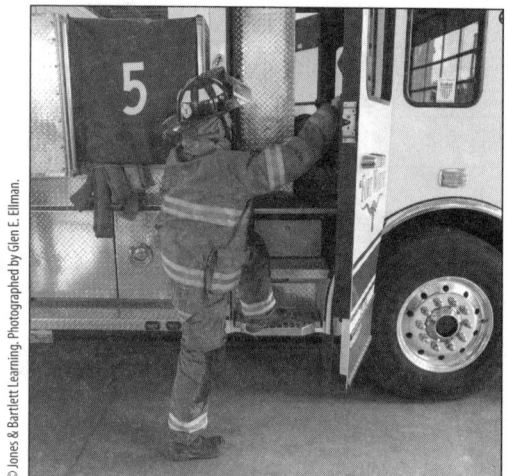

1. When mounting (climbing aboard) fire apparatus, always have at least one hand firmly grasping a _____ at least one foot firmly placed on a _____ surface. Maintain the one-hand-and-one-foot placement until you are _____.

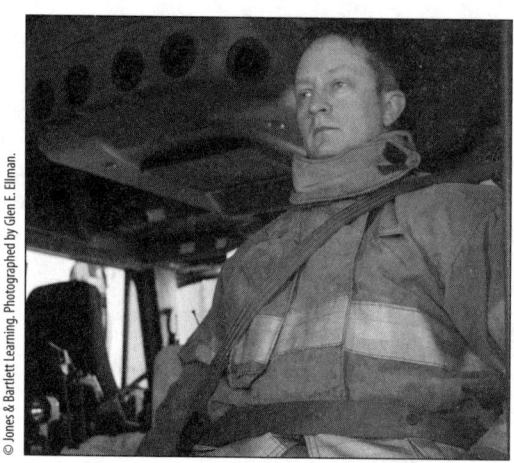

2. Fasten your _____ and leave it fastened until the apparatus is stopped at its destination. Don any other required safety equipment for the response, such as _____ protection and intercom systems.

Skill Drill 2-2: Dismounting a Stopped Apparatus Fire Fighter I, NFPA 1001: 4.3.2
Test your knowledge of the skill drill by filling in the correct words in the photo captions.

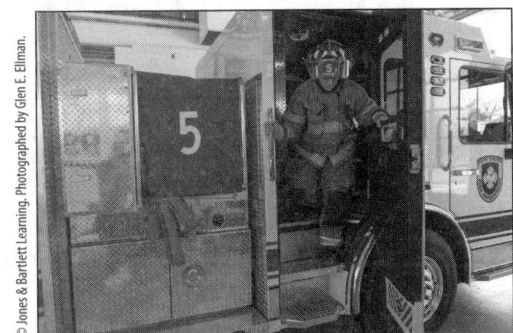

1. Become familiar with your riding _____ and the safest way to dismount.

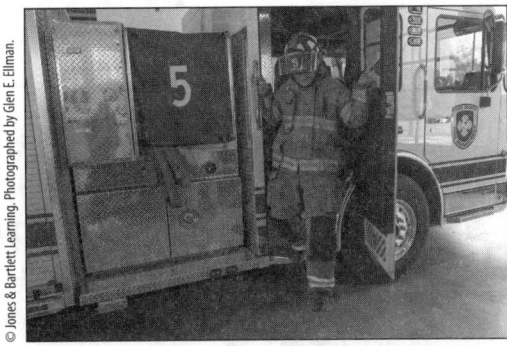

2. Maintain the one-hand-and-one-foot placement when leaving the apparatus, especially on _____ or potentially icy roadway surfaces.

Personal Protective Equipment

Workbook Activities

The following activities have been designed to help you. Your instructor may require you to complete some or all of these activities as a regular part of your fire fighter training program. You are encouraged to complete any activity your instructor does not assign to you, as a way to enhance your learning in the classroom.

Chapter Review

The following exercises provide an opportunity to refresh your knowledge of this chapter.

Matching
Match each of the terms in the left column to the appropriate definition in the right column.

_____ 1. Personal alert safety system
_____ 2. Cascade system
_____ 3. Self-contained breathing apparatus (SCBA)
_____ 4. Nomex®
_____ 5. IDLH
_____ 6. Don
_____ 7. Doff
_____ 8. Compressor
_____ 9. Open-circuit breathing apparatus
_____ 10. Full Face piece

A. A flame-resistant synthetic material
B. To put on an item of clothing or equipment
C. To take off an item of clothing or equipment
D. Several large storage cylinders of compressed breathing air connected by a high-pressure manifold system
E. Filters atmospheric air, compresses it to a high pressure, and transfers it to the SCBA cylinders
F. An electronic device that sounds a loud audible signal when a fire fighter becomes trapped or injured
G. An apparatus in which a tank of compressed air provides the breathing air supply for the user, and exhaled air is released into the atmosphere through a one-way valve
H. A component of the SCBA that covers the entire face
I. Provides respiratory protection by giving the fire fighter an independent, limited air supply
J. Any condition that would pose an immediate or delayed threat to life, cause irreversible adverse health effects, or interfere with an individual's ability to escape unaided from a hazardous environment

Multiple Choice
Read each item carefully, and then select the best response.

_____ 1. An electronic semiconductor that emits a single-color light when activated is an LED, which is an acronym for
   A. light-emergent device.
   B. light-exiting device.
   C. light-emitting diode.
   D. laser-emitting diode.

CHAPTER 3

_____ 2. PBI®, Kevlar®, and Nomex® are materials used in the construction of
   A. personal protective clothing.
   B. firefighting ropes.
   C. communications equipment.
   D. the buddy system.

_____ 3. In general, an SCBA weighs at least
   A. 25 pounds (11.34 kilograms).
   B. 30 pounds (13.61 kilograms).
   C. 40 pounds (18.14 kilograms).
   D. 45 pounds (20.41 kilograms).

_____ 4. An SCBA in which exhaled air is released into the atmosphere and is not reused is a(n)
   A. closed-circuit breathing apparatus.
   B. cascade system.
   C. open-circuit breathing apparatus.
   D. supplied-air apparatus.

_____ 5. What provides the frame for mounting the other working parts of the SCBA?
   A. Regulator
   B. Backpack
   C. Harness
   D. Straps and belt

_____ 6. During operating mode, if the SCBA regulator fails to function properly, what releases a constant flow of breathing air into the face piece?
   A. Respirator
   B. Air line
   C. Purge valve
   D. PBI®

_____ 7. Putting on an item of clothing or equipment is called
   A. doffing.
   B. freelancing.
   C. prepping.
   D. donning.

_____ 8. Which NFPA standard applies to turnout coats used for structural firefighting?
   A. NFPA 1776
   B. NFPA 1492
   C. NFPA 1971
   D. NFPA 1963

_____ 9. Which of the following is designed to help colleagues locate a downed fire fighter by sending out a loud audible signal?
   A. Respirator
   B. PASS device
   C. SCBA regulator
   D. LED

_____ 10. Oxygen deficiency occurs when the atmosphere's oxygen level drops below
   A. 19.5 percent.
   B. 21 percent.
   C. 9 percent.
   D. 6 percent.

_____ 11. Donning SCBA must be done in a specific order, and quickly. Fire fighters should be able to don their SCBA in
   A. 30 seconds.
   B. 45 seconds.
   C. 60 seconds.
   D. 120 seconds.

_____ 12. Most fire deaths are caused by
   A. smoke inhalation.
   B. burns.
   C. poisonous gases.
   D. disorientation.

_____ 13. The part of the SCBA face piece that comes in contact with the skin is made of
   A. rubber or silicon.
   B. PBI Kevlar®.
   C. cotton.
   D. Nomex®.

_____ 14. The U.S. Department of Transportation requires this kind of testing on a periodic basis to ensure that SCBA cylinders are in good working condition.
   A. Thread
   B. Hydrostatic
   C. NIOSH
   D. Standard operating procedure

_____ 15. An SCBA designed to recycle the user's exhaled air is a(n)
   A. closed-circuit breathing apparatus.
   B. cascade system.
   C. open-circuit breathing apparatus.
   D. supplied-air apparatus.

_____ 16. The interior atmosphere of a burning building is considered to be
   A. safe.
   B. warm.
   C. NIMS.
   D. IDLH.

_____ 17. Which part of the personal protective equipment is worn over the head and under the helmet to protect the neck and ears?
   A. Helmet shell
   B. Protective hood
   C. Bunker hood
   D. Face piece

_____ 18. The straps and fasteners used to attach the SCBA to the fire fighter are part of the
   A. face piece.
   B. backpack.
   C. bunker coat.
   D. harness.

_____ 19. The device on an SCBA that measures and displays the amount of pressure currently in the cylinder is the
   A. personal safety gauge.
   B. pressure gauge.
   C. SCBA regulator.
   D. air line.

_____ 20. What very toxic gas is commonly present in smoke?
  A. Carbon monoxide
  B. Hydrogen cyanide
  C. Phosgene
  D. All of the above

Vocabulary

Define the following terms using the space provided.

1. Smoke particles:

   _____
   _____
   _____

2. Oxygen deficiency:

   _____
   _____
   _____

3. National Institute for Occupational Safety and Health (NIOSH):

   _____
   _____
   _____

4. PASS device:

   _____
   _____
   _____

5. Supplied-air respirator (SAR):

   _____
   _____
   _____

6. End-of-service-time indicator (EOSTI):

   _____
   _____
   _____

7. Hydrostatic testing:

   _____
   _____
   _____

8. Cascade system:
   _____
   _____
   _____

Fill-In
Read each item carefully, and then complete the statement by filling in the missing word(s).

1. A(n) _____ is a breathing apparatus that uses an external source for the breathing air.

2. Due to the risk of fire at the scene of a vehicle extrication incident, members of the emergency team will wear _____.

3. A(n) _____-_____ breathing apparatus is typically used for structural firefighting.

4. Smoke contains _____, substances capable of causing cancer.

5. _____ protective clothing must be worn in a specific order to obtain maximum protection.

6. The temperature of smoke varies depending on the _____, _____ and the fire conditions.

7. A fire fighter should always carry a(n) _____, given that most interior firefighting takes place in near-dark, zero-visibility conditions.

8. An atmosphere is described as _____ when the oxygen level is 19.5 percent or less.

9. A fire fighter's _____ must provide full-body coverage and protection from a variety of hazards.

10. Composite-fiber-wrapped SCBA cylinders must be replaced every _____.

True/False
If you believe the statement to be more true than false, write the letter "T" in the space provided. If you believe the statement to be more false than true, write the letter "F."

1. _____ Wearing PPE decreases normal sensory abilities.
2. _____ Newer synthetic fabrics such as nylon provide added protection to fire fighters from thermal burns.
3. _____ A complete annual inspection and maintenance procedure must be performed on each SCBA unit.
4. _____ Carbon monoxide is a toxic gas that is often present in smoke.
5. _____ Structural firefighting gear is not designed for extended wildland firefighting.
6. _____ A structural firefighting ensemble protects against many of the hazards present at a vehicle extrication incident, such as broken glass and sharp metal objects.
7. _____ Some of the toxic droplets in smoke can cause poisoning if they are absorbed through the skin.
8. _____ Phosgene gas is a dangerous by-product of incomplete combustion.
9. _____ At 21-percent oxygen concentration in air, judgment and coordination is impaired and a fire fighter will have a lack of muscle control.
10. _____ Most regular washing machines are capable of also washing fire fighter protective clothing.

Short Answer

Complete this section with short written answers using the space provided.

1. What are the six types of protection provided by PPE?

2. Identify three types of flame-resistant material commonly used in the construction of firefighting PPE.

3. List three reasons why fire fighters need respiratory protection during fire incidents.

4. List the physiological effects of reduced oxygen concentrations.

5. Identify five limitations of PPE.

Fire Alarms

The following real case scenarios will give you an opportunity to explore the concerns associated with fire fighter qualifications and safety. Read each scenario, and then answer each question in detail.

1. It is just after dinner when your ladder truck company is dispatched to an apartment fire. Upon arrival, you are assigned to search and rescue on the second floor. You have just completed searching the first apartment when your SCBA regulator malfunctions. How should you proceed?

   _____
   _____
   _____
   _____
   _____
   _____

2. You have just returned from a commercial structure fire at a mattress store. Your PPE is soiled with the products of combustion. Although you were sprayed off with water at the scene, your gear is still very dirty. How should you proceed?

   _____
   _____
   _____
   _____
   _____
   _____

Skill Drills

Skill Drill 3-1: Donning Personal Protective Clothing Fire Fighter I, NFPA 1001: 4.1.2
Test your knowledge of this skill drill by placing the photos below in the correct order. Number the first step with a "1," the second step with a "2," and so on.

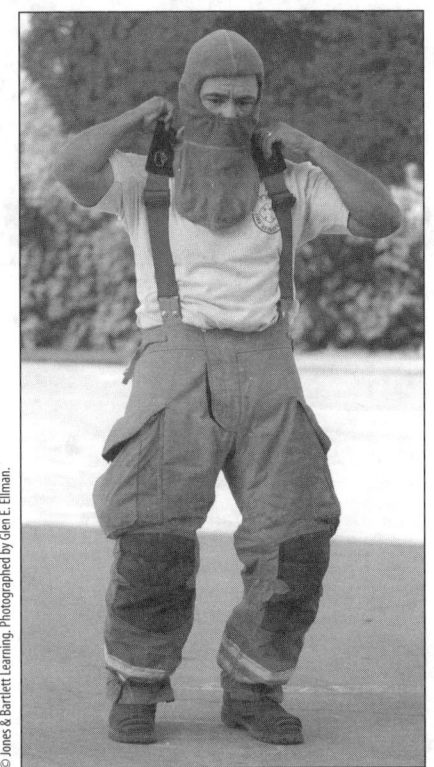

_____ Put on your boots, and pull up your protective pants. Place the suspenders over your shoulders, and secure the front of the pants.

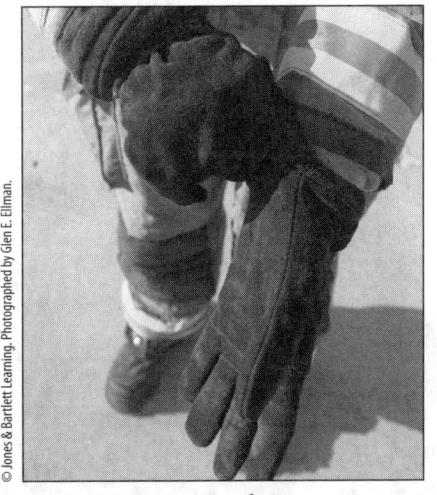

_____ Put on your gloves.

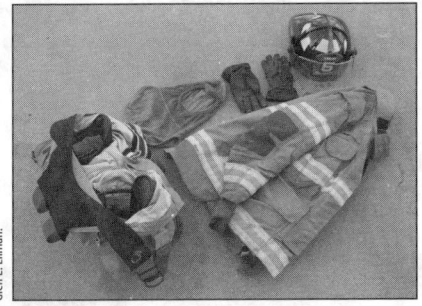

_____ Place your equipment in a logical order for donning.

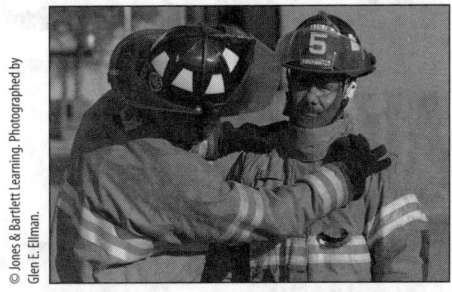

_____ Have your partner check your clothing.

24 Fundamentals of Fire Fighter Skills

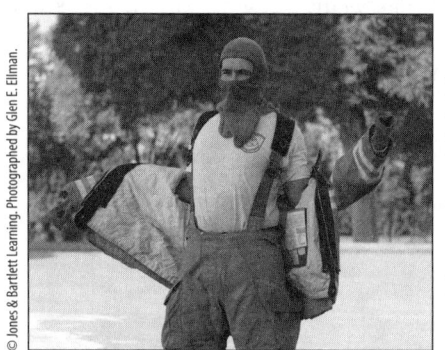
_____ Put on your protective coat, and close the front of the coat.

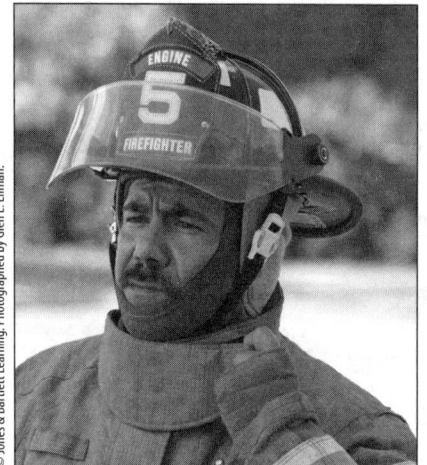
_____ Place your helmet on your head and adjust the chin strap securely. Turn up your coat collar, and secure it in front.

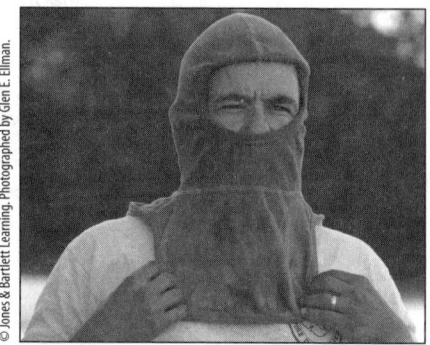
_____ Place your protective hood over your head and down around your neck.

Skill Drill 3-2: Doffing Personal Protective Clothing Fire Fighter I, NFPA 1001: 4.1.2
Test your knowledge of this skill drill by placing the photos below in the correct order. Number the first step with a "1," the second step with a "2," and so on.

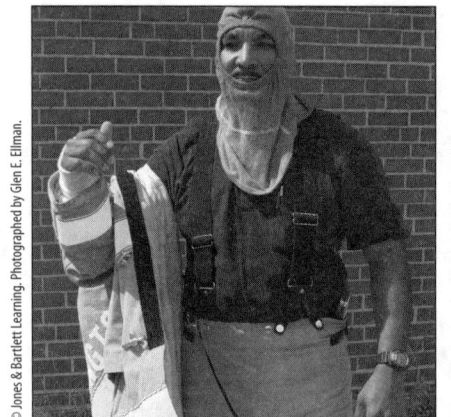
_____ Remove your protective coat.

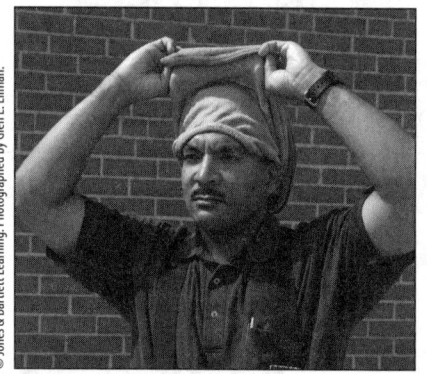
_____ Remove your protective hood.

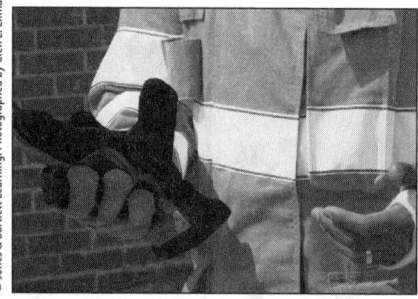
_____ Remove your gloves.

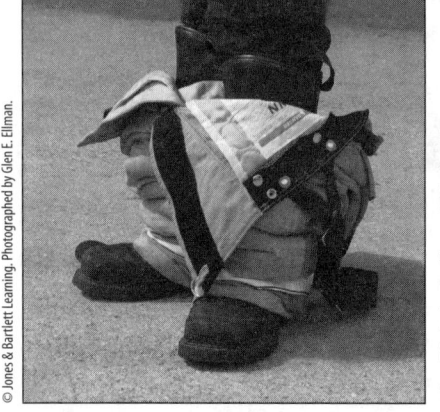
_____ Remove your protective pants and boots.

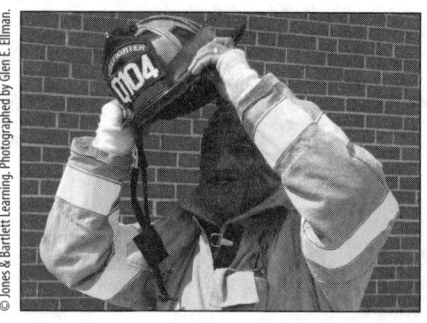
_____ Release the helmet chin strap, and remove your helmet.

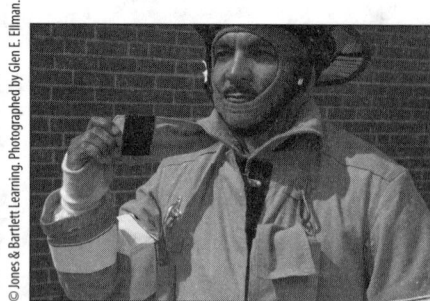
_____ Open the collar of your protective coat.

Skill Drill 3-3: Donning an SCBA from an Apparatus Seat Mount Fire Fighter I, NFPA 1001: 4.3.1

Test your knowledge of this skill drill by placing the photos below in the correct order. Number the first step with a "1," the second step with a "2," and so on.

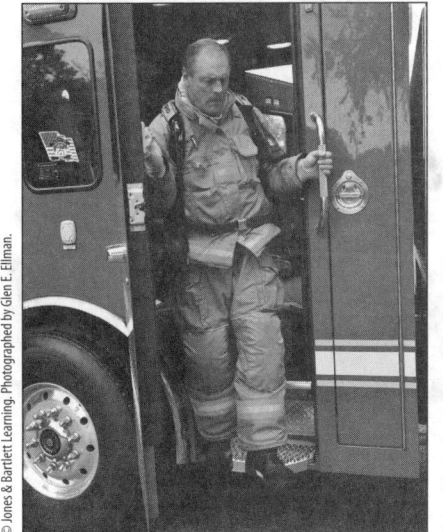

_____ Carefully exit the apparatus. Maintain three points of contact with the vehicle while exiting.

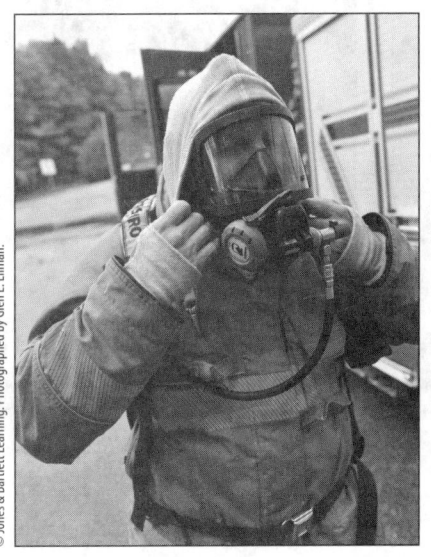

_____ Don the face piece, and check for leaks. Pull the protective hood up over your head, put the helmet on, and secure the chin strap.

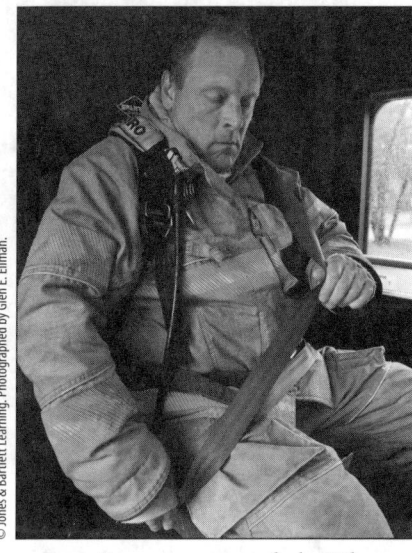

_____ Fasten your seat belt. When the apparatus stops at the emergency scene, release the seat belt, and release the SCBA from its brackets. If the apparatus has an SCBA locking device, detach the SCBA from the locking device.

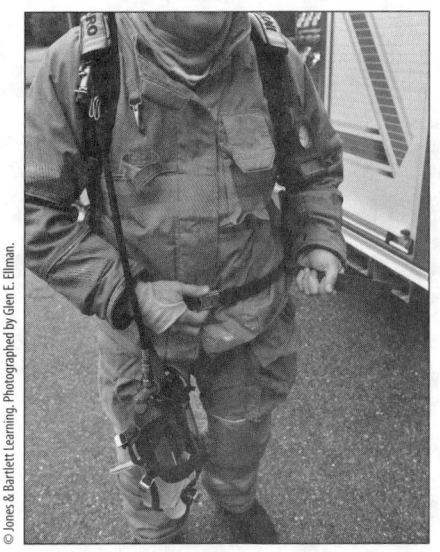

_____ Cinch down the SCBA waist belt.

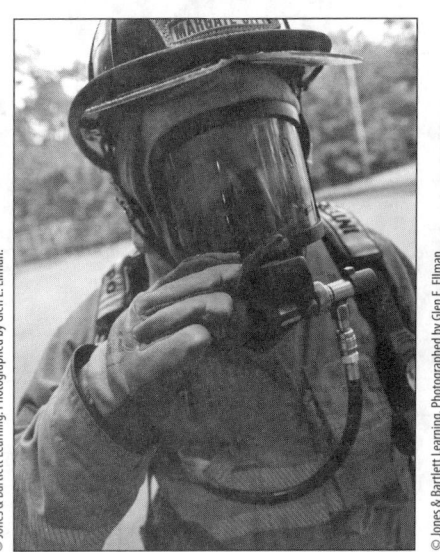

_____ If necessary, connect the regulator to the face piece or attach the low-pressure air supply hose to the regulator. Activate the air flow and ensure that the PASS device alarm is operating.

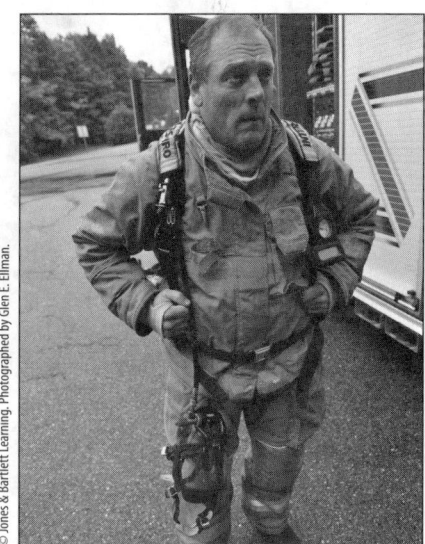

_____ Adjust shoulder straps until they are snug.

26 FUNDAMENTALS OF FIRE FIGHTER SKILLS

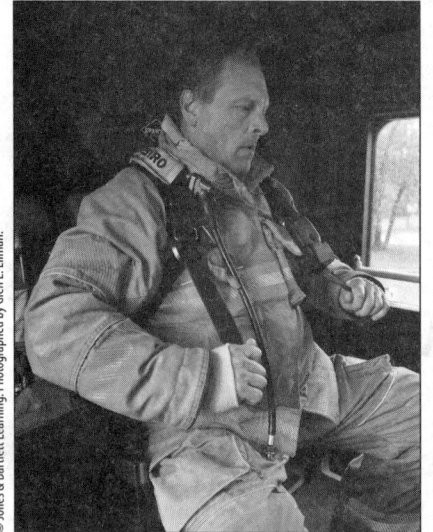

_____ Don your protective hood, pants, boots, and coat. Safely mount the apparatus, and sit on the seat. Place your arms through the SCBA shoulder straps. Partially tighten the shoulder straps; do not fully tighten them.

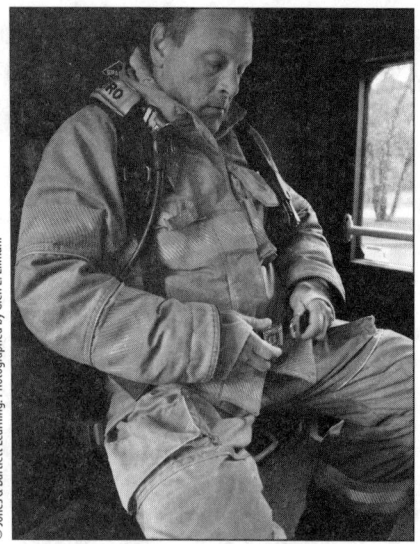

_____ Fasten your SCBA waist belt.

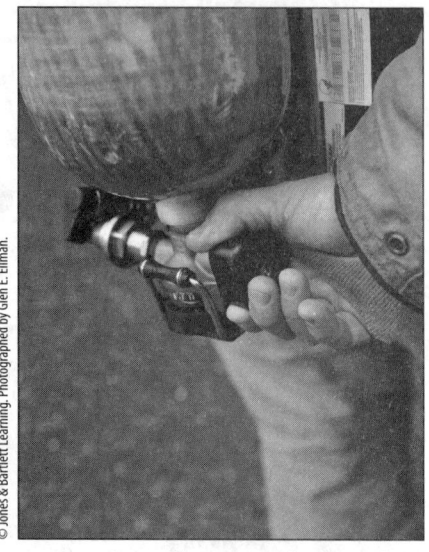

_____ Open the main cylinder valve. Activate the air saver/donning switch to prevent the flow of air, if needed.

Skill Drill 3-5: Donning an SCBA Using the Over-the-Head Method Fire Fighter I, NFPA 1001: 4.3.1
Test your knowledge of this skill drill by filling in the correct words in the photo captions.

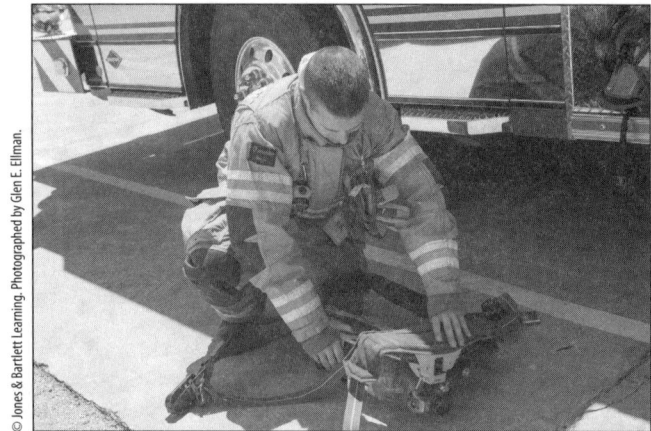

1. Lay out the SCBA so that the _____ is resting on the floor or ground, the _____ is facing up, and the _____ is facing away from you. Move the shoulder straps to the sides.

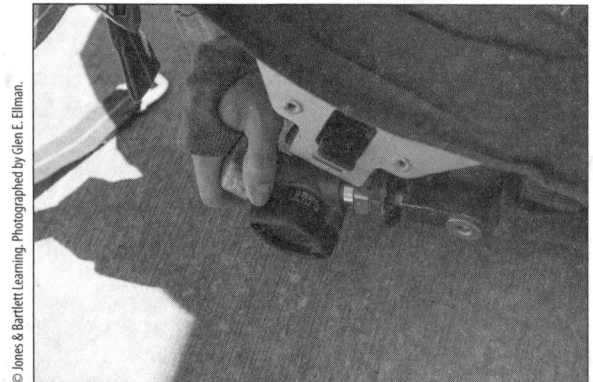

2. Fully open the main air cylinder valve. Activate the _____ / _____ to prevent the flow of air, if needed.

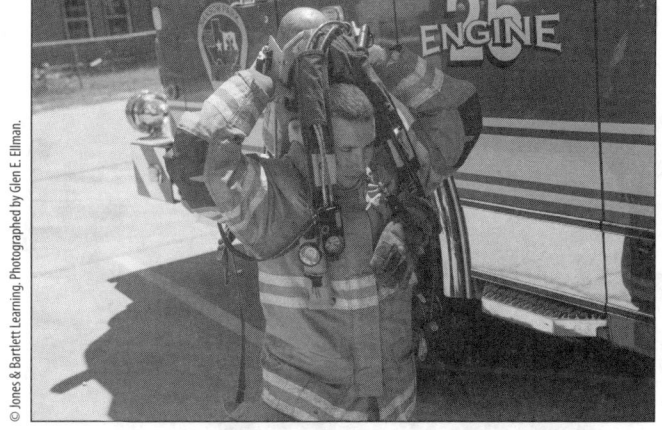

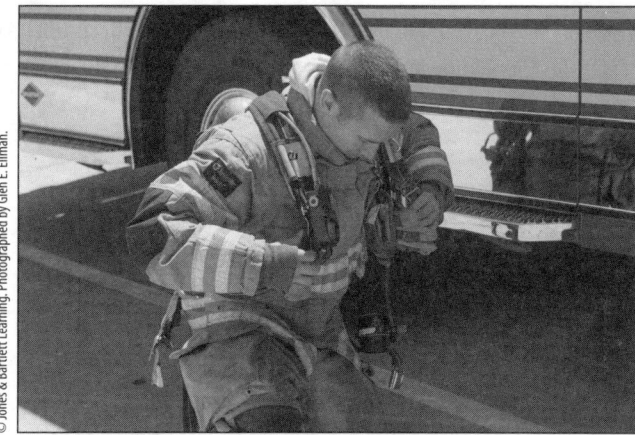

3. Bend down and grasp the SCBA _____ with both hands. Using your knees to support and lift the extra weight, lift the SCBA up and over your head. Once the SCBA clears your head, rotate it _____ so that the waist belt straps are pointed toward the ground.

4. Slowly slide the pack down your back. Make sure your arms slide into the shoulder straps. Once the SCBA is in place, tighten the shoulder straps and secure the _____.

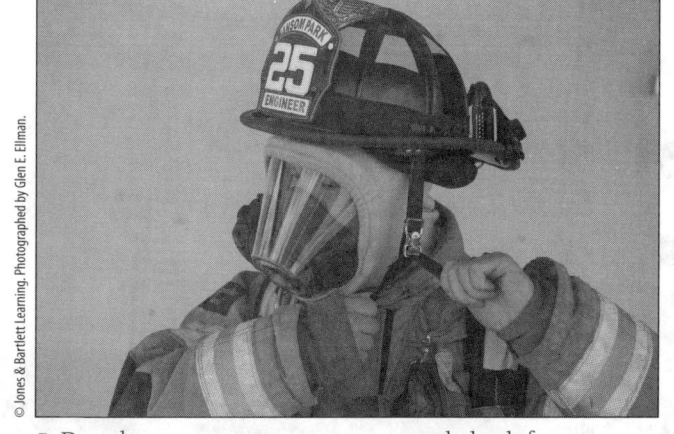

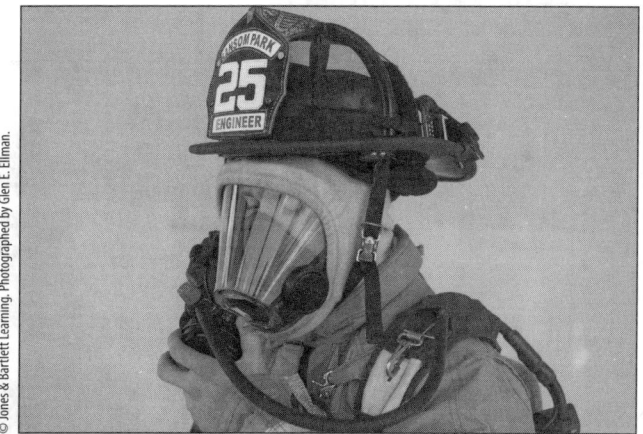

5. Don the _____, and check for an adequate _____. Pull your protective hood into position on your head, don your helmet, and secure the chin strap.

6. If necessary, connect the _____ to the face piece, or attach the low-pressure air supply hose to the regulator. Activate the air flow, and ensure that the _____ is operating.

Skill Drill 3-7: Donning a Face Piece Fire Fighter I, NFPA 1001: 4.3.1
Test your knowledge of this skill drill by filling in the correct words in the photo captions.

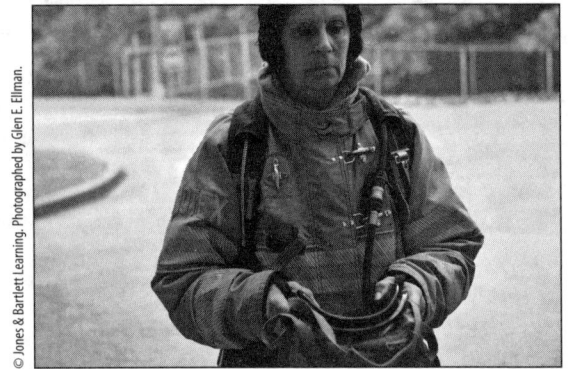

1. Fully extend the _____ straps on the face piece.

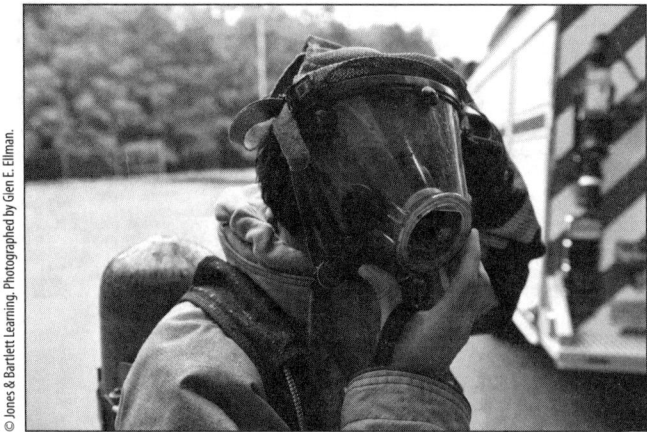

2. Rest your chin in the _____ at the bottom of the face mask. Fit the face piece to your face, bringing the straps or _____ over your head.

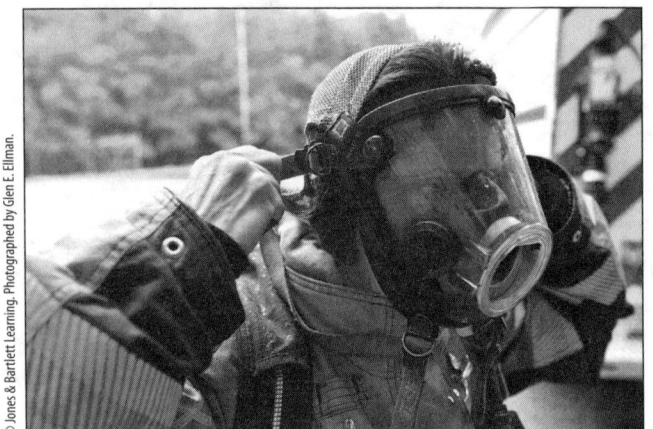

3. Tighten the lowest two straps. To tighten them, pull the straps straight back, rather than out and away from your head. Check the _____ to make sure it is lying flat against the back of your head. Tighten the pair of straps at your temple, if these straps are present. If your model has additional straps, tighten the _____ last.

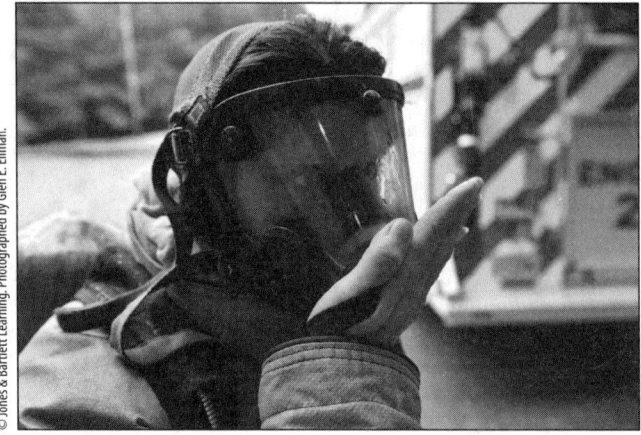

4. Check for a _____. This process depends on the model and type of face piece you use. Confirm that your nose fits in the nose cup.

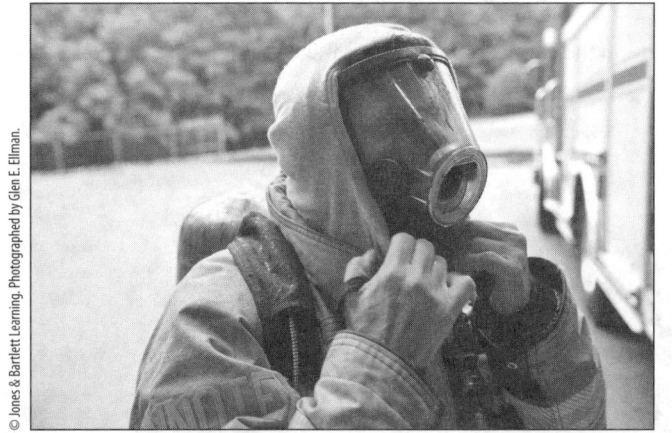

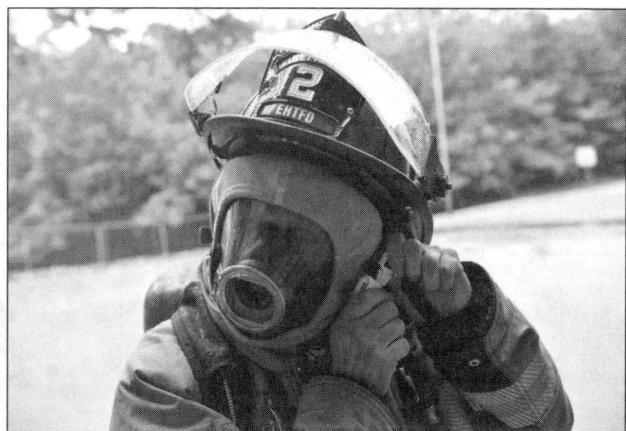

5. Pull the protective hood into position on your head. Make sure it does not get _____ your face piece or obscure your _____.

6. Don your helmet, and secure the _____.

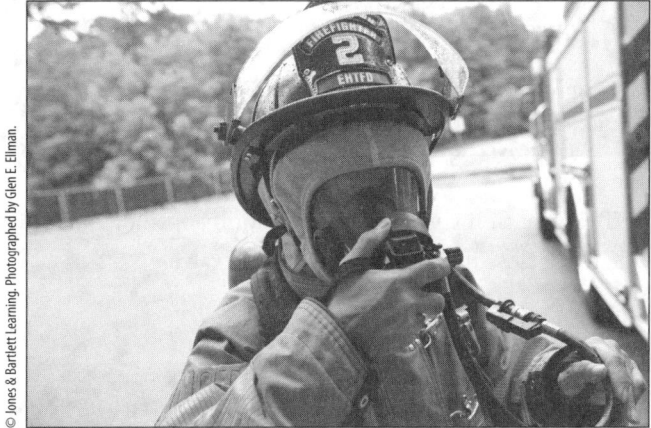

7. If needed, attach the regulator to your _____, or attach the low-pressure air supply hose to the _____.

Skill Drill 3-8: Doffing an SCBA Fire Fighter I, NFPA 1001:4.3.1

Test your knowledge of this skill drill by placing the photos below in the correct order. Number the first step with a "1," the second step with a "2," and so on.

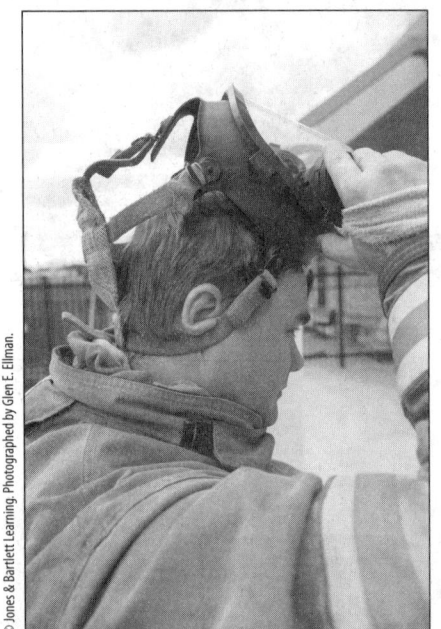
_____ Remove your face piece.

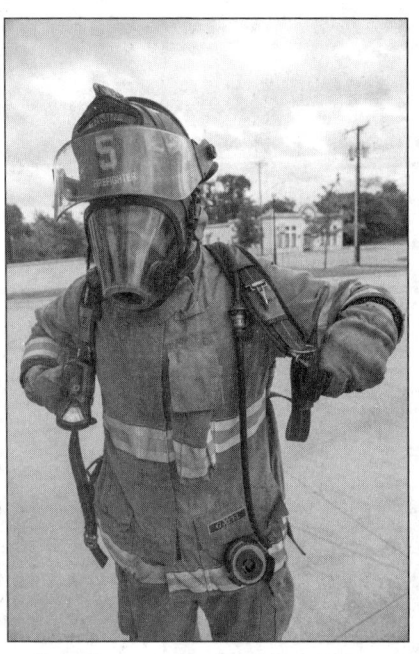
_____ Loosen the shoulder straps, and remove the SCBA harness. If you have not already done so, close the air cylinder valve.

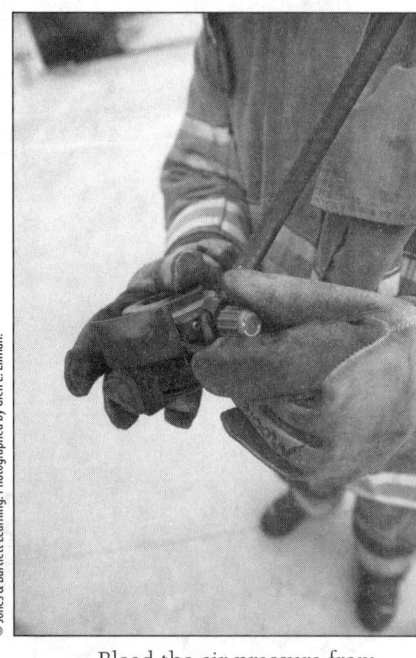
_____ Bleed the air pressure from the regulator by opening the regulator purge/bypass valve.

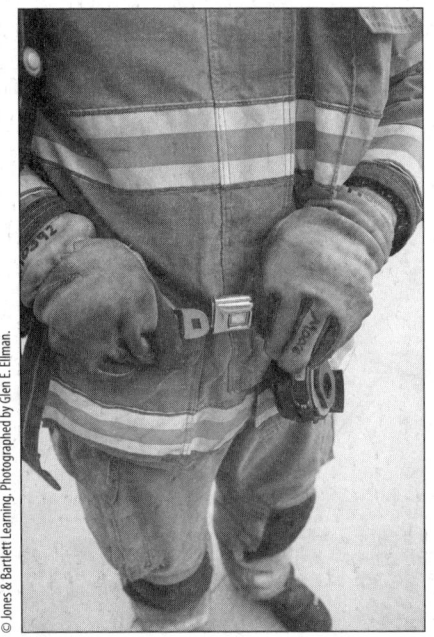
_____ Release your waist belt.

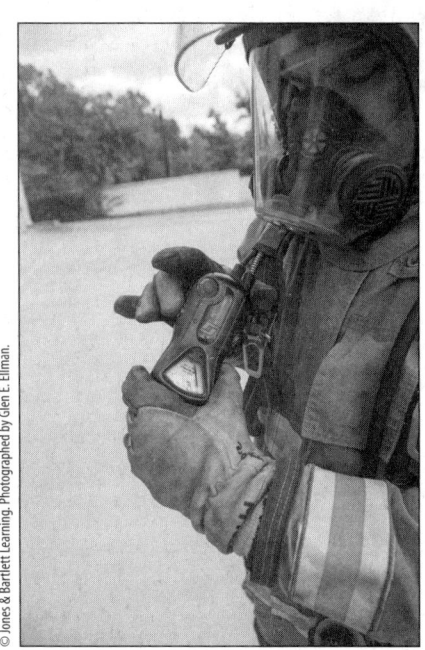
_____ Ensure that the PASS device is turned off. Place the SCBA in a safe location. Clean your SCBA as soon as possible, following the manufacturer's instructions.

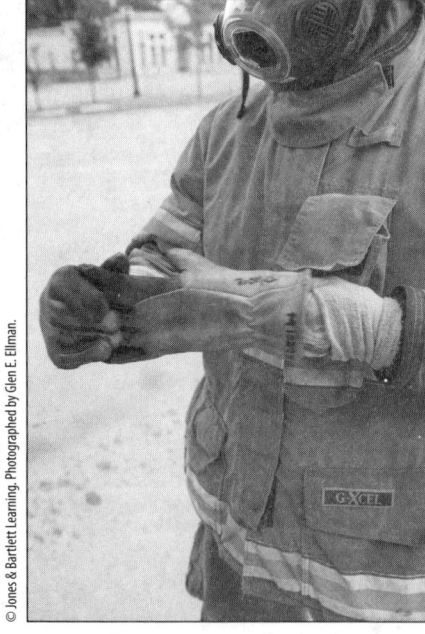
_____ Remove your gloves. Remove your helmet, and pull your protective hood down around your neck. Loosen the straps on your face piece.

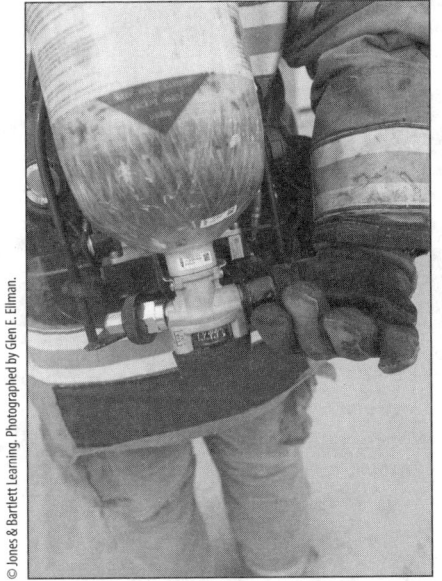

_____ Close the air cylinder valve, or fully depress the air saver/donning switch to stop the flow of air.

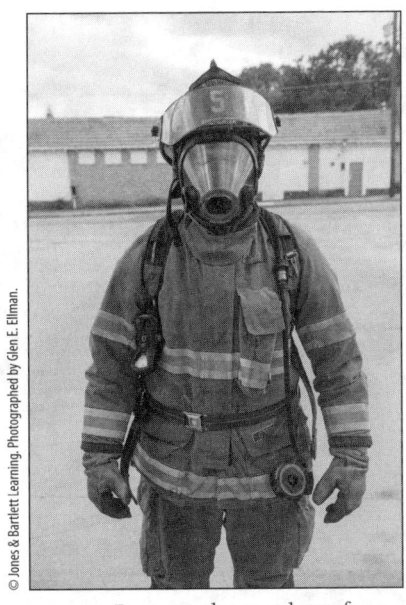

_____ Remove the regulator from your face piece, or disconnect the low-pressure air supply hose from the regulator.

Skill Drill 3-9: Visible SCBA Inspection Fire Fighter I, NFPA 1001: 4.5.1

Test your knowledge of this skill drill by placing the photos below in the correct order. Number the first step with a "1," the second step with a "2," and so on.

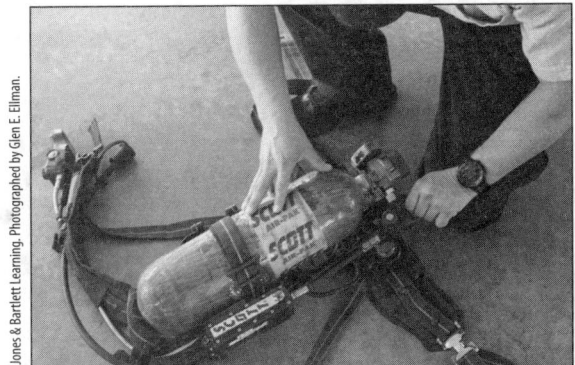

_____ Visually inspect the air cylinder and valve assembly for dents and gouges. Look for black or discolored areas that indicate exposure to flame.

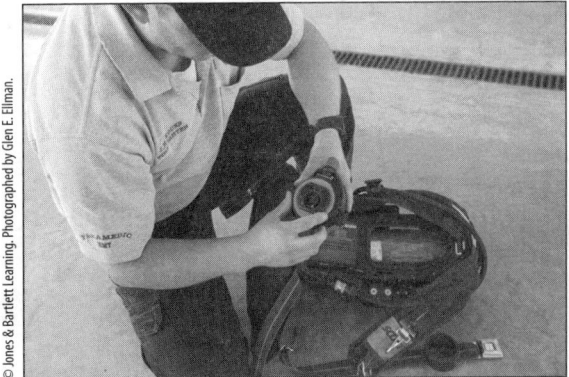

_____ Verify that the SCBA has been cleaned according to the manufacturer's and department's recommendations. Inspect the regulator for intact gaskets and visible damage.

32 Fundamentals of Fire Fighter Skills

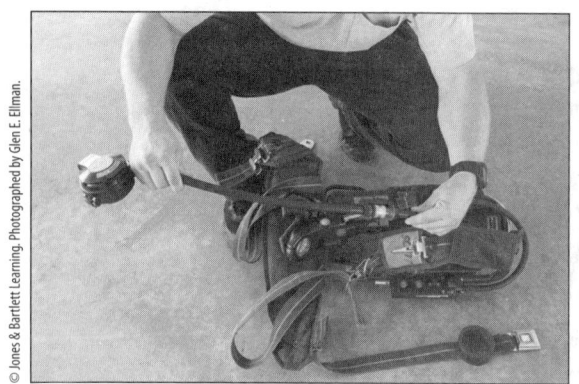

_____ Inspect hose and rubber parts for damage or deterioration.

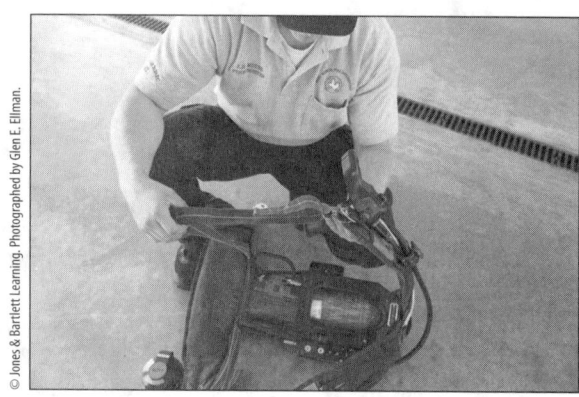

_____ Inspect the SCBA harness, webbing, buckles, fasteners, and cylinder retention system for damage.

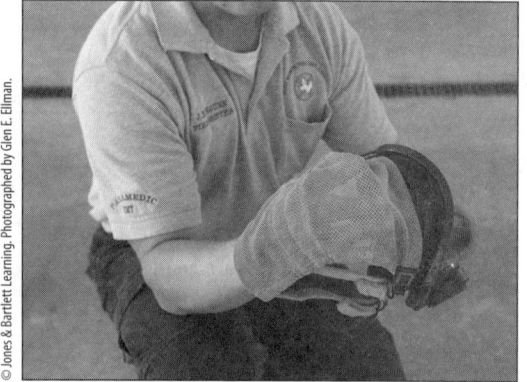

_____ Inspect the head harness to confirm that all parts are present and working properly.

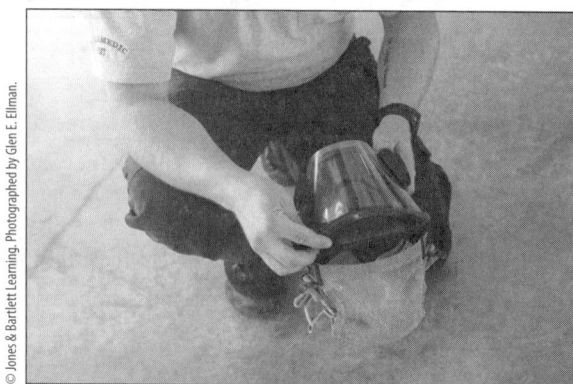

_____ Inspect the face piece for damage and worn components. Look for damage to the lenses and check for the presence of a nose cup.

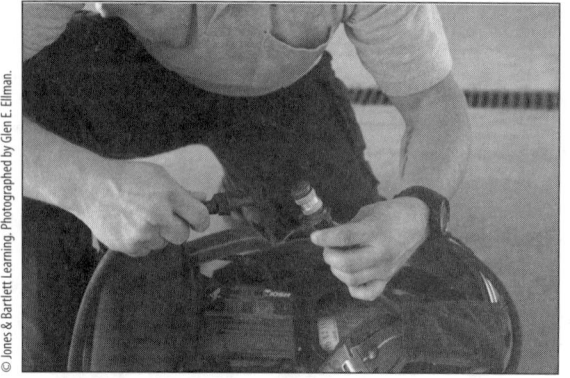

_____ Check the quick disconnects and the RIC UAC to make sure they are not damaged, that they are operating properly, and that the dust cap is in place.

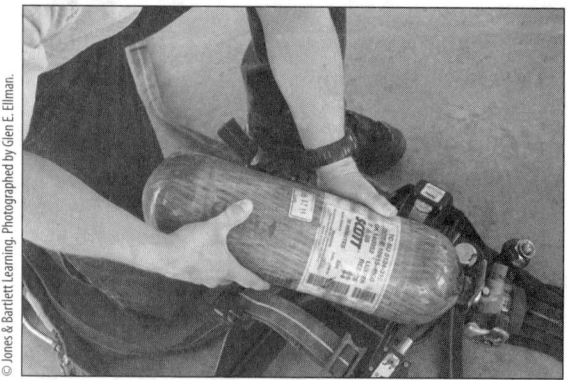

_____ Check the cylinder for the current hydrostatic test date and date of manufacture. Check the air-cylinder pressure gauge to be sure it is full.

Skill Drill 3-10: SCBA Operational Inspection Piece Fire Fighter I, NFPA 1001: 4.5.1

Test your knowledge of this skill drill by filling in the correct words in the photo captions.

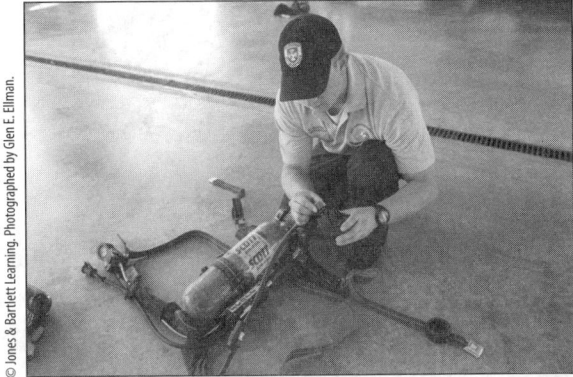

1. Check the regulator _____ / _____ valve to be sure it is closed.

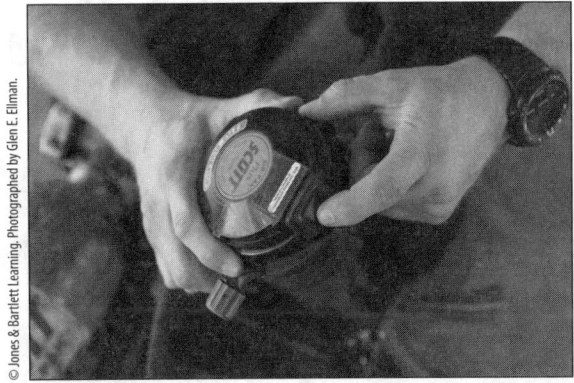

2. Depress the _____ / _____ switch, if present, to start the flow of air.

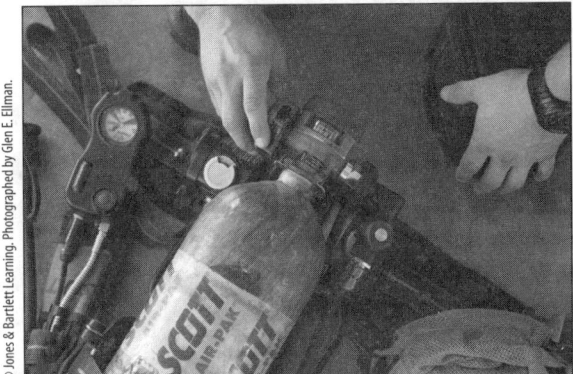

3. Slowly open the _____ valve. Check for proper operation of the heads-up display and of the low-battery indicator. Confirm that the _____-_____ and _____ devices are working.

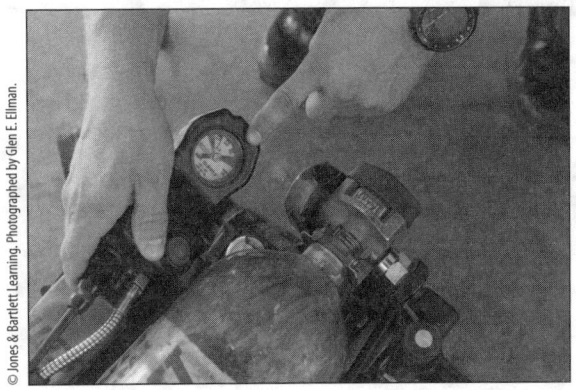

4. Check the _____ for proper operation.

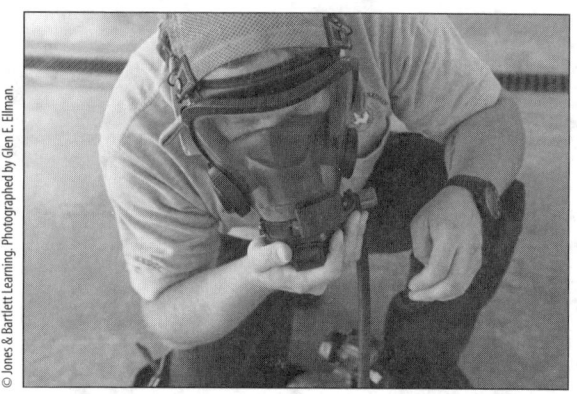

5. Don the _____. Adjust it to obtain a good seal. Inhale sharply to start the flow of air. Breathe normally to check for proper operation.

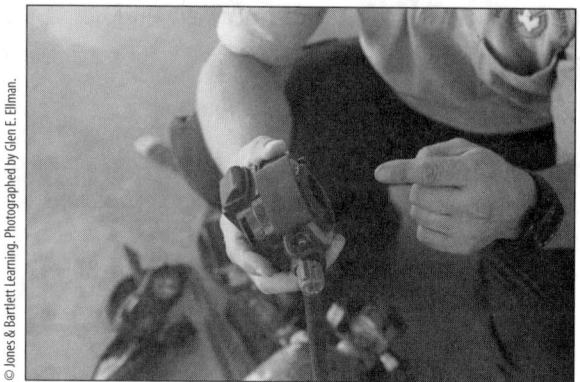

6. Remove the regulator or face piece; air should flow _____.

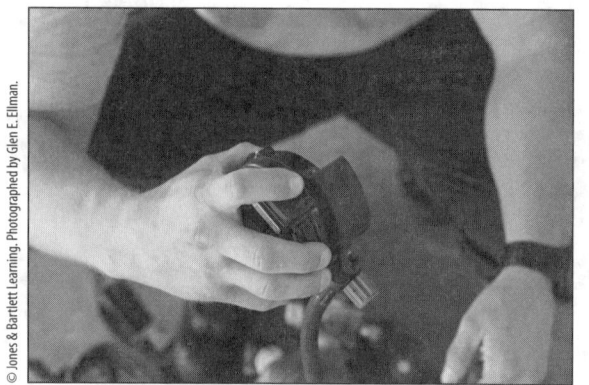

7. Depress the _____ / _____ switch to stop the flow of air.

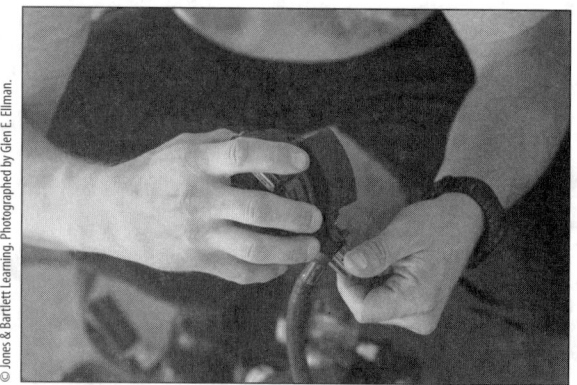

8. Open the _____ / _____ valve to check for air flow.

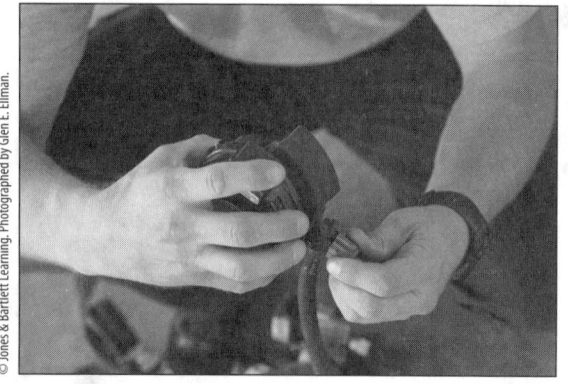

9. Close the _____ / _____ valve to stop the flow of air.

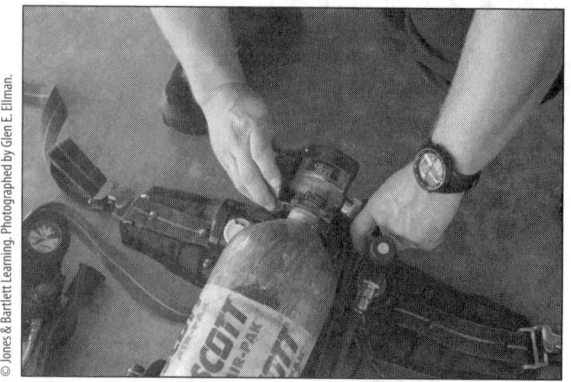

10. Rotate the _____ valve to close it.

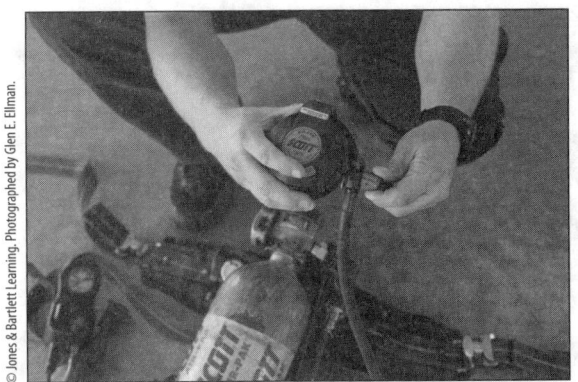

11. Open the regulator purge/bypass valve slightly to vent _____ from the system. Watch the _____-_____ display to verify its proper operation as the air pressure is exhausted.

12. Once the air flow _____, close the regulator purge/bypass valve. Complete any _____ that is required.

Skill Drill 3-11: Replacing an SCBA Cylinder Fire Fighter I, NFPA 1001: 4.5.1
Test your knowledge of this skill drill by filling in the correct words in the photo captions.

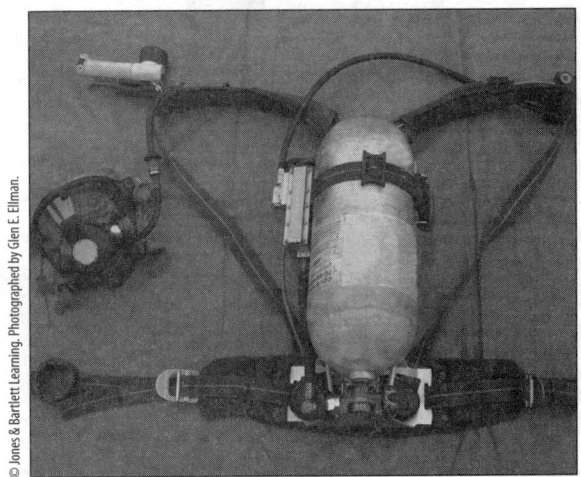

1. Place the SCBA on the _____ or a _____.

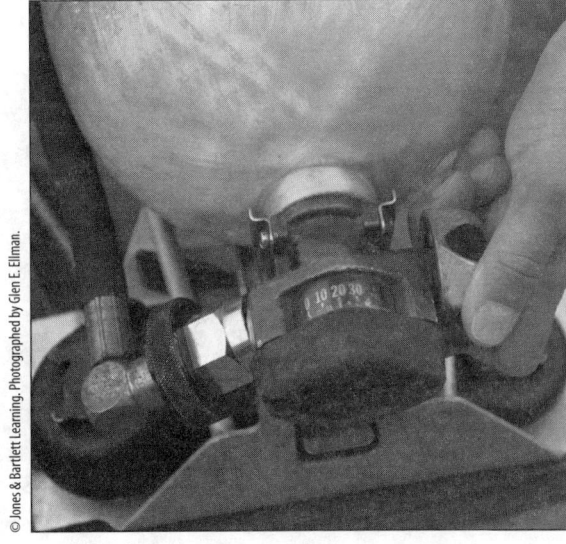

2. Close the _____

36 Fundamentals of Fire Fighter Skills

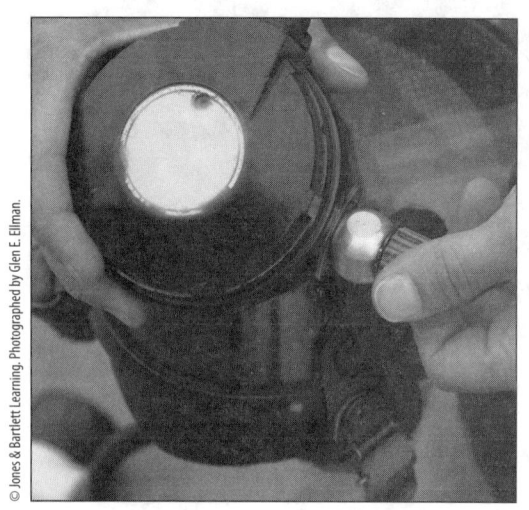

3. Open the regulator purge/bypass valve to _____ the pressure.

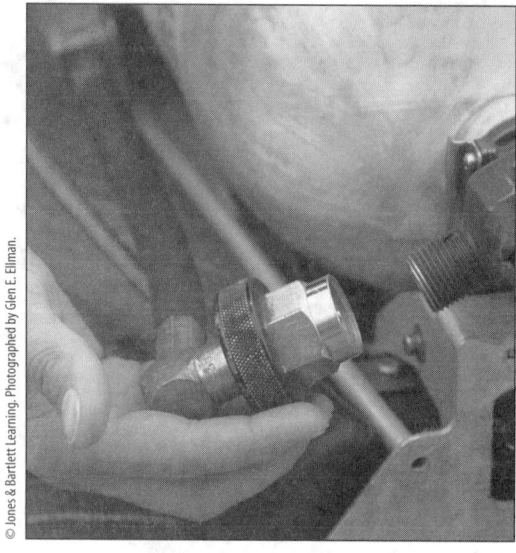

4. Disconnect the _____-_____ supply hose. Keep the ends _____.

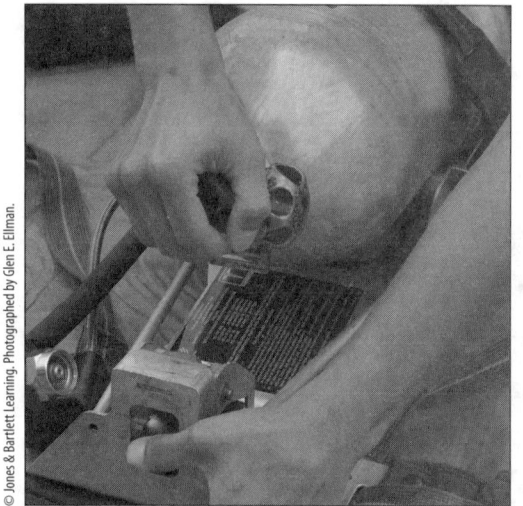

5. Release the air cylinder from the SCBA harness, and remove the _____.

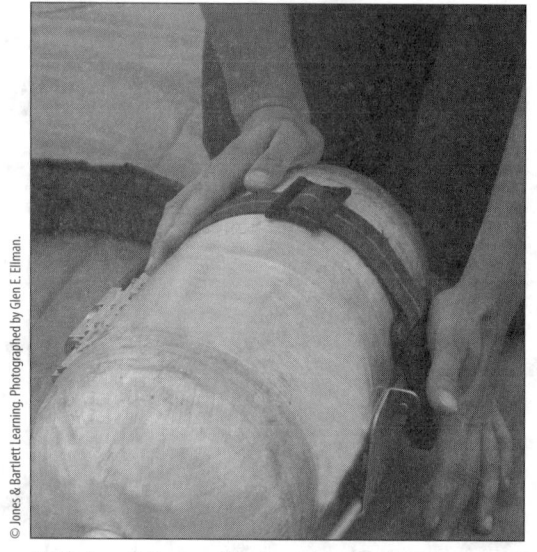

6. Slide a full air cylinder into the SCBA harness. Align the _____ to the _____. Lock the air cylinder in place.

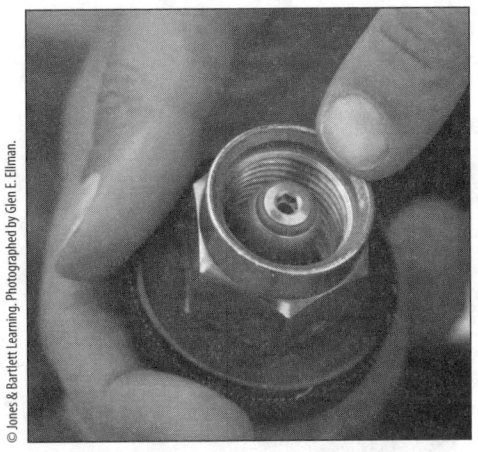

7. Check that the _____ is present and in good shape.

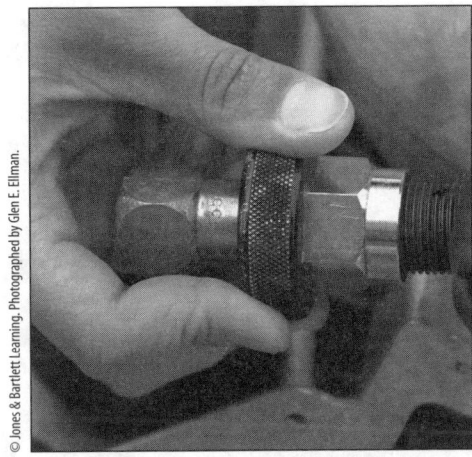

8. Connect the high-pressure hose to the _____. Hand-tighten only.

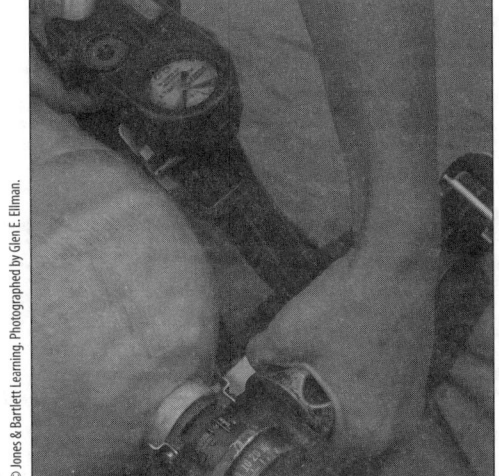

9. Open the air cylinder valve. Check the air-cylinder _____ and the _____ pressure gauge.

Skill Drill 3-14: Cleaning an SCBA Fire Fighter I, NFPA 1001: 4.5.1

Test your knowledge of this skill drill by filling in the correct words in the photo captions.

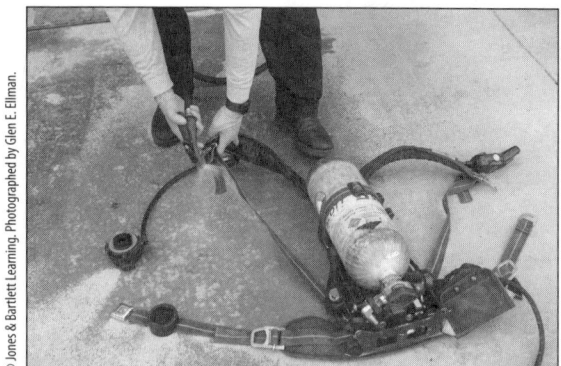

1. Rinse the entire unit using a hose with _____. Inspect the SCBA for any damage that might have occurred before cleaning.

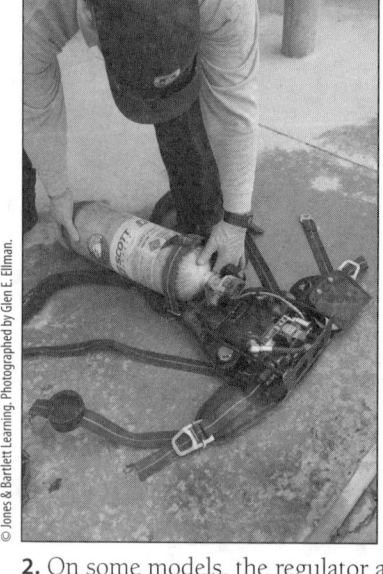

2. On some models, the regulator also can be removed from the _____. Detach the SCBA air cylinder from the _____.

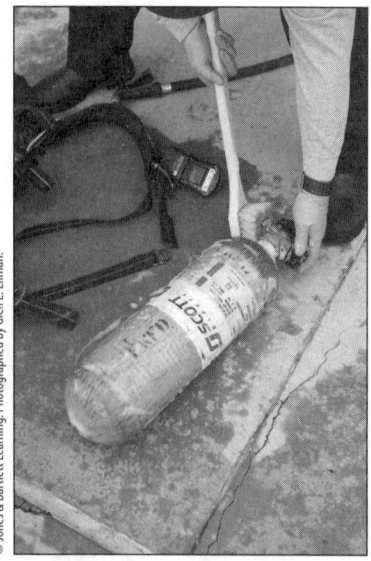

3. Using a _____, along with a mild detergent/soap-and-water solution, scrub the SCBA air cylinder and harness. Rinse and set these pieces aside to dry.

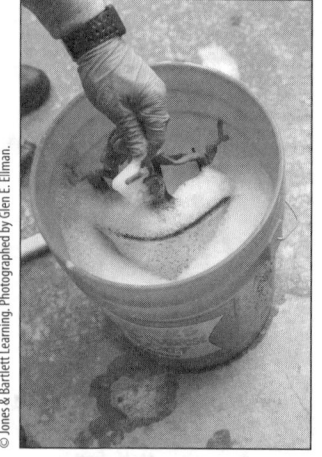

4. In a _____-_____ bucket, make a mixture of mild detergent/soap-and-water solution; alternatively, use the manufacturer's recommended cleaning and disinfecting solution and water. Submerge the SCBA face piece in the soapy water or cleaning solution. For heavier cleaning, allow the face piece to _____.

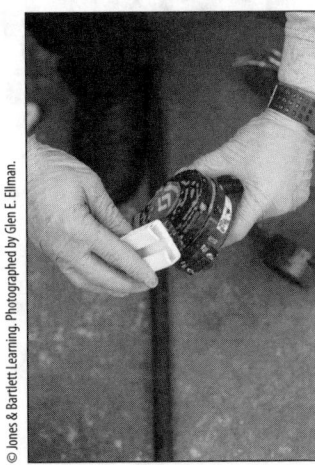

5. Clean the _____ with the soapy water or cleaning solution, following the manufacturer's instructions. Use a _____, if necessary, to scrub contaminants from the face piece and regulator.

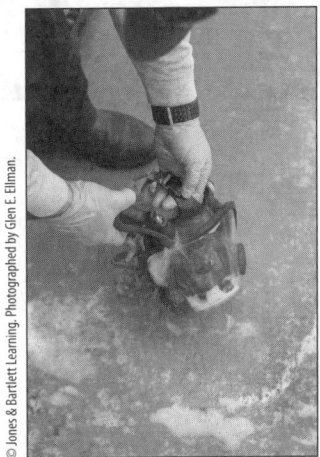

6. Completely rinse the face piece and the regulator with clean water. Do not _____ the regulator. Set them aside and allow them to dry. Reassemble and inspect the entire SCBA before _____ it back in service.

Fire Service Communications

Workbook Activities

The following activities have been designed to help you. Your instructor may require you to complete some or all of these activities as a regular part of your fire fighter training program. You are encouraged to complete any activity your instructor does not assign to you, as a way to enhance your learning in the classroom.

Chapter Review

The following exercises provide an opportunity to refresh your knowledge of this chapter.

Matching

Match each of the terms in the left column to the appropriate definition in the right column.

_____ 1. Time marks
_____ 2. CAD
_____ 3. Mobile data terminals
_____ 4. Portable radio
_____ 5. Radio repeater system
_____ 6. ANI
_____ 7. Duplex channel
_____ 8. Talk-around channel
_____ 9. Simplex channel
_____ 10. Mayday

A. A battery-operated, hand-held transceiver
B. Update that should include the type of operation, the progress of the incident, the anticipated actions, and the need for additional resources
C. Allows fire fighters to receive information on the apparatus or at the station
D. Code indicating that a fire fighter is lost, is missing, or requires immediate assistance
E. A radio channel using two frequencies
F. Automated systems used by telecommunicators to obtain and assess dispatch information
G. A radio system that automatically retransmits a radio signal on a different frequency
H. A radio channel using one frequency
I. A radio channel that bypasses a repeater system
J. Automatic number identification

Multiple Choice

Read each item carefully, and then select the best response.

_____ 1. The process of assigning a response category is based on the nature of the reported problem or
   A. classification and prioritization.
   B. location validation.
   C. unit selection.
   D. dispatch directive.

_____ 2. Some dispatch centers are equipped with automatic vehicle locator systems that track apparatus by using
   A. GPS devices.
   B. CAD systems.
   C. FCC-regulated technology.
   D. TDD systems.

_____ 3. Two-way radios that are permanently mounted in vehicles are called
   A. portable radios.
   B. base stations.
   C. simplex channel radios.
   D. mobile radios.

_____ 4. Telecommunicators must follow standard operating procedures (SOPs) and use
   A. the incident management system.
   B. active listening.
   C. FCC guidelines.
   D. talk-around channels.

_____ 5. One of the first things you should learn when assigned to a fire station is how to use the
   A. personal protective equipment (PPE).
   B. response vehicles.
   C. incident management system.
   D. telephone and intercom system.

_____ 6. The central processing point for all information relating to an emergency incident is the
   A. incident commander.
   B. communications center.
   C. fire department.
   D. computer-aided dispatch.

_____ 7. The first-arriving unit at an incident should always give a brief initial report and
   A. control traffic.
   B. determine the duration of the ongoing incident.
   C. establish command.
   D. prepare an offensive attack unit.

_____ 8. Unit selection is the process of determining exactly which
   A. radio frequency to assign.
   B. equipment will be needed in the response.
   C. attack strategy will be assigned.
   D. unit(s) to dispatch.

_____ 9. A CAD system helps meet the most important objective in processing an emergency call, which is
   A. recording communications messages.
   B. documenting the incident.
   C. sending the appropriate units to the correct location as quickly as possible.
   D. identifying the potential casualties.

_____ 10. The telecommunicator can initiate a response after determining the
   A. location and nature of the problem.
   B. time of the communication and nature of the problem.
   C. urgency of the response.
   D. fire department location.

_____ 11. Someone in the communications center must remain in contact with the responding units
   A. until an incident commander is on the scene.
   B. throughout the incident.
   C. throughout the on-site scene assessment.
   D. until the incident is under control.

_____ 12. A call box connects a person directly to a(n)
   A. fire department.
   B. police station.
   C. incident commander.
   D. telecommunicator.

_____ 13. The first-arriving unit at an incident should
   A. give a brief initial radio report.
   B. establish command.
   C. tell other responding units what is happening.
   D. All of the above.

_____ 14. Radio codes, such as "ten codes,"
   A. are widely used and popular.
   B. are understood by all radio operators.
   C. can be problematic.
   D. work well when responding with other jurisdictions.

_____ 15. When you speak into the microphone, always speak across the microphone
   A. at a 90-degree angle.
   B. at a 45-degree angle, holding the microphone 1 to 2 inches (2.5 to 5 cm) from the mouth.
   C. as loudly as possible.
   D. without background interference.

_____ 16. A group of shared frequencies controlled by a computer is called a
   A. trunking system.
   B. mobile radio system.
   C. radio repeater system.
   D. base station system.

_____ 17. Call classification determines the
   A. incident management system.
   B. equipment to transport to the incident.
   C. record documentation format.
   D. number and types of units that are dispatched.

_____ 18. Urgent messages that take priority over all other communications are known as
   A. time marks.
   B. dispatch information.
   C. emergency traffic.
   D. ten-code communications.

_____ 19. Which of the following is used to warn all fire personnel to pull back to a safe location?
   A. Evacuation signal
   B. Mayday
   C. Retreat signal
   D. PAR

_____ 20. Some communities estimate that about _____ percent of their emergency calls are reported using cellular phones.
   A. 25
   B. 50
   C. 70
   D. 90

Vocabulary

Define the following terms using the space provided.

1. Automatic location identification:

2. Run cards:

3. TDD/TTY/text phone:

4. Ten-codes:

5. Time marks:

6. Activity logging system:

7. Computer-aided dispatch (CAD):

8. Evacuation signal:

Fill-In
Read each item carefully, and then complete the statement by filling in the missing word(s).

1. A(n) _____ sends out emergency response resources promptly to an address or incident location for a specific purpose.

2. Radio systems that use one frequency to transmit and receive all messages are called _____ channels.

3. A(n) _____ channel radio utilizes two frequencies per channel.

4. A(n) _____ radio is a two-way radio that is permanently mounted in a fire apparatus.

5. A(n) _____ system uses a shared bank of frequencies to make the most efficient use of radio resources.

6. The facility that receives the emergency reports and is responsible for dispatching fire department units is the _____.

7. The _____ is a trained individual responsible for answering requests for emergency assistance from citizens.

8. _____ provide status updates to the communications center at predetermined intervals.

9. _____ is an emergency code indicating that a fire fighter is missing or requires immediate assistance.

10. A(n) _____ signal warns all personnel to pull back to a safe location.

True/False
If you believe the statement to be more true than false, write the letter "T" in the space provided. If you believe the statement to be more false than true, write the letter "F."

1. _____ Size-up should be transmitted by the second-arriving unit at an incident.
2. _____ Individuals with speech or hearing impairments can access the 911 system through telephones.
3. _____ All calls to 911 are directed to a designated public safety answering point for that jurisdiction.
4. _____ The telecommunicator who takes a call must conduct a "telephone interrogation."
5. _____ A telecommunicator can initiate a response with just two pieces of information: the location and a list of available units to dispatch.
6. _____ Before transmitting over a radio, push and hold the PTT button for at least 2 seconds.
7. _____ Most fire departments use plain English for radio communications.
8. _____ Automatic number identification displays the address where the call originated.
9. _____ The police, fire, and EMS departments must always have separate communication centers.
10. _____ Municipal fire alarm boxes have been discontinued in many communities due to high maintenance costs.

Short Answer
Complete this section with short written answers using the space provided.

1. What are five of the basic functions performed in a communications center?

_____

_____

_____

_____

2. Explain the term *LUNAR*.

3. Identify the five major steps in processing an emergency incident.

4. Why have many communities eliminated their municipal fire alarm systems or fire alarm boxes?

5. Define *emergency traffic*.

6. Describe common evacuation signals.

7. Explain how to initiate a mayday call.

Fire Alarms

The following real case scenarios will give you an opportunity to explore the concerns associated with fire service communications. Read each scenario, and then answer each question in detail.

1. You are sitting in the report room finishing up paperwork from an earlier call when the phone rings. You answer the phone using your department's standard operating procedures (SOPs). The caller states that her neighbor's burn pile has grown out of control and that it is rapidly getting larger. The caller further reports that her neighbor is chasing the fire with a garden hose. How should you proceed?

   _____
   _____
   _____
   _____
   _____
   _____

2. Your engine company is dispatched to a commercial structure fire in a large grocery store. This is the second fire to which you have responded on your shift. You and your crew are assigned to a search-and-rescue team in the storage area of the store. While there, you become disoriented and cannot find your way out. You have your radio and need to contact the IC to let him know you are lost. How should you proceed?

   _____
   _____
   _____
   _____
   _____
   _____

Skill Drills

Skill Drill 4-1: Receiving a Call and Initiating a Response to an Emergency Fire Fighter I, NFPA 1001: 4.2.1 and 4.2.2
Test your knowledge of this skill drill by filling in the correct words in the photo captions.

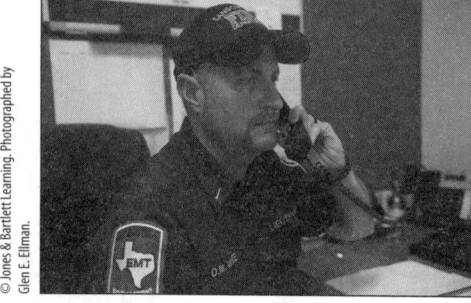

1. Answer _____ and professionally. Identify yourself, your agency, and your location. Determine immediately whether there is an emergency. If the call involves an emergency, follow your department _____. Organize your questions to get the following information:

   • _____ (including cross streets and identifying landmarks)
   • Type of _____ / _____
   • _____ information
   • _____ the incident occurred
   • Caller's _____
   • _____ of the caller, if different from the incident location
   • Caller's _____

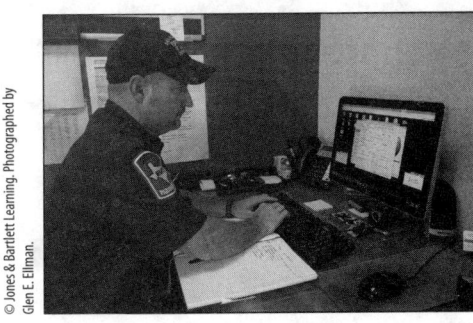

2. Record the information needed, including the date and time of the call. Initiate a response following the _____ of your communications center. The protocols in your department may vary from the steps listed here. Follow the protocols of the agency having jurisdiction for your department's communications.

Skill Drill 4-2: Touring the Communications Center
Test your knowledge of this skill drill by filling in the correct words in the photo captions.

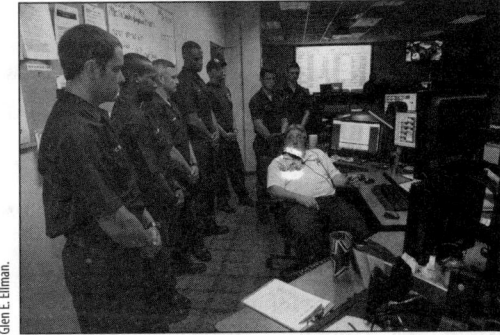

1. Arrange for a tour. Conduct yourself in a _____ manner. Observe the use of equipment.

2. Observe the _____ of a reported emergency. Differentiate the needs of fire, police, and emergency medical services (EMS) personnel. Understand the _____ job.

Fire Behavior

Workbook Activities

The following activities have been designed to help you. Your instructor may require you to complete some or all of these activities as a regular part of your fire fighter training program. You are encouraged to complete any activity that your instructor does not assign to you, as a way to enhance your learning in the classroom.

Chapter Review

The following exercises provide an opportunity to refresh your knowledge of this chapter.

Matching

Match each of the terms in the left column to the appropriate definition in the right column.

_____ 1. Endothermic

_____ 2. Gas

_____ 3. Decay

_____ 4. Oxidation

_____ 5. Conduction

_____ 6. Radiation

_____ 7. Plume

_____ 8. Convection

_____ 9. Nuclear fission

_____ 10. Hypoxia

_____ 11. Flash point

_____ 12. Heat flux

_____ 13. Incipient stage

_____ 14. Smoke explosion

_____ 15. Ventilation limited

A. The process of transferring heat through matter by movement of the kinetic energy from one particle to another

B. The column of hot gases, flames, and smoke rising above a fire; also called convection column, thermal updraft, or thermal column

C. One of the three states of matter

D. Transfer of heat through the emission of energy in the form of invisible waves

E. The process in which oxygen combines chemically with another substance to create a new compound

F. The stage of fire where the fire is running out of fuel or oxygen

G. Reactions that absorb heat or require heat to be added

H. Heat transfer by circulation within a medium such as a gas or a liquid

I. A state of inadequate oxygenation of the blood and tissue

J. Created by splitting the nucleus of an atom

K. A fire in an enclosed building that is restricted because there is insufficient oxygen available for the fire to burn as rapidly as it would with an unlimited supply of oxygen

L. The measure of the rate of heat transfer from one surface to another

M. A violent release of confined energy that occurs when a mixture of flammable gases and oxygen, usually in a void or other area separate from the fire compartment, come in contact with a source of ignition

N. The lowest temperature at which a liquid produces a flammable vapor

O. The stage of fire development where the fire has not progressed beyond a size that can be extinguished with a portable fire extinguisher

CHAPTER 5

Multiple Choice

Read each item carefully, and then select the best response.

_____ 1. A thin piece of wood burns quickly due to its
   A. mass.
   B. composition.
   C. weight-to-mass ratio.
   D. large surface area.

_____ 2. Which class of fires involves ordinary combustibles such as wood?
   A. Class A fires
   B. Class B fires
   C. Class C fires
   D. Class D fires

_____ 3. A high-volume, high-velocity, turbulent, ultra-dense black smoke that may exist in a structure fire is known as
   A. wet smoke.
   B. temperature-enriched smoke.
   C. liquid fire.
   D. black fire.

_____ 4. A very rapid chemical process that combines oxygen with another substance and results in the release of heat and light is called
   A. oxidization.
   B. combustion.
   C. pyrolysis.
   D. decomposition.

_____ 5. Which class of fires involves flammable or combustible liquids such as gasoline?
   A. Class A fires
   B. Class B fires
   C. Class C fires
   D. Class D fires

_____ 6. The initial growth of a fire is largely dependent on
   A. the type of fuel.
   B. the amount of fuel being pyrolyzed into vapor.
   C. thermal layering.
   D. A and B.

_____ 7. The movement of heat through a fluid medium such as air or a liquid is
   A. convection.
   B. endothermic.
   C. exothermic.
   D. conduction.

_____ 8. The phenomenon of gases forming into layers according to temperature is called
   A. thermal differentiation.
   B. thermal division.
   C. thermal layering.
   D. thermal balance.

_____ 9. The lowest temperature at which a liquid produces a flammable vapor is the
   A. flame point.
   B. fire point.
   C. ignition temperature.
   D. flash point.

_____ 10. In which stage of the fire does hot smoke and gases start to rise because of heating and becoming lighter?
   A. Ignition stage
   B. Growth stage
   C. Fully developed stage
   D. Decay stage

_____ 11. Which class of fires involves combustible metals?
   A. Class A fires
   B. Class B fires
   C. Class C fires
   D. Class D fires

_____ 12. Incomplete combustion produces
   A. pure air.
   B. solids.
   C. smoke.
   D. oxidizers.

_____ 13. The weight of a gaseous fuel is the
   A. gas mass.
   B. vapor density.
   C. explosive limit.
   D. BLEVE.

_____ 14. When reading smoke, the smoke density is an indication of
   A. where the fire is traveling.
   B. the amount of moisture in the smoke.
   C. how much fuel is in the smoke.
   D. None of the above.

_____ 15. The transfer of heat energy in the form of invisible waves is called
   A. radiation.
   B. oxidization.
   C. volatility.
   D. transpiration.

_____ 16. The four conditions that must be present for fire to take place are represented in the
   A. fire tetrahedron.
   B. fire square.
   C. fire triangle.
   D. fire rectangle.

_____ 17. Particles, vapors, and gases are the three major components of
   A. fumes.
   B. silt.
   C. smoke.
   D. exhaust.

_____ 18. The key to preventing a BLEVE is to
   A. flush the spill.
   B. ventilate the area.
   C. cool the top of the tank.
   D. apply an oxidizing agent.

_____ 19. A fire requires fuel that is in the form of
   A. combustible vapors.
   B. solid.
   C. liquid.
   D. particles.

_____ 20. The range of gas-air mixtures that will burn varies
   A. from one fuel to another.
   B. with the amount of energy present.
   C. with the vapor pressure.
   D. with the vapor density.

Labeling
Label the following diagram with the correct terms.

1. The fire tetrahedron

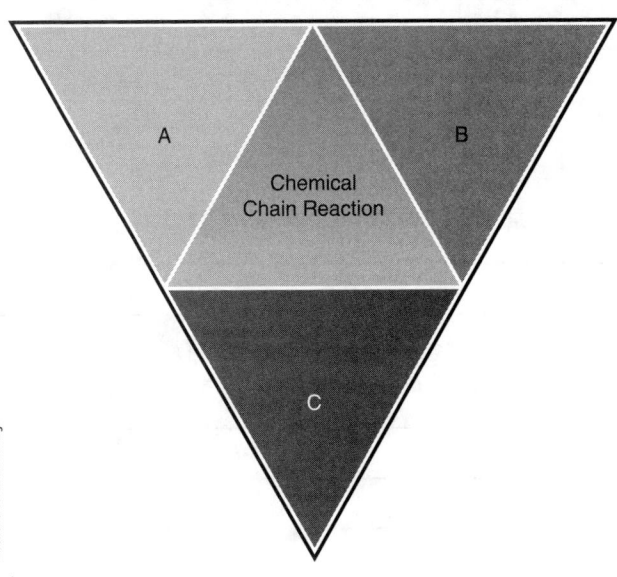

Vocabulary
Define the following terms using the space provided.

1. Lower explosive limit:
_____
_____
_____

2. Ignition temperature:
_____
_____
_____

3. Flash point:

4. BLEVE:

5. Thermal layering:

6. Fire triangle:

7. Flashover:

8. Fully developed stage:

9. Roll-over:

10. Smoke explosion:

Fill-In
Read each item carefully, and then complete the statement by filling in the missing word(s).

1. A fire involving a liquid fuel can be extinguished by shutting off the _____ of fuel, or using _____ to exclude oxygen from the fuel.

2. Carbon _____ is deadly in small quantities.

3. Research indicates that fires in modern residential occupancies are likely to enter a _____ _____ decay stage prior to the arrival of the first engine company.

4. For a fuel to burn, it must be changed into a _____.

5. Because smoke is the product of incomplete combustion and contains unburned hydrocarbons, we need to remember that it is a form of _____.

6. When hot fire gases are exhausted from a fire building, if they are above the _____ of the gases, they may ignite upon mixing with a fresh supply of oxygen.

7. Matter exists in three states: _____, _____, and _____.

8. _____ is a high-volume, high-density, high-velocity, turbulent, ultra-dense black smoke.

9. The amount of liquid that is vaporized when it is heated relates to the _____ of the liquid.

10. Reactions that produce heat are referred to as _____ reactions.

True/False
If you believe the statement to be more true than false, write the letter "T" in the space provided. If you believe the statement to be more false than true, write the letter "F."

1. _____ The size and shape of the fuel will greatly impact the ability of the fuel to ignite.
2. _____ A roll-over is when smoke traveling some distance from the fire comes in contact with a source of ignition, often in a violent manner.
3. _____ Flashover is a slow change or transition from the growth stage to the fully developed stage.
4. _____ A column of hot black smoke coming into contact with an adequate supply of oxygen and an ignition source can ignite suddenly and violently.
5. _____ The flash point is the lowest temperature at which a liquid produces enough vapor to sustain a continuous fire.
6. _____ A backdraft can occur when oxygen is introduced into a closed, superheated room.
7. _____ The three basic ingredients required to create a fire are fuel, oxygen, and air.
8. _____ Gas has neither independent shape nor volume and tends to expand indefinitely.
9. _____ A smoke explosion usually occurs when a mixture of flammable gases and oxygen are present in the fire compartment.
10. _____ Mechanical, electrical, and chemical energy can be converted to heat.

Short Answer

Complete this section with short written answers using the space provided.

1. List the four key attributes of smoke that must be considered when reading smoke.

   _____
   _____
   _____
   _____

2. Explain how the color of smoke may provide an indication as to the location of the fire.

   _____
   _____
   _____
   _____
   _____

3. Explain how the widespread use of plastics in modern structures has affected fire behavior.

   _____
   _____
   _____
   _____
   _____

4. Identify the four basic methods of extinguishing fires.

   _____
   _____
   _____
   _____
   _____

Fire Alarms

The following real case scenarios will give you an opportunity to explore the concerns associated with fire behavior. Read each scenario, and then answer each question in detail.

1. It is 3:00 in the afternoon when your engine company is dispatched to a kitchen fire in a multifamily condominium unit. You and your Lieutenant enter the unit, and it appears that the kitchen has flashed over. You are on the nozzle, and your Lieutenant tells you this is a hot fire and not to disrupt the thermal balance. How should you proceed?

   _____
   _____
   _____
   _____
   _____

2. Your engine company is dispatched to a two-story, single-family home in a newer development. Upon arrival, you find there is no flame visible and the window glass is smoke-stained with a lot of heat inside. Upon investigation, you see smoke emanating under pressure from cracks. The smoke is puffing and being drawn back as if it were breathing. How should you proceed?

___
___
___
___
___
___

Building Construction

Workbook Activities

The following activities have been designed to help you. Your instructor may require you to complete some or all of these activities as a regular part of your fire fighter training program. You are encouraged to complete any activity your instructor does not assign to you, as a way to enhance your learning in the classroom.

Chapter Review

The following exercises provide an opportunity to refresh your knowledge of this chapter.

Matching

Match each of the terms in the left column to the appropriate definition in the right column.

_____ 1. Combustibility A. A natural material composed of calcium sulfate and water molecules
_____ 2. Thermal conductivity B. Interior walls extending from the floor to the underside of the floor above
_____ 3. Fire window C. Built-up unit of construction materials set in mortar
_____ 4. Fire barrier wall D. Walls designed for structural support
_____ 5. Gypsum E. The weight of the building contents
_____ 6. Occupancy F. How a building is used
_____ 7. Live load G. Describes how readily a material will conduct heat
_____ 8. Load-bearing walls H. Used when a window is needed in a required fire-resistant wall
_____ 9. Spalling I. Determines whether a material will burn
_____ 10. Masonry J. Chipping or pitting of concrete or masonry surfaces

Multiple Choice

Read each item carefully, and then select the best response.

_____ 1. Thermoplastic materials melt and drip when exposed to high temperatures, some even as low as
   A. 100°F (37.8°C).
   B. 250°F (121.1°C).
   C. 500°F (260°C).
   D. 650°F (343.3°C).

CHAPTER 6

_____ 2. What is another term for wood-frame construction?
   A. Type I
   B. Type II
   C. Type IV
   D. Type V

_____ 3. A steel bar joist is an example of a
   A. bowstring truss.
   B. pitched chord truss.
   C. parallel chord truss.
   D. flat chord truss.

_____ 4. When selecting materials for building construction, architects most often place a priority on
   A. price and ease of construction.
   B. functionality and aesthetics.
   C. availability of materials and price.
   D. durability and maintenance expenses.

_____ 5. How many layers will a typical built-up roof covering have?
   A. 3
   B. 5
   C. 7
   D. 9

_____ 6. Which of the following materials will expand at extremely high temperatures, conduct heat well, and lose its strength as the temperature increases?
   A. Steel
   B. Concrete
   C. Masonry
   D. Gypsum

_____ 7. Fire doors and fire windows are rated for a particular duration of
   A. heat resistance to controlled temperatures.
   B. internal temperature compliance.
   C. standard fire resistance.
   D. fire resistance to a standard test fire.

_____ 8. The weight of the building is called the
   A. live load.
   B. total load.
   C. dead load.
   D. structural load.

FUNDAMENTALS OF FIRE FIGHTER SKILLS

_____ 9. Which type of glass consists of a thin sheet of plastic between two sheets of glass?
   A. Tempered glass
   B. Wired glass
   C. Laminated glass
   D. Glass blocks

_____ 10. Walls that are constructed on the line between two properties and are shared by a building on each side of the line are called
   A. fire walls.
   B. fire partitions.
   C. curtain walls.
   D. party walls.

_____ 11. The exposed interior surfaces of a building are commonly referred to as the
   A. interior finish.
   B. building surfaces.
   C. structural surfaces.
   D. structural finish.

_____ 12. Which of the following is a commonly used building material?
   A. Steel
   B. Concrete
   C. Aluminum
   D. All of the above

_____ 13. Pitched, curved, and flat are types of
   A. awnings.
   B. roofs.
   C. stairways.
   D. rafters.

_____ 14. Which synthetic material is found in many products and may be transparent or opaque, stiff or flexible, and tough or brittle?
   A. Glass
   B. Plastic
   C. Aluminum
   D. Copper

_____ 15. Trusses are used extensively in support systems for
   A. both floors and roofs.
   B. floors.
   C. roofs.
   D. roofs, with the exception of flat roofs.

_____ 16. What term describes the length of time a building or building components can withstand a fire before igniting?
   A. Pyrolysis
   B. Thermal resistance
   C. Fire retardance
   D. Fire resistance

_____ 17. Lightweight and heavy timber construction are examples of
   A. Type I construction.
   B. window frames.
   C. wood floor structures.
   D. roofs.

_____ 18. Which type of building construction has two separate fire loads?
   A. Type II
   B. Type III
   C. Type IV
   D. Type V

_____ 19. Which type of building construction provides the highest degree of safety and is usually made of reinforced concrete and protected steel-frame construction?
   A. Type I
   B. Type II
   C. Type IV
   D. Type V

_____ 20. Buildings having masonry exterior walls, and interior walls, floors, and roofs made of wood, are considered to be
   A. Type II construction.
   B. Type III construction.
   C. Type IV construction.
   D. Type V construction.

Vocabulary

Define the following terms using the space provided.

1. Hybrid building:

   _____
   _____
   _____

2. Platform frame:

   _____
   _____
   _____

3. Balloon-frame construction:

   _____
   _____
   _____

4. Bowstring truss:

   _____
   _____
   _____

5. Thermoplastic materials:
   _____
   _____
   _____

6. Heavy timber construction:
   _____
   _____
   _____

Fill-In
Read each item carefully, and then complete the statement by filling in the missing word(s).

1. A building with a(n) _____ will have a distinctive curved roof.

2. When wood is exposed to high temperatures, its strength can be decreased through the process of _____.

3. Type _____ construction was commonly used to build mills in the 1800s.

4. A(n) _____ chord truss is typically used to support a sloping roof.

5. A(n) _____ helps prevent the spread of a fire from one side to the other side of the wall.

6. The term _____ refers to how a building is used.

7. Type _____ is the most fire-resistive category of building construction.

8. Fire severity in a Type II building is determined by the _____.

9. _____-frame construction is used for almost all modern wood-frame construction.

10. The weight of the building's contents is called _____.

True/False
If you believe the statement to be more true than false, write the letter "T" in the space provided. If you believe the statement to be more false than true, write the letter "F."

1. _____ The structural components and building contents in Type III and Type IV construction are considered noncombustible.

2. _____ Aluminum is more expensive than, and not as strong as, steel.

3. _____ The entire structure of a manufactured (mobile) home can be destroyed by fire within a few minutes.

4. _____ Trusses are used in support systems for both floors and roofs.

5. _____ Fire doors and fire windows are rated for a particular duration of fire resistance to a standard fire test.
6. _____ Most doors are constructed of aluminum.
7. _____ Concrete is one of the most commonly used building materials.
8. _____ Aluminum floors are common in fire-resistive construction.
9. _____ Type I building construction provides the highest degree of safety.
10. _____ The support systems for most flat roofs are constructed of aluminum.

Short Answer

Complete this section with short written answers using the space provided.

1. List the five factors that affect how fast wood ignites, burns, and decomposes.

   _____
   _____
   _____
   _____

2. Identify and briefly describe the five types of building construction.

   _____
   _____
   _____
   _____

3. What problems must be anticipated when considering the fire risks associated with a construction or demolition site?

   _____
   _____
   _____
   _____

4. List the four key factors that affect building materials under fire.

   _____
   _____
   _____
   _____

5. Briefly describe gusset plates and how they respond when heated.

_____

_____

_____

_____

6. List some of the building construction–related questions that should be asked during preincident planning.

_____

_____

_____

_____

Fire Alarms

The following real case scenarios will give you an opportunity to explore the concerns associated with building construction. Read each scenario, and then answer each question in detail.

1. Your ladder truck company is dispatched to a structure fire at a three-story Type III construction nursing home.

The fire is reported in the kitchen. You start to think about the contents and the building construction. What are your concerns?

_____

_____

_____

_____

_____

_____

2. It is 10:00 on Friday night when your engine is dispatched to a fire at a bowling alley. Upon arrival, you find a masonry building with a curved roof and the rear exterior wall leaning out. The fire has involved the office area in the rear of the building. How should you proceed?

_____
_____
_____
_____
_____
_____

Portable Fire Extinguishers

Workbook Activities

The following activities have been designed to help you. Your instructor may require you to complete some or all of these activities as a regular part of your fire fighter training program. You are encouraged to complete any activity your instructor does not assign to you, as a way to enhance your learning in the classroom.

Chapter Review

The following exercises provide an opportunity to refresh your knowledge of this chapter.

Matching

Match each of the terms in the left column to the appropriate definition in the right column.

_____ 1. Extinguishing agent   **A.** Periodic testing of an extinguisher to verify it has sufficient strength to withstand internal pressures

_____ 2. Aqueous film-forming foam   **B.** Very cold, forms a dense cloud that displaces the air surrounding the fuel

_____ 3. Incipient   **C.** An extinguishing agent used on Class B fires that forms a foam layer over the liquid and stops the production of flammable vapors

_____ 4. Hydrostatic testing   **D.** The weight of combustibles in a fire area or on a floor in buildings and structures

_____ 5. Pressure indicator   **E.** A retaining device that breaks when the locking mechanism is released

_____ 6. Ammonium phosphate   **F.** The initial stage of a fire

_____ 7. FFFP   **G.** An extinguishing agent used in dry chemical fire extinguishers that can be used on Class A, B, and C fires

_____ 8. Carbon dioxide   **H.** A material used to stop the combustion process

_____ 9. Tamper seal   **I.** Film-forming fluoroprotein foam, a Class B foam additive

_____ 10. Fire load   **J.** A gauge on a pressurized portable fire extinguisher that indicates the internal pressure of the expellant

Multiple Choice

Read each item carefully, and then select the best response.

_____ 1. The sodium chloride–based extinguishing agent that is used in portable fire extinguishers can be
    A. stored in liquid form.
    B. harmful to the environment.
    C. used in all portable fire extinguishers.
    D. applied by hand.

CHAPTER 7

_____ 2. Fire extinguishers weighing more than 40 lb (18.1 kg) should be mounted so that the top of the extinguisher is not more than
   A. 5 ft above the floor.
   B. 3 ft above the floor.
   C. 2 ft above the floor.
   D. 6 ft above the floor.

_____ 3. The best method of transporting a hand-held portable fire extinguisher depends on the
   A. training level of the operator.
   B. size, weight, and design of the extinguisher.
   C. type of extinguishing agent.
   D. size and type of fire.

_____ 4. All fires require
   A. fuel, heat, and oxygen.
   B. fuel and oxygen.
   C. an ignition source.
   D. fuel, heat, oxygen, and carelessness.

_____ 5. Class A fire extinguishers include a number. This number is related to the
   A. type of fuel the fire extinguisher can extinguish.
   B. size of the discharge field.
   C. approximate area of burning fuel the fire extinguisher can extinguish.
   D. amount of water the fire extinguisher holds.

_____ 6. The safest and surest way to extinguish a Class C fire is to turn off the power and
   A. treat it like a Class A or B fire.
   B. treat it like a Class D fire.
   C. treat it like a Class K fire.
   D. treat it like a Class A, B, or D fire.

_____ 7. Class D fires are most often encountered in
   A. kitchens or restaurants.
   B. offices or schools.
   C. machine or repair shops.
   D. hayfields or woodland areas.

_____ 8. Where is the extinguishing agent in a fire extinguisher stored?
   A. Trigger
   B. Nozzle
   C. Cylinder
   D. Handle

_____ 9. Carbon dioxide is a gas that is 1.5 times heavier than
   A. water.
   B. most extinguishing agents.
   C. air.
   D. carbon monoxide.

_____ 10. Two factors to consider when determining the number and types of fire extinguishers that should be placed in each area of occupancy are the
   A. quality and quantities of the fuels.
   B. fuels and ignition sources.
   C. types of fuels and area traffic.
   D. types and quantities of the fuels.

_____ 11. Fires that have not spread past their point of origin are
   A. called introductory fires.
   B. called incipient-stage fires.
   C. easily suppressed.
   D. most often suppressed with an exterior attack.

_____ 12. What is the only dry chemical extinguishing agent rated as suitable for Class A fires?
   A. Potassium chloride
   B. Potassium bicarbonate
   C. Ammonium phosphate
   D. Ammonium bicarbonate

_____ 13. An extinguisher rated 40-B should be able to control a liquid pan fire
   A. with a surface area of 40 ft^2 (3.7 m^2).
   B. within 40 seconds.
   C. 40 times more effectively than a normal Class B extinguisher.
   D. 4 times more effectively than a normal Class B extinguisher.

_____ 14. The three risk classifications according to the amount and type of combustibles that are present in an area are
   A. light, ordinary, and extra hazards.
   B. light, medium, and extra hazards.
   C. normal, light, and extra hazards.
   D. normal, average, and extra hazards.

_____ 15. Class A fires involve
   A. combustible metal fires.
   B. ordinary combustibles.
   C. vegetable oils.
   D. electrically charged materials.

_____ 16. Self-expelling agents do not require
   A. regular maintenance.
   B. tamper seals on the cylinders.
   C. a separate gas cartridge.
   D. maintenance personnel to be specially trained in their use.

_____ 17. Carbon dioxide extinguishers have relatively short discharge ranges of
   A. 1 to 3 ft (0.3 to 0.9 m).
   B. 3 to 8 ft (0.9 to 2.4 m).
   C. 10 to 15 ft (3 to 4.6 m).
   D. 15 to 30 ft (4.6 to 9.1 m).

_____ 18. Which lever is used to discharge the agent from a portable fire extinguisher?
   A. Trigger
   B. Nozzle
   C. Cylinder
   D. Handle

_____ 19. Vegetable oil fires are classified as
   A. Class A fires.
   B. Class B fires.
   C. Class C fires.
   D. Class K fires.

_______ **20.** Class B fire extinguishers can be identified by the
A. solid red square.
B. solid blue square.
C. solid red circle.
D. solid yellow five-point star.

_______ **21.** Carbon dioxide extinguishers are not recommended for
A. Class B fires.
B. Class C fires.
C. outdoor use.
D. use in kitchens or laboratories.

_______ **22.** Electrical rooms should have extinguishers that are approved for use on
A. Class K fires.
B. Class A fires.
C. Class B fires.
D. Class C fires.

Labeling

Label the following diagram with the correct terms.

1. Basic parts of a portable fire extinguisher.

Courtesy of Amerex Corporation.

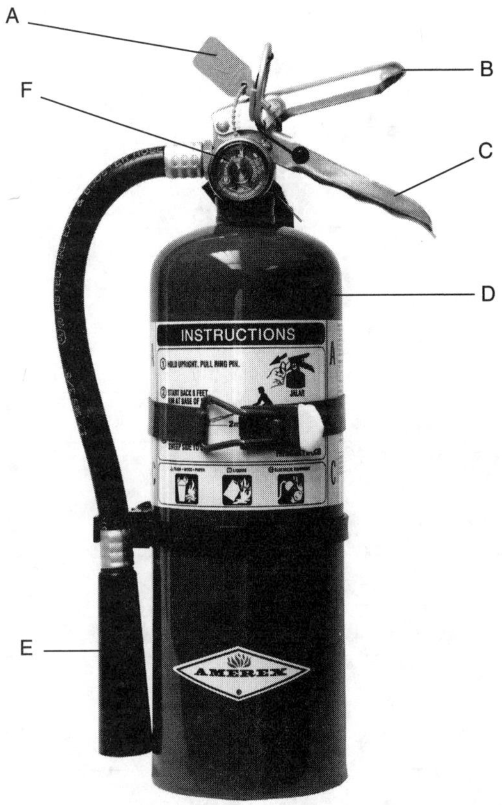

A. ______________________________

B. ______________________________

C. ______________________________

D. ______________________________

E. ______________________________

F. ______________________________

Vocabulary

Define the following terms using the space provided.

1. Polar solvent:

2. Extra hazard locations:

3. Extinguishing agent:

4. Cartridge/cylinder fire extinguisher:

5. Underwriters Laboratories, Inc. (UL):

6. Class K fires:

7. Oxidation:

8. Multipurpose dry chemical extinguisher:

Fill-In
Read each item carefully, and then complete the statement by filling in the missing word(s).

1. _____ extinguishers have a short discharge range.
2. The extinguishing agent of a portable extinguisher is discharged through a(n) _____ or horn.
3. An individual with _____ training should be able to use most fire extinguishers effectively.
4. _____ is a fire extinguishing agent that does not leave a residue when it evaporates.
5. _____ extinguishers are used primarily outdoors for fighting brush and grass fires.
6. Class _____ labels are represented by a solid blue circle.
7. A Class _____ fire is one that involves wood, cloth, rubber, household rubbish, and some plastics.
8. _____ is a colorless, odorless, electronically nonconductive gas that puts out Class B and C fires by displacing oxygen and cooling the fuel.
9. A fire extinguisher must be _____ after each and every use.
10. The ignition point is the _____ at which a substance will burn.

True/False
If you believe the statement to be more true than false, write the letter "T" in the space provided. If you believe the statement to be more false than true, write the letter "F."

1. _____ Class K extinguishers are identified by a solid yellow five-point star.
2. _____ Halon should be used with care in confined areas.
3. _____ "Press the trigger" is the first step of PASS.
4. _____ The bottom of an extinguisher should be mounted at least 4 in. (10.2 cm) above the floor.
5. _____ A Class B extinguisher with a 10-B rating indicates it is capable of extinguishing the highest level of Class B fires.
6. _____ Most offices or classrooms would be examples of light hazard areas.
7. _____ The primary disadvantage of fire extinguishers is their effectiveness.
8. _____ All fire fighters are trained to perform fire extinguisher maintenance.
9. _____ Time intervals for testing requirements for an extinguisher are based on construction material and vessel type.
10. _____ Fire extinguishers can contain several hundred pounds of extinguishing agent.

Short Answer
Complete this section with short written answers using the space provided.

1. Identify the six basic steps in extinguishing a fire with a portable fire extinguisher.

_____
_____
_____
_____
_____

70   FUNDAMENTALS OF FIRE FIGHTER SKILLS

2. Describe the PASS acronym used for fire extinguisher operations.

3. List five typical examples of occupancies that would be classified as ordinary (moderate) hazards.

4. Identify the seven types of fire extinguishers.

Fire Alarms

The following real case scenarios will give you an opportunity to explore the concerns associated with portable fire extinguishers. Read each scenario, and then answer each question in detail.

1. It is 7:00 on a Thursday evening when your engine is dispatched to a chimney fire. Upon arrival, you find a two-story, wood-frame residential structure with nothing showing. Upon further investigation, you confirm there is a fire in the chimney. Your Lieutenant tells you to extinguish the fire in the fireplace with an extinguisher. How should you proceed?

2. It is 8:00 on Saturday morning, and your Lieutenant is conducting the morning shift meeting. Saturday's duties are to do a detailed inspection of all equipment. The Lieutenant assigns you to inspect all of the extinguishers on the apparatus and report any that need maintenance. How should you proceed?

Skill Drills

Skill Drill 7-1: Transporting a Fire Extinguisher Fire Fighter I, NFPA 1001: 4.3.16
Test your knowledge of this skill drill by filling in the correct words in the photo captions.

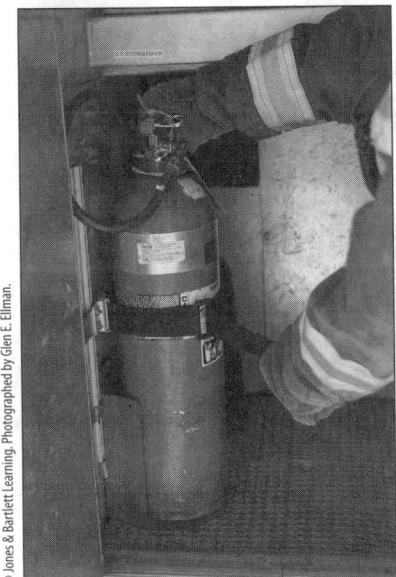

1. Locate the closest _____.

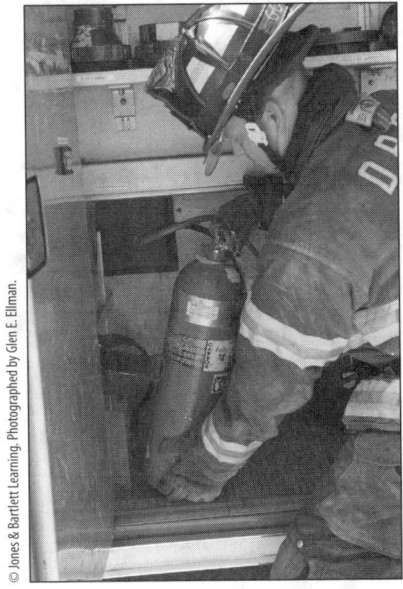

2. Assess that the fire extinguisher is safe and effective for the type of fire being attacked. Release the _____.

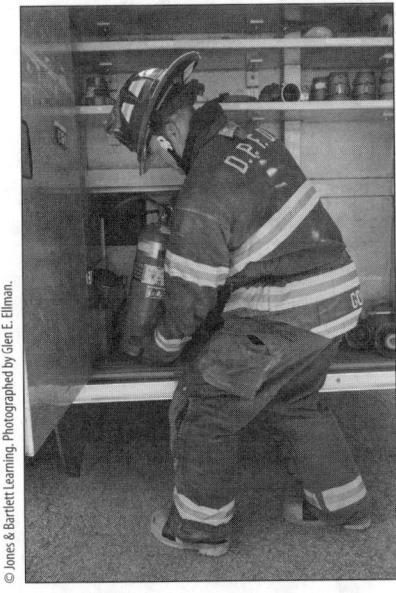

3. Lift the fire extinguisher using good body mechanics. Lift small fire extinguishers with _____ and large extinguishers with _____.

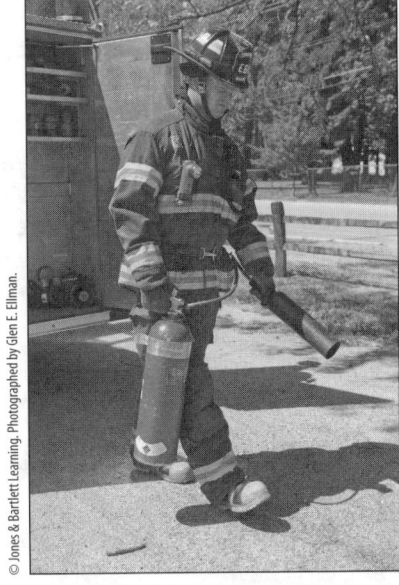

4. Walk briskly—do not run—toward the fire. If the fire extinguisher has a hose and _____, carry the extinguisher with one hand, and grasp the _____ with the other hand.

Skill Drill 7-2: Extinguishing a Class A Fire with a Stored-Pressure Water-Type Fire Extinguisher Fire Fighter I, NFPA 1001: 4.3.16
Test your knowledge of this skill drill by filling in the correct words in the photo captions.

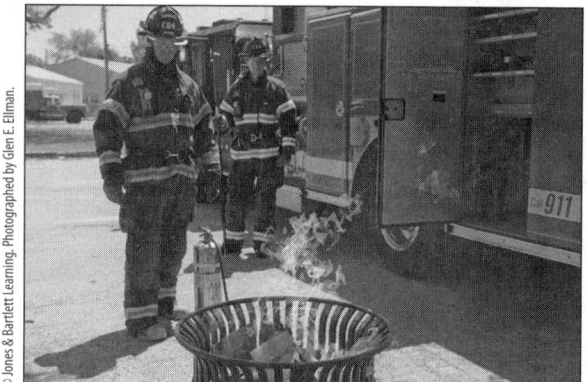

1. Size up the fire to determine whether a stored-pressure water-type fire extinguisher is safe and effective for the fire. Ensure the fire extinguisher is large enough to be safe and effective. Ensure your safety. Make sure you have a(n) _____ from the fire. Do not turn your back on a fire.

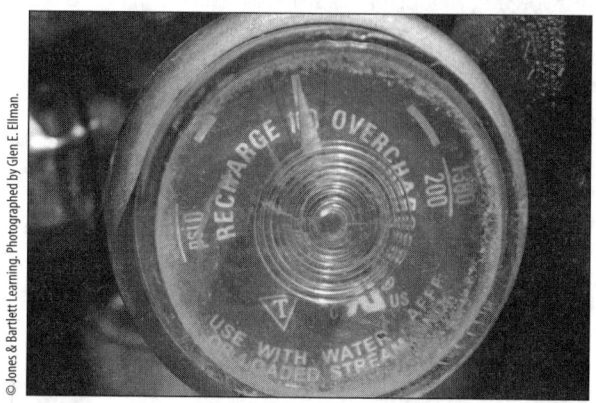

2. Remove the hose and nozzle. Quickly check the _____ to verify that the fire extinguisher is adequately charged.

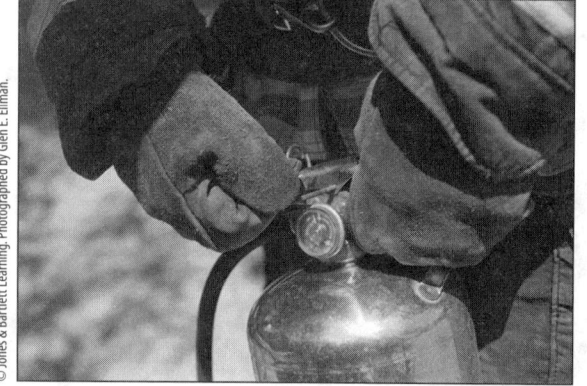

3. Pull the _____ to release the fire extinguisher control valve. You must be within 35 to 40 ft (11 to 12 m) of the fire to be effective.

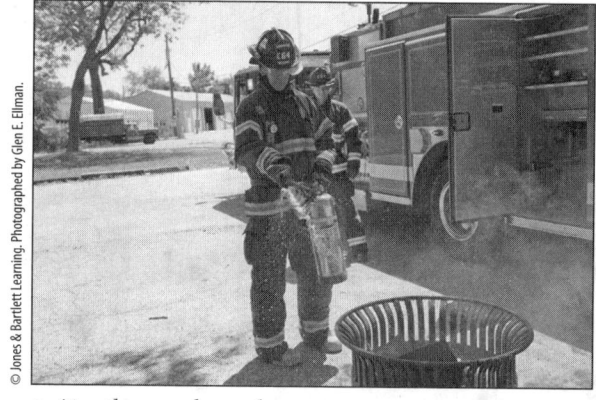

4. Aim the nozzle, and _____ the water stream at the base of the flames.

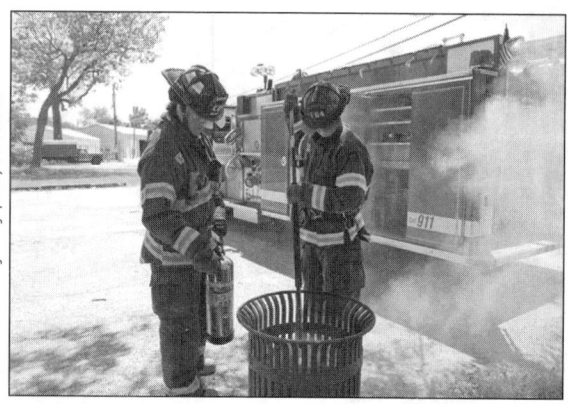

5. Overhaul the fire. Take steps to prevent _____, break apart tightly packed fuel, and summon additional help if needed.

Skill Drill 7-3: Extinguishing a Class A Fire with a Multipurpose Dry-Chemical Fire Extinguisher Fire Fighter I, NFPA 1001: 4.3.16

Test your knowledge of this skill drill by placing the tasks below in the correct order. Number the first step with a "1," the second step with a "2," and so on.

1. _____ Overhaul the fire; take steps to prevent rekindling, break apart tightly packed fuel, and summon additional help if needed.

2. _____ Pull the pin to release the fire extinguisher control valve. Depending on the size of the fire and fire extinguisher, you must be within 5 to 45 ft (2 to 14 m) of the fire to be effective.

3. _____ Remove the hose and nozzle. Quickly check the pressure gauge to verify that the fire extinguisher is adequately charged.

4. _____ Aim the nozzle, and sweep the dry-chemical discharge at the base of the flames. Coat the burning fuel with dry chemical.

5. _____ Size up the fire to determine whether a multipurpose dry-chemical fire extinguisher is safe and effective for this fire. Ensure the fire extinguisher is large enough to be safe and effective. Ensure your safety. Make sure you have an exit route from the fire. Do not turn your back on a fire.

Skill Drill 7-4: Extinguishing a Class B Flammable Liquid Fire with a Dry-Chemical Fire Extinguisher Fire Fighter I, NFPA 1001: 4.3.16

Test your knowledge of this skill drill by placing the photos below in the correct order. Number the first step with a "1," the second step with a "2," and so on.

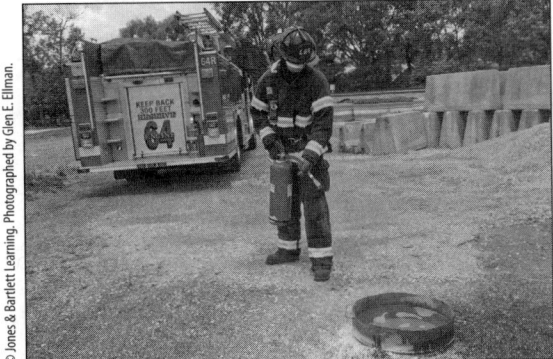

_____ Overhaul the fire; take steps to prevent rekindling, keep a blanket of dry chemical over the fuel, and summon additional help if needed.

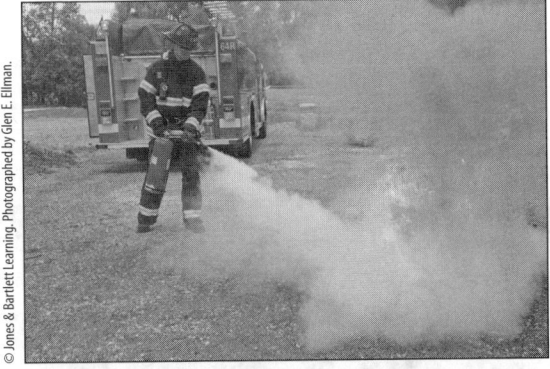

_____ Aim the nozzle, and sweep the dry-chemical discharge across the surface of the burning liquid. Start at the near edge of the fire, and work toward the back.

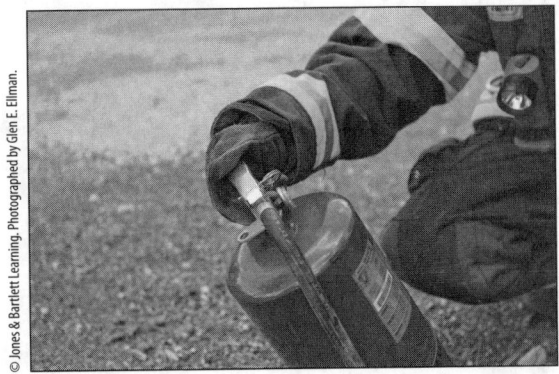

_____ Pull the pin to release the fire extinguisher valve. Depending on the size of the fire and fire extinguisher, you must be within 5 to 45 ft of the fire to be effective.

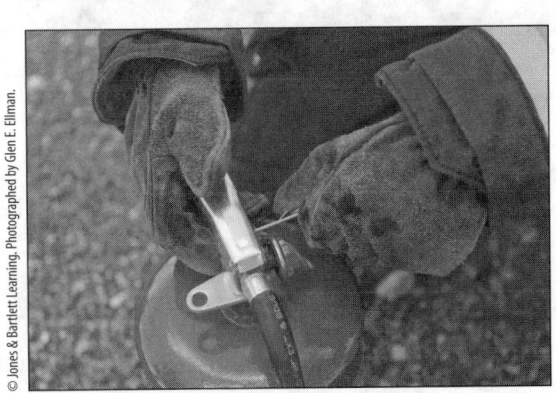

_____ Size up the fire, and ensure your safety. Check the pressure gauge.

Skill Drill 7-5: Extinguishing a Class B Flammable Liquid Fire with a Stored-Pressure Foam Fire Extinguisher (AFFF or FFFP) Fire Fighter I, NFPA 1001: 4.3.16

Test your knowledge of this skill drill by filling in the correct words in the photo captions.

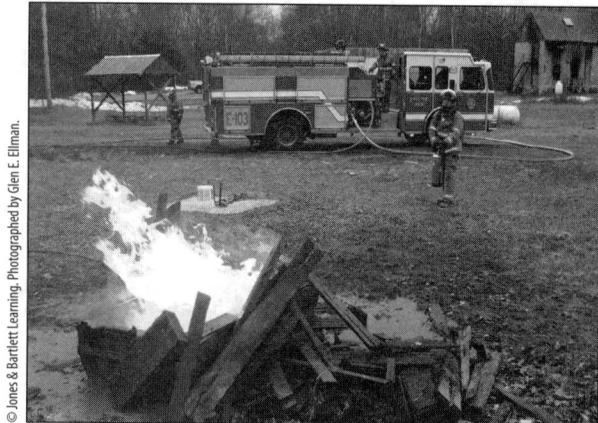

1. Size up the fire, and ensure your safety. Remove the hose and nozzle. Quickly check the pressure gauge to verify that the fire extinguisher is adequately _____. Pull the pin to release the fire extinguisher control valve. You must be within 20 to 25 ft (6 to 8 m) of the fire to be effective.

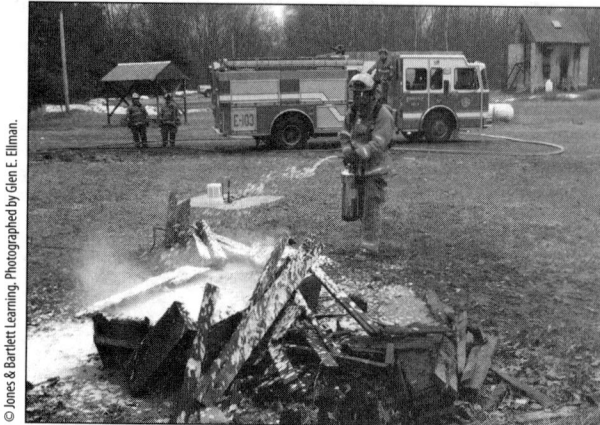

2. Aim the nozzle, and discharge the stream of foam so the foam drops gently onto the surface of the burning liquid at the front or the back of the container. Let the _____ flow across the surface of the burning liquid. Avoid splashing foam on the burning liquid, because it can cause the burning fuel to splatter.

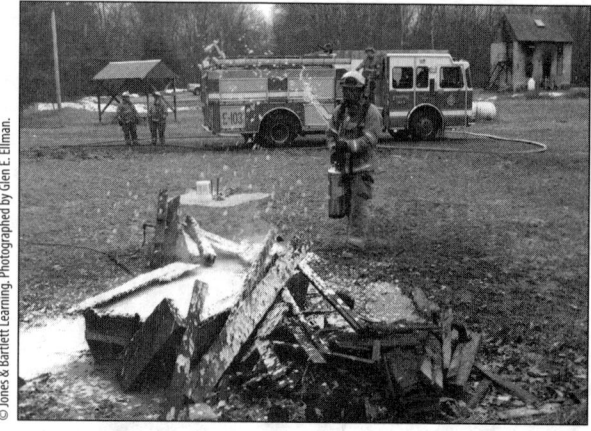

3. Overhaul the fire. Keep a thick blanket of foam intact over the hot liquid, reapply foam over any _____, and summon additional help if needed.

Skill Drill 7-6: Operating a Carbon Dioxide Fire Extinguisher Fire Fighter I, NFPA 1001: 4.3.16
Test your knowledge of this skill drill by filling in the correct words in the photo captions.

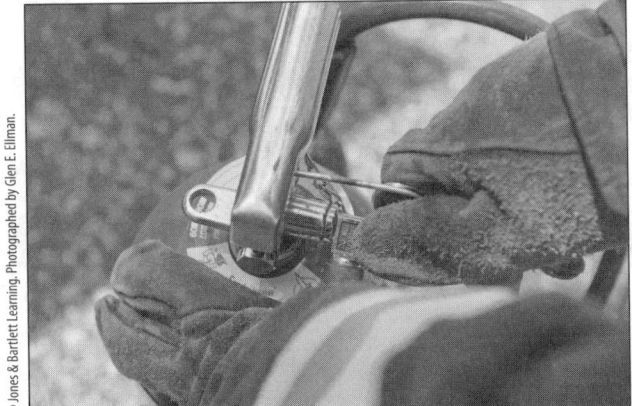

1. Size up the fire to determine whether _____ is a safe and effective agent for this fire. Ensure the fire extinguisher is large enough to be safe and effective. Ensure your safety. Make sure you have an exit route from the fire. Do not turn your back on a fire. Remove the horn or nozzle. Pull the pin to release the fire extinguisher control valve.

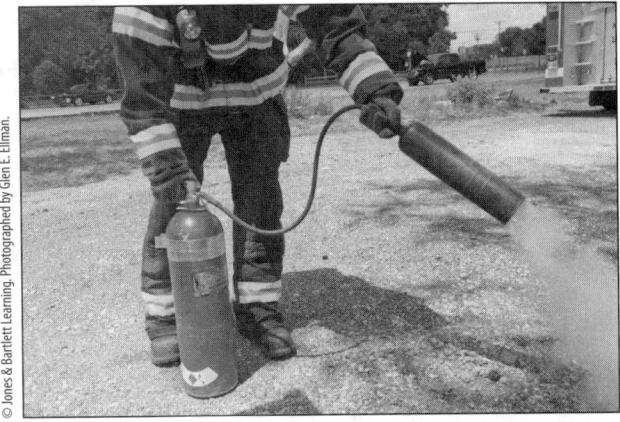

2. Quickly squeeze to verify that the fire extinguisher is charged; CO_2 fire extinguishers do not have _____. You must be within 3 to 8 ft (1 to 2.5 m) of the fire to be effective.

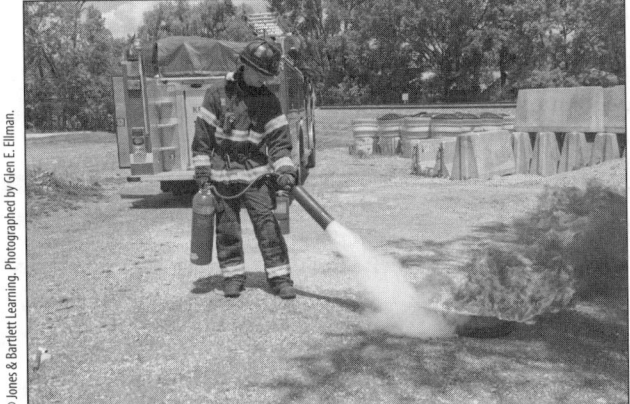

3. Aim the horn or nozzle, and sweep at the _____ of the flames.

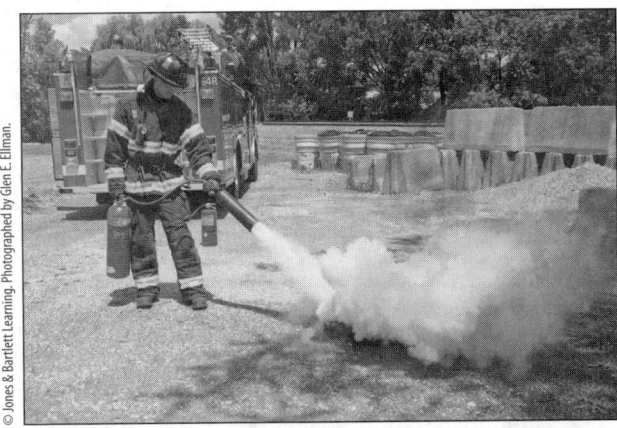

4. Overhaul the fire. Take steps to prevent _____, and summon additional help if needed.

Skill Drill 7-7: Operating a Halogenated Stored-Pressure Fire Extinguisher Fire Fighter I, NFPA 1001: 4.3.16

Test your knowledge of this skill drill by placing the tasks below in the correct order. Number the first step with a "1," the second step with a "2," and so on.

1. _____ Size up the fire to determine whether a halogenated stored-pressure fire extinguisher is safe and effective for this fire. Ensure the fire extinguisher is large enough to be safe and effective.

2. _____ Remove the hose and nozzle. Quickly check the pressure gauge to verify that the fire extinguisher is adequately charged.

3. _____ Ensure your safety. Turn off electricity if possible. Make sure you have an exit route from the fire. Do not turn your back on a fire.

4. _____ Overhaul the fire; take steps to prevent rekindling, continue to apply the extinguishing agent to cool the fuel, and summon additional help if needed.

5. _____ Aim the nozzle at the base of the flames to sweep the flames off the surface starting at the near edge of the flames.

6. _____ Pull the pin to release the fire extinguisher control valve. Depending on the size of the fire and fire extinguisher, you must be within 3 to 35 ft (1 to 11 m) of the fire to be effective.

Skill Drill 7-8: Operating a Dry-Powder Fire Extinguisher Fire Fighter I, NFPA 1001: 4.3.16

Test your knowledge of this skill drill by placing the tasks below in the correct order. Number the first step with a "1," the second step with a "2," and so on.

1. _____ Pull the pin to release the control valve. You must be within 6 to 8 ft (2 to 2.5 m) of the fire to be effective.

2. _____ Remove the hose and nozzle. Quickly check the pressure gauge to ensure the fire extinguisher is charged.

3. _____ Ensure your safety. Make sure you have an exit route from the fire. Do not turn your back on a fire.

4. _____ Size up the fire to determine whether a dry-powder fire extinguisher is safe and effective for this fire. Ensure the fire extinguisher is large enough to be safe and effective. Avoid water or other extinguishing agents that might react with the combustible metals.

5. _____ Overhaul the fire; take steps to prevent rekindling, continue to place a thick layer of the extinguishing agent over the hot metal to form an airtight blanket, allow the hot metal to cool, and summon additional help if needed.

6. _____ Aim the nozzle, and fully open the valve to provide a maximum range, and then reduce the valve to produce a soft, heavy flow down to completely cover the burning metal. The method of application may vary depending on the type of metal burning and the extinguishing agent.

Skill Drill 7-9: Operating a Wet-Chemical Fire Extinguisher Fire Fighter I, NFPA 1001: 4.3.16
Test your knowledge of this skill drill by filling in the correct words in the photo captions.

1. Size up the fire, and ensure your _____.

2. Remove the hose and nozzle. Quickly check the _____ to verify that the fire extinguisher is adequately charged.

3. Pull the _____ to release the fire extinguisher control valve. You must be within 8 to 12 ft (2.5 to 4 m) of the fire to be effective.

4. Aim the nozzle and discharge so the stream of wet chemical drops gently into the _____ of the burning liquid at the front or back of the deep-fat fryer.

5. Let the deep foam blanket flow across the surface of the burning liquid. Avoid _____ on the burning liquid.

6. Continue to apply the agent until the foam blanket has extinguished _____ of the flames.

7. Do not disturb the foam blanket even after all of the flames have been suppressed. If _____ occurs, repeat these steps.

Fire Fighter Tools and Equipment

Workbook Activities

The following activities have been designed to help you. Your instructor may require you to complete some or all of these activities as a regular part of your fire fighter training program. You are encouraged to complete any activity your instructor does not assign to you, as a way to enhance your learning in the classroom.

Chapter Review

The following exercises provide an opportunity to refresh your knowledge of this chapter.

Matching

Match each of the terms in the left column to the appropriate definition in the right column.

_____ 1. Roofman's hook
_____ 2. Multipurpose hook
_____ 3. Size-up
_____ 4. Ventilation
_____ 5. Rapid intervention
_____ 6. Box-end wrench
_____ 7. Sledgehammer
_____ 8. Hydraulic spreader
_____ 9. Battering ram
_____ 10. Thermal imaging device

A. A long pole with a wooden or fiberglass handle and a metal hook on one end used for pulling
B. The process of making openings so that the smoke, heat, and gases can escape vertically from a structure
C. A team of fire fighters designated to stand by, in a ready state, for immediate rescue of injured or trapped fire fighters
D. A long, heavy hammer that requires the use of both hands
E. A long pole with a solid metal hook used for pulling
F. A tool made of hardened steel with handles on the sides used to force doors and to breach walls
G. A hand tool with a closed end used to tighten or loosen bolts
H. A lightweight, hand-operated tool that can produce up to 10,000 pounds of prying and spreading force
I. The observation and evaluation of existing factors that are used to develop objectives, strategy, and tactics for fire suppression
J. Electronic devices that detect differences in temperature based on infrared energy and then generate images based on those data

Multiple Choice

Read each item carefully, and then select the best response.

_____ 1. A pike pole
   A. is a lever used for prying.
   B. is used for rotating.
   C. is a pulling tool.
   D. is a cutting tool.

CHAPTER 8

_____ 2. Which tool heats metal until it melts?
   A. Hydraulic spreader
   B. Power saw
   C. Air bag
   D. Cutting torch

_____ 3. Proper personal protective equipment (PPE) includes
   A. approved helmet.
   B. eye protection.
   C. firefighting gloves.
   D. All of the above.

_____ 4. Tools used for vertical roof ventilation include
   A. shovels and brooms.
   B. power saws and axes.
   C. negative-pressure fans.
   D. rakes and buckets.

_____ 5. Which of the following is not considered part of a fire fighter's PPE?
   A. Boots
   B. Approved firefighting gloves
   C. Approved firefighting prying tool
   D. Personal alert safety system

_____ 6. Which of these are prying tools?
   A. Sledgehammer
   B. Halligan bar and crowbar
   C. K tool and chisel
   D. Bucket and shovel

_____ 7. Pike poles are commonly used for
   A. pulling ceilings.
   B. opening floors.
   C. popping doors off hinges.
   D. car fires.

_____ 8. Which of the following tools is often used in vehicular crashes to gain access to a victim who needs care?
   A. Spring-loaded center punch
   B. Sledgehammer
   C. Chainsaw
   D. Crowbar

_____ 9. After use, all hand tools should be completely cleaned and
   A. scientifically tested.
   B. inspected.
   C. sharpened.
   D. placed in the tool cabinet.

_____ 10. Which of the following is considered a tool for cutting metal?
   A. Crowbar
   B. Drywall hook
   C. Pick-head axe
   D. Hacksaw

_____ 11. Which of the following is considered a rotating tool?
   A. Claw bar
   B. Ceiling hook
   C. Axe
   D. Screwdriver

_____ 12. Wood handles on tools should be
   A. sanded and painted.
   B. sanded and varnished.
   C. sanded and have linseed oil applied.
   D. left alone.

_____ 13. Which of the following is a basic piece of equipment for interior firefighting?
   A. Hand light or portable light
   B. Thermal imaging device
   C. Chain saw
   D. Exhaust fan

_____ 14. Which tool is used to cut chains or padlocks?
   A. Bolt cutter
   B. Battering ram
   C. Flat-head axe
   D. K tool

_____ 15. Which of the following is not a mechanical saw?
   A. Chain saw
   B. Rotary saw
   C. Reciprocating saw
   D. Hacksaw

_____ 16. Which of the following is considered a tool for striking?
   A. Crowbar
   B. Drywall hook
   C. Pick-head axe
   D. Hacksaw

_____ 17. Special equipment to be carried by a rapid intervention crew (RIC) should include
   A. a thermal imager.
   B. prying tools.
   C. striking tools.
   D. All of the above.

_____ 18. Which of the following is an example of a special use tool?
   A. Multipurpose hook
   B. Air bags
   C. Sledgehammer
   D. Cutting torch

_____ 19. Which of the following is not a basic search and rescue hand tool?
   A. Halligan tool
   B. Axe
   C. Hand light
   D. K tool

_____ 20. All power equipment should be left in a ready state, which includes
   A. fuel tanks filled completely with fresh fuel.
   B. hydraulic hoses, if applicable, cleaned and inspected.
   C. the removal and replacement of any dull or damaged blades.
   D. All of the above.

Vocabulary

Define the following terms using the space provided.

1. Claw bar:

   _____
   _____
   _____

2. Reciprocating saw:

   _____
   _____
   _____

3. Overhaul:

   _____
   _____
   _____

4. Gripping pliers:

   _____
   _____
   _____

5. Crowbar:

   _____
   _____
   _____

6. Seat belt cutter:

   _____
   _____
   _____

7. Spanner wrench:

   _____
   _____
   _____

Fundamentals of Fire Fighter Skills

8. Kelly tool:
   _____
   _____
   _____

9. Cutting torch:
   _____
   _____
   _____

10. Hydrant wrench:
    _____
    _____
    _____

11. Ceiling hook:
    _____
    _____
    _____

12. Pike pole:
    _____
    _____
    _____

Fill-In

Read each item carefully, and then complete the statement by filling in the missing word(s).

1. A fire fighter must know how to use tools _____, efficiently, and safely.

2. _____ is the phase during which fire fighters start thinking about the possible tools or equipment they may need during an incident.

3. _____ is a prime consideration when using any tools and equipment.

4. A(n) _____ is a specialized striking tool with an axe on one end of the head and a sledgehammer on the other end.

5. _____ or _____ tools allow a fire fighter to increase the power exerted upon an object and extend the fire fighter's reach.

6. A(n) _____ has a pointed "pick" on one end of the head and an axe blade on the other end.

7. To reduce the total number of tools needed to achieve a goal, a fire fighter may carry a tool that has a number of uses. This tool is categorized as a(n) _____ tool.

8. _____ are tools that use extremely high-temperature flames to cut through an object.

9. A salvage tool known as a _____ is designed to cover a section of carpet or hardwood flooring.

10. A flat-head axes and a Halligan tool are collectively called the _____.

True/False

If you believe the statement to be more true than false, write the letter "T" in the space provided. If you believe the statement to be more false than true, write the letter "F."

1. _____ One of the most popular prying tools is the Halligan tool.
2. _____ One of the three primary types of mechanical saws is the combination saw.
3. _____ Department guidelines or standard operating procedures usually guide the decision for which tool to use during an incident.
4. _____ Air bags can be used to lift heavy objects.
5. _____ Striking tools should be assigned to crews only during the forcible entry phase of a response.
6. _____ The K tool is used to pull the lock cylinder out of a door.
7. _____ Interior attack can be orchestrated by any response member at any time during an emergency response.
8. _____ Mechanically powered equipment is more powerful than manually powered equipment.
9. _____ New fire fighters are often surprised by the strength and energy required to perform many tasks.
10. _____ A RIC should carry self-contained breathing apparatus (SCBA) and spare air cylinders.

Short Answer

Complete this section with short written answers using the space provided.

1. What are two advantages of using pushing/pulling tools? Give five examples of pushing/pulling tools.

   _____
   _____
   _____
   _____

2. Why is it important to know which tools are needed for each phase of an incident?

   _____
   _____
   _____
   _____

3. Identify the tools used during salvage and overhaul operations.

   _____
   _____
   _____
   _____

Fundamentals of Fire Fighter Skills

4. Identify the basic set of tools used for interior firefighting.
   _____
   _____
   _____
   _____

5. Identify the basic set of tools used for search and rescue.
   _____
   _____
   _____
   _____

Fire Alarms
The following real case scenarios will give you an opportunity to explore the concerns associated with fire fighter tools and equipment. Read each scenario, and then answer each question in detail.

1. It is 6:00 on a Monday morning when your engine is dispatched to a commercial structure fire in a warehouse.

   You are the fifth engine to arrive at the scene. The IC assigns your engine to the RIC group. Your Lieutenant tells you to gather the RIC equipment and place it in the staging area. How should you proceed?
   _____
   _____
   _____
   _____
   _____
   _____

2. It is 7:30 on a Sunday morning and your Lieutenant is conducting a shift meeting. The Lieutenant tells you to ensure the power tools and equipment are clean and inspected. After the meeting, you start with the ladder truck by pulling off the chainsaws. How should you proceed?
   _____
   _____
   _____
   _____
   _____
   _____

Skill Drills

Skill Drill 8-1: Cleaning and Inspecting Hand Tools Fire Fighter I, NFPA 1001: 4.5.1
Test your knowledge of this skill drill by filling in the correct words in the photo captions.

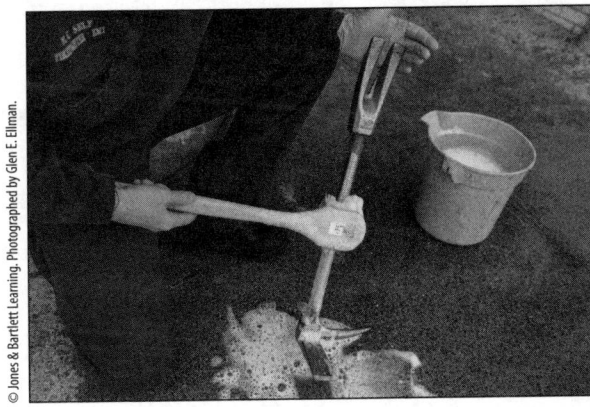

1. Clean and dry all _____ parts. Metal tools must be dried completely, either by _____ or by _____, before being returned to the apparatus. Remove _____ with steel wool. Coat unpainted metal surfaces with a light film of _____ to help prevent rusting. Do not _____ the striking surface of metal tools, as this treatment may cause them to slip.

2. Inspect _____ handles for damage such as cracks and splinters. Repair or replace any damaged handles. _____ the handle if necessary. Do not paint or varnish a wood handle; instead, apply a coat of _____. Check that the tool head is tightly fixed to the handle.

3. Clean _____ handles with soap and water. Inspect for damage. Repair or replace any damaged handles. Check that the tool head is tightly fixed to the handle.

4. Inspect _____ for nicks or other damage. Cutting tools should be sharpened after each use. File and sharpen as needed. _____ may weaken some tools, so hand sharpening may be required.

Ropes and Knots

Workbook Activities

The following activities have been designed to help you. Your instructor may require you to complete some or all of these activities as a regular part of your fire fighter training program. You are encouraged to complete any activity your instructor does not assign to you, as a way to enhance your learning in the classroom.

Chapter Review

The following exercises provide an opportunity to refresh your knowledge of this chapter.

Matching

Match each of the terms in the left column to the appropriate definition in the right column.

_____ 1. Safety knot
_____ 2. Twisted rope
_____ 3. Standing part
_____ 4. Hitches
_____ 5. Block creel construction
_____ 6. Dynamic rope
_____ 7. Escape rope
_____ 8. Bight
_____ 9. Static rope
_____ 10. Clove hitch

A. The part of a rope between the working end and the running end
B. Rope constructed without knots or splices in the yarns, ply yarns, strands, braids, or rope
C. A knot used to attach a rope firmly to a round object, such as a tree or fencepost
D. A U-shape created by bending a rope with the two sides parallel
E. A knot used to secure the leftover working end of the rope; also known as an overhand knot or keeper knot
F. A rope generally made out of synthetic material that stretches very little under load
G. Rope constructed of fibers twisted into strands, which are then twisted together
H. An emergency-use rope designed to carry the weight of only one person and to be used only once
I. Knots that wrap around an object
J. A rope generally made out of synthetic materials that is designed to be elastic and stretch when loaded

Multiple Choice

Read each item carefully, and then select the best response.

_____ 1. What is the working end of the rope used for?
  A. Lifting or hoisting
  B. Securing the knot
  C. Carrying the rope
  D. Forming the knot

_____ 2. What are three primary types of rope used in the fire service?
  A. Polypropylene, synthetic, and nylon
  B. Natural fiber, manila, and sisal
  C. Life safety, utility, and escape
  D. Hauling, securing, and towing

CHAPTER 9

_____ 3. The running end is the part of the rope used for
   A. forming the knot.
   B. life safety.
   C. securing the knot.
   D. lifting or hoisting.

_____ 4. The knot used to secure the leftover working end of a rope is called a
   A. granny knot and severe tangle.
   B. becket bend.
   C. slip knot.
   D. safety knot.

_____ 5. Natural fiber ropes
   A. lose their load-carrying ability over time.
   B. absorb water.
   C. degrade quickly.
   D. All of the above.

_____ 6. A pike pole is hoisted using
   A. a figure eight and a clove hitch.
   B. clove and half hitches.
   C. a figure eight on a bight.
   D. a safety knot and bowline.

_____ 7. Life safety rope is used solely for
   A. sectioning off safety areas.
   B. supporting people.
   C. medical response.
   D. hoisting equipment.

_____ 8. Synthetic ropes
   A. absorb more water than natural fiber ropes.
   B. cannot be used as a life safety rope.
   C. can be damaged by ultraviolet light.
   D. will not be damaged by acids.

_____ 9. Fire department ropes may be cleaned by using
   A. mild alkali solution.
   B. mild acid solution.
   C. mild soap and water.
   D. window cleaner.

_____ 10. Life safety rope is made of
   A. continuous filament virgin fiber and woven of block creel construction.
   B. the strongest natural fiber available.
   C. lightweight water-resistant fibers.
   D. fibers tested by the NFPA.

88 FUNDAMENTALS OF FIRE FIGHTER SKILLS

_____ 11. Polypropylene rope is often used in water rescue because
   A. it is light, does not absorb water, and floats.
   B. it is less expensive than natural rope.
   C. it is light and has built-in water repellents.
   D. it is easier to control.

_____ 12. The load-carrying capacity or strength of the rope will be
   A. increased by any knot.
   B. reduced by any knot.
   C. maintained by any knot.
   D. maintained by a bend or hitch.

_____ 13. Utility ropes
   A. may be used for a personal safety rope.
   B. can bear a single person (300 lb [136.1 kg]).
   C. can bear two persons (600 lb [272.2 kg]).
   D. are not to be used as a life safety rope.

_____ 14. How is a loop formed?
   A. By using the standing part of the rope
   B. By rolling from the end of the rope
   C. By making a circle in the rope
   D. By using the standing part of the knot

_____ 15. When hoisting an axe, a good rule of thumb is to
   A. hoist the equipment in a vertical position.
   B. use a one-person rope.
   C. use dynamic rope.
   D. execute the hoist as quickly as possible.

_____ 16. Life safety ropes are rated under the minimum requirements set by the
   A. NRA.
   B. NFPA.
   C. NIOSH.
   D. CDC.

Labeling

Label the following diagram with the correct terms.

1. Sections of a rope used in tying knots.

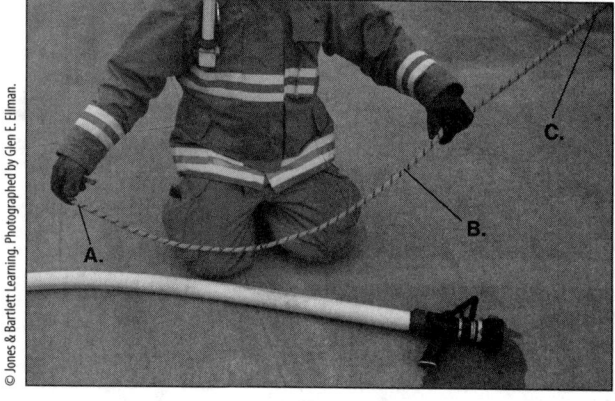

A. _____

B. _____

C. _____

Vocabulary

Define the following terms using the space provided.

1. Running end:

2. Knot:

3. Braided rope:

4. Rope bag:

5. Depressions:

6. Shock load:

7. Kernmantle rope:

8. Working end:

9. Round turn:

_____
_____
_____

10. Bight:

_____
_____
_____

Fill-In

Read each item carefully, and then complete the statement by filling in the missing word(s).

1. _____ are used to fasten rope or webbing to objects or to each other.

2. A(n) _____ is formed by reversing the direction of the rope to form a U bend with two parallel ends.

3. _____ are knots that wrap around an object such as a pike pole or fencepost.

4. Any knot will _____ the load-carrying capacity or strength of the rope.

5. A(n) _____ is used to secure the leftover working end of the rope to the standing part of the rope.

6. The figure eight on a bight knot creates _____ at the working end of a rope.

7. A(n) _____ is formed by making a loop and then bringing the two ends of the rope parallel to each other.

8. Each piece of rope must have a(n) _____ that details its history, usage, type of use, and loads applied.

9. A(n) _____ is a knot that can be used to form a loop. This type of knot is frequently used to secure the end or a rope to an object or anchor point.

10. A _____ knot is used to join webbing of the same or different sizes together.

True/False

If you believe the statement to be more true than false, write the letter "T" in the space provided. If you believe the statement to be more false than true, write the letter "F."

1. _____ Escape ropes can be used only once.
2. _____ A safety knot should always be used to finish other knots.
3. _____ Kernmantle ropes are the only ropes subject to being shock-loaded.
4. _____ Hitches are used to attach a rope around an object.
5. _____ Life safety ropes must be inspected after each use.
6. _____ Life safety ropes can be made of natural fibers if properly inspected, recorded, and maintained.
7. _____ All knots reduce the load-carrying capacity of a rope.
8. _____ A static rope is better suited for most fire rescue situations.
9. _____ A disadvantage of a loop knot is that it can easily slip.
10. _____ Bends are used to join two ropes together.

Short Answer

Complete this section by writing short answers in the spaces provided.

1. Identify the four parts of the rope maintenance formula.
   _____
   _____
   _____
   _____

2. List and describe the three types of rope construction.
   _____
   _____
   _____
   _____

3. List and describe the most common synthetic fiber ropes used for fire department operations.
   _____
   _____
   _____
   _____

4. What are some of the drawbacks of using natural fiber ropes?
   _____
   _____
   _____
   _____

5. List the principles to preserve the strength and integrity of rope.
   _____
   _____
   _____
   _____

Fire Alarms

The following real case scenarios will give you an opportunity to explore the concerns associated with ropes and knots. Read each scenario, and then answer each question in detail.

1. It is 9:00 on a Thursday evening when your engine company is dispatched to a structure fire at a three-story townhouse. Upon arrival, you are assigned to staging. The fire has been extinguished on the third floor. The IC assigns you and your partner to retrieve a ventilation fan from your engine and secure it to the rope that is deployed from the third floor. How should you proceed?

   _____
   _____
   _____
   _____
   _____
   _____

2. You have just returned from an apartment fire. During the fire, you used some of the utility rope off your engine to raise and lower equipment from the roof. While using the rope, it became dirty and needs to be cleaned and inspected. How should you proceed?

   _____
   _____
   _____
   _____
   _____
   _____

Skill Drills

Skill Drill 9-1: Caring for Life Safety Ropes Fire Fighter I, NFPA 1001: 4.5.1

Test your knowledge of this skill drill by filling in the correct words in the photo captions.

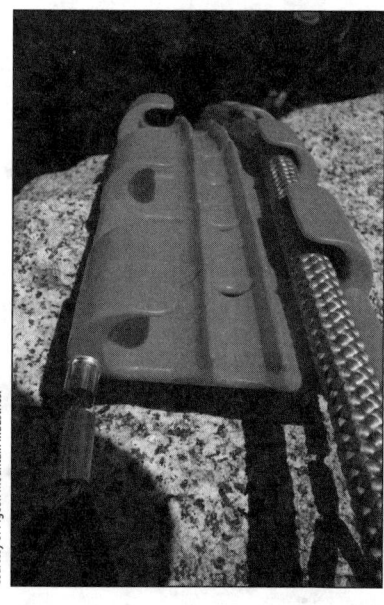

1. Protect the rope from _____ and _____ edges; use edge protectors.
2. Protect the rope from _____ against other ropes.
3. Protect the rope from _____, _____, _____, and _____.
4. Avoid _____ on the rope.

Skill Drill 9-7: Tying a Clove Hitch in the Open Fire Fighter I, NFPA 1001: 4.1.2, 4.3.20

Test your knowledge of this skill drill by placing the photos below in the correct order. Number the first step with a "1," the second step with a "2," and so on.

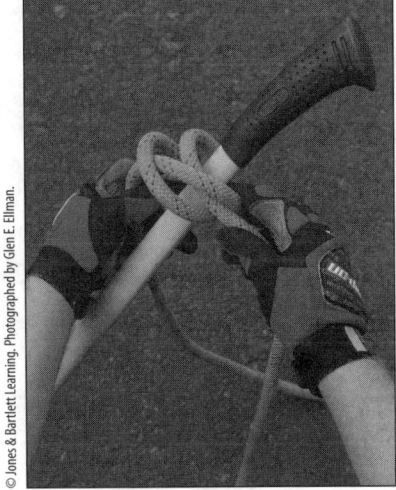
_____ Slide both loops over the object.

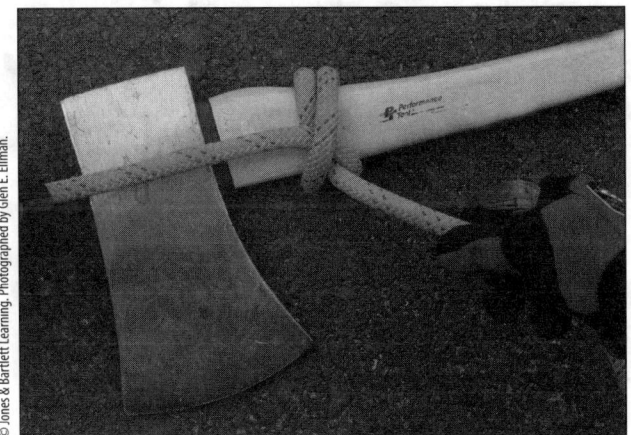
_____ Pull in opposite directions to tighten the clove hitch. Tie a safety knot in the working end of the rope.

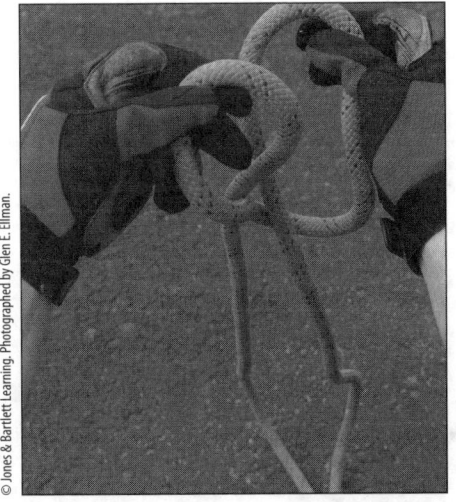
_____ Slide the right-hand loop behind the left-hand loop.

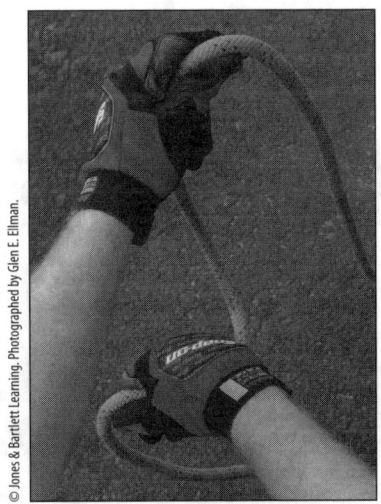
_____ Starting from left to right on the rope, grab the rope with crossed hands with the left positioned higher than the right.

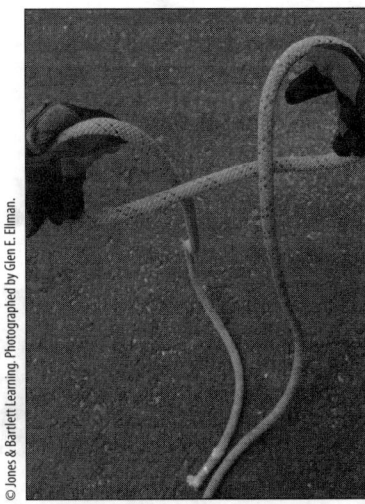
_____ Holding on to the rope, uncross your hands. This will create a loop in each hand.

Skill Drill 9-8: Tying a Clove Hitch Around an Object Fire Fighter I, NFPA 1001: 4.1.2, 4.3.20
Test your knowledge of this skill drill by placing the photos below in the correct order. Number the first step with a "1," the second step with a "2," and so on.

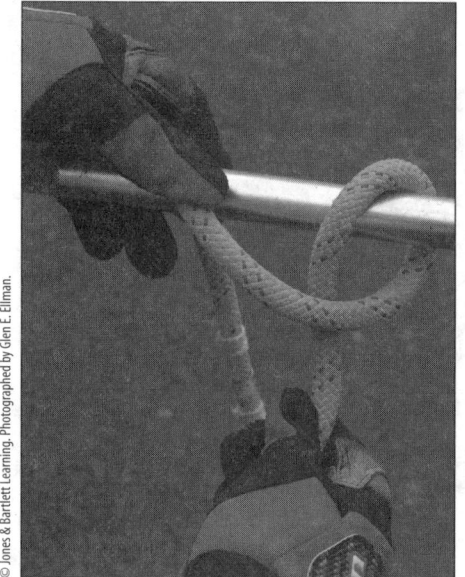
_____ Make a complete loop around the object, working end down.

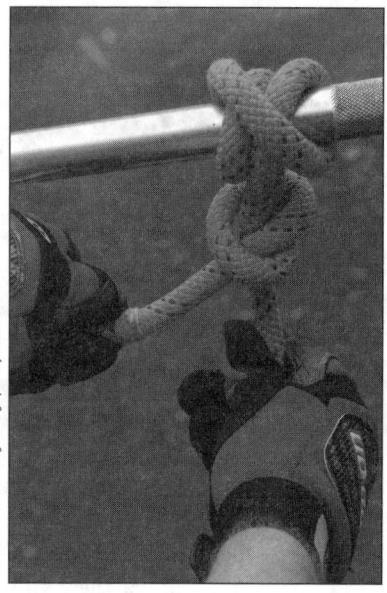
_____ Tie a safety knot in the working end of the rope.

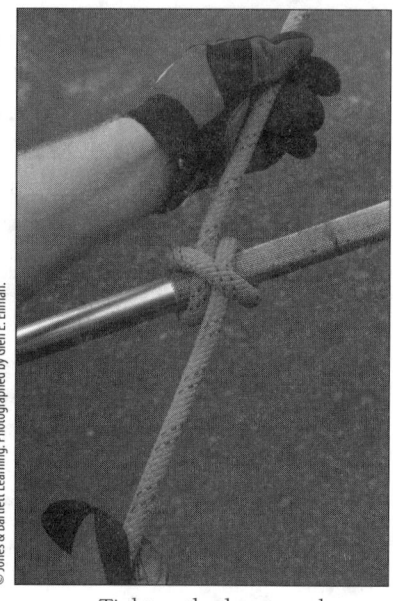
_____ Tighten the knot, and secure it by pulling on both ends.

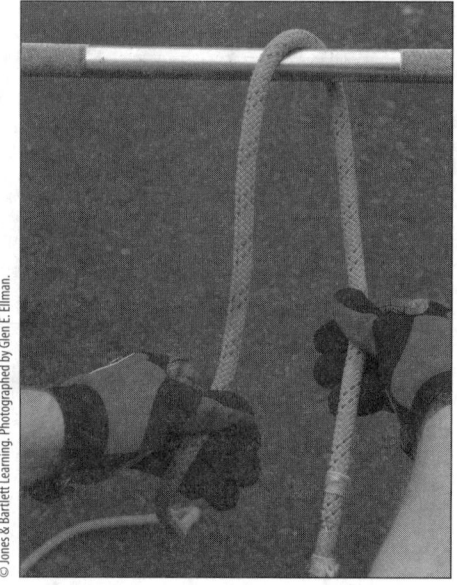
_____ Place the working end of the rope over the object.

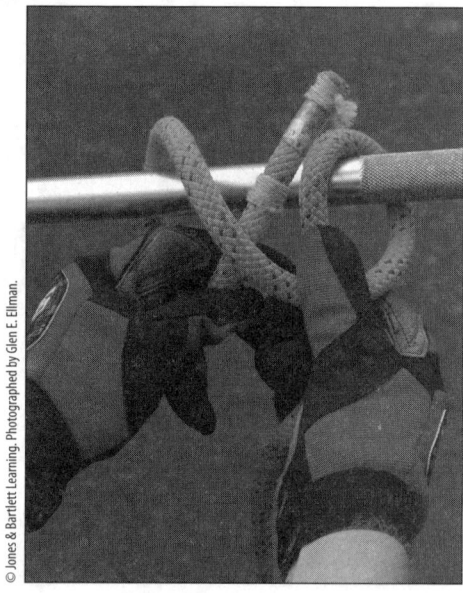
_____ Make a second loop around the object a short distance above the first loop. Pass the working end of the rope under the second loop, above the point where the second loop crosses over the first loop.

Skill Drill 9-12: Tying a Figure Eight Bend Fire Fighter 1, NFPA 1001: 4.1.2, 4.3.20
Test your knowledge of this skill drill by filling in the correct words in the photo captions.

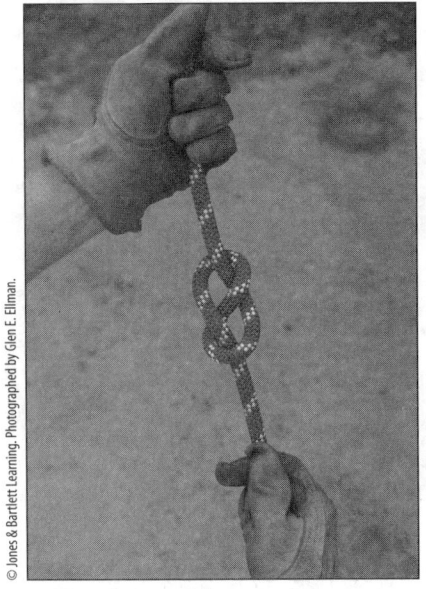 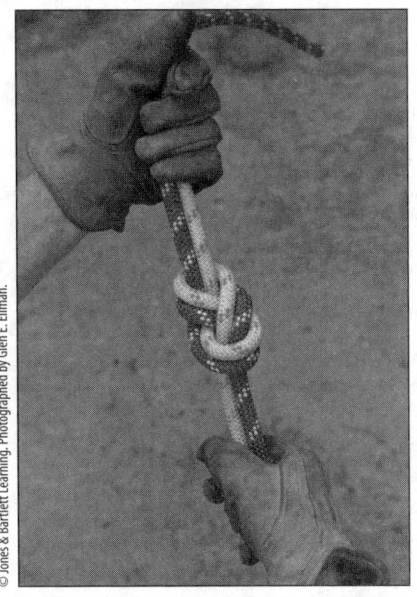 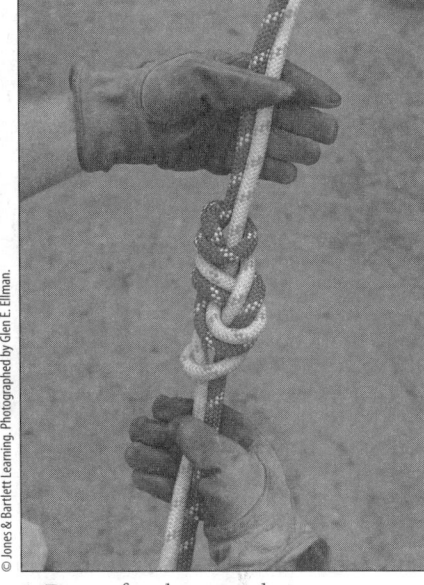

1. Tie a figure eight near the _____ of one rope.

2. Thread the end of the second rope completely through the knot from the _____ end. Pull the knot tight.

3. Tie a safety knot on the _____ end of each rope to the standing part of the other.

Skill Drill 9-13: Tying a Bowline Fire Fighter I, NFPA 1001: 4.1.2, 4.3.20
Test your knowledge of this skill drill by placing the photos below in the correct order. Number the first step with a "1," the second step with a "2," and so on.

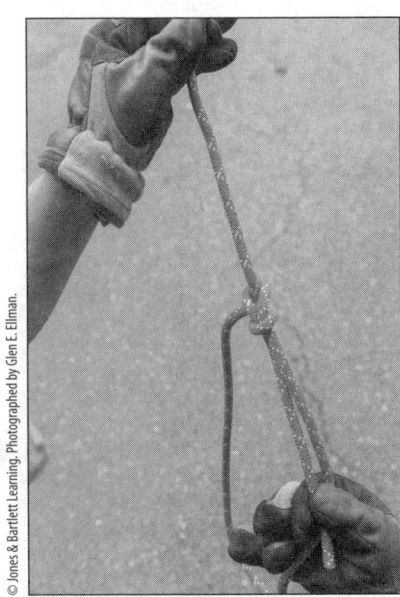 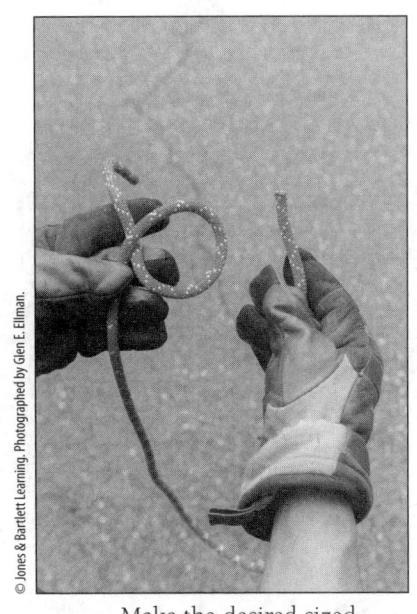 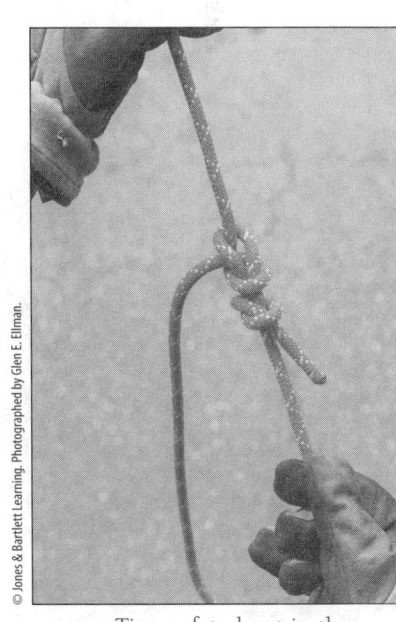

_____ Tighten the knot by holding the working end and pulling the standing part of the rope backward.

_____ Make the desired sized loop, and bring the working end back to the standing part.

_____ Tie a safety knot in the working end of the rope.

96 FUNDAMENTALS OF FIRE FIGHTER SKILLS

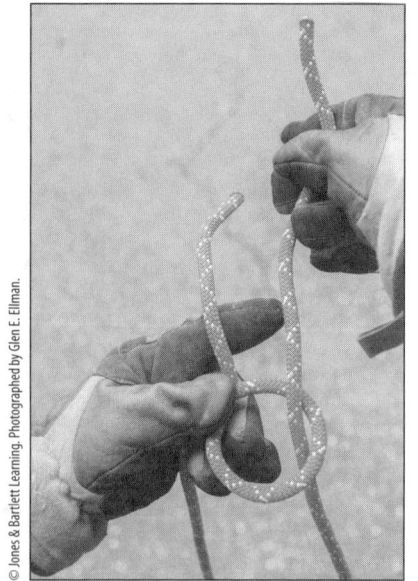

_____ Form another small loop in the standing part of the rope with the section close to the working end on top. Thread the working end up through this loop from the bottom.

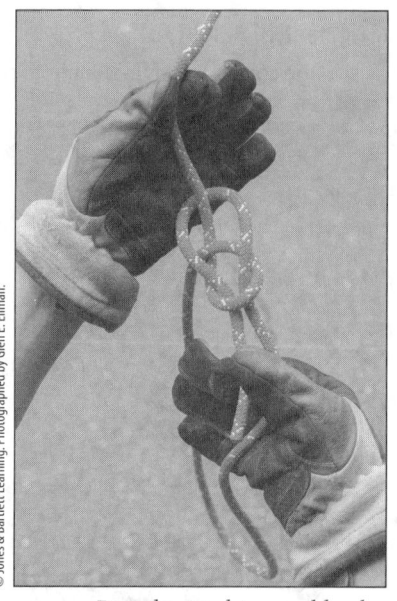

_____ Pass the working end back down through the same opening.

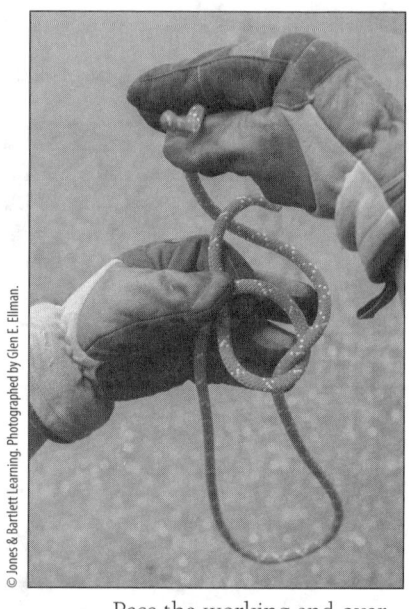

_____ Pass the working end over the loop and around and under the standing part.

Skill Drill 9-14: Tying a Sheet or Becket Bend Fire Fighter I, NFPA 1001: 4.1.2, 4.3.20
Test your knowledge of the skill drill by filling in the correct words in the photo captions.

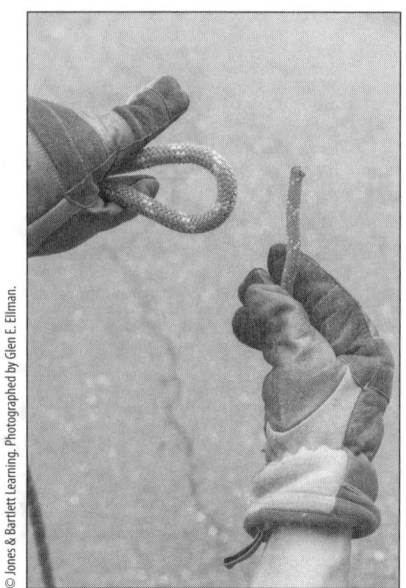

1. Using your left hand, form a _____ at the working end of one rope. If the ropes are of unequal size, the _____ should be made in the larger rope.

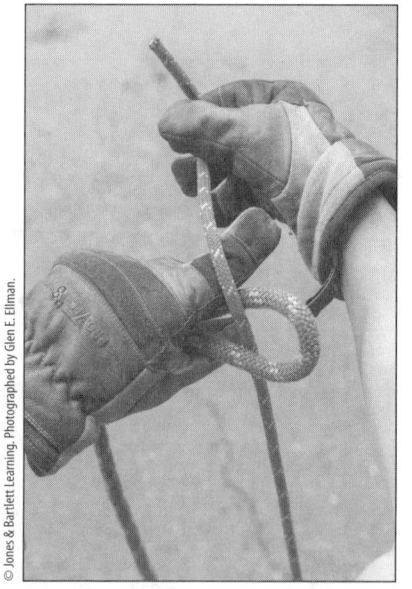

2. Thread the _____ end of the second rope up through the opening of the bight, between two _____ sections of the first rope.

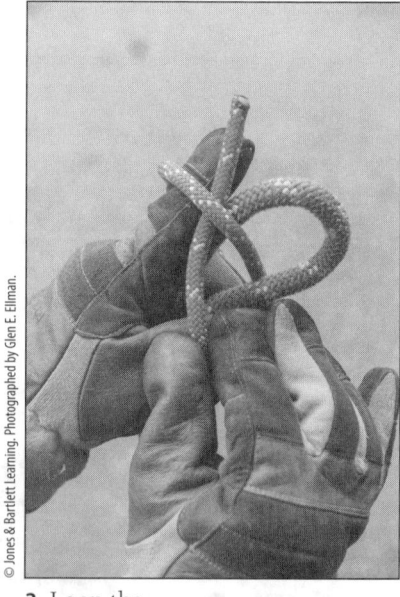

3. Loop the _____ rope completely around both sides of the bight. Pass the working end of the second rope between the original bight and under the second rope.

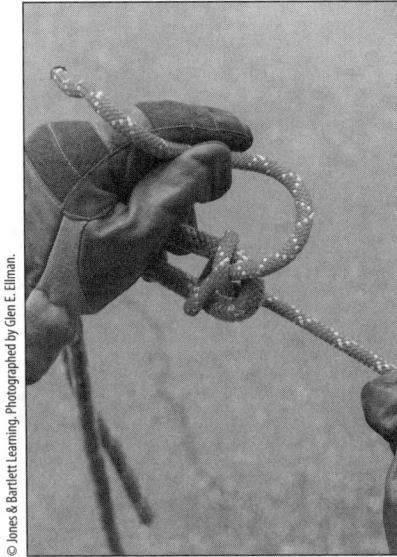

4. Tighten the knot by holding the _____ rope firmly while pulling back on the _____ rope.

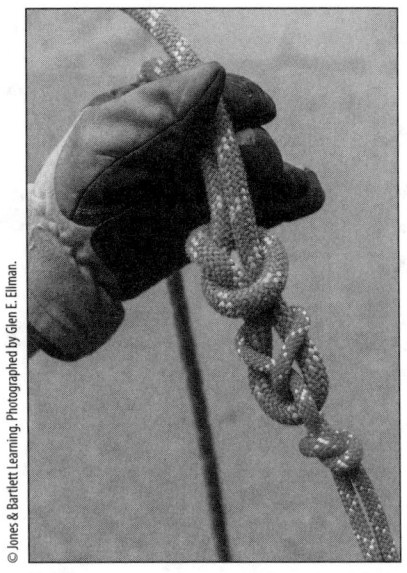

5. Tie a _____ in the working end of each rope.

Skill Drill 9-16: Hoisting an Axe Fire Fighter I, NFPA 1001: 4.1.2, 4.3.20

Test your knowledge of this skill drill by placing the photos below in the correct order. Number the first step with a "1," the second step with a "2," and so on.

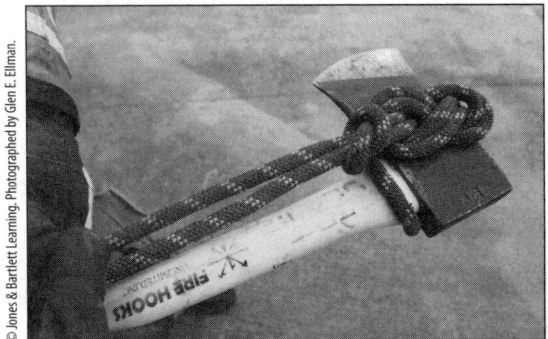

_____ Place the standing part of the rope parallel to the axe handle.

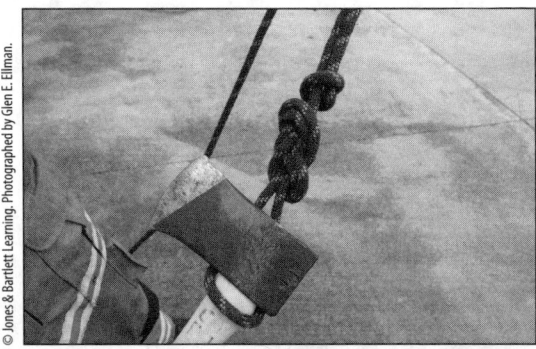

_____ Loop the standing part of the rope under the head.

98　FUNDAMENTALS OF FIRE FIGHTER SKILLS

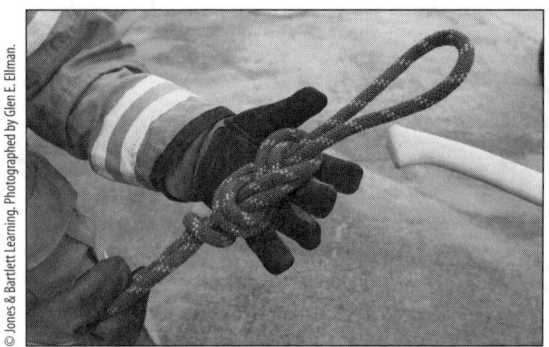

_____ Tie the end of the hoisting rope around the handle of the axe near the head using either a figure eight on a bight or a clove hitch. Slip the knot down the handle from the end to the head.

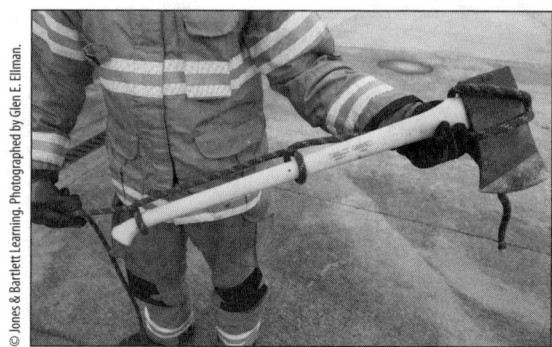

_____ Communicate with the fire fighter above that the axe is ready to raise.

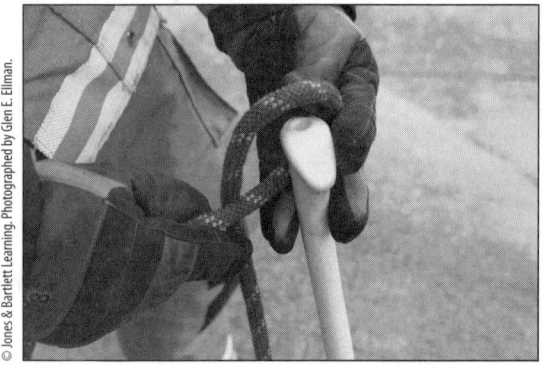

_____ Use one or two half hitches along the axe handle to keep the handle parallel to the rope.

Skill Drill 9-17: Hoisting a Pike Pole Fire Fighter I, NFPA 1001: 4.1.2, 4.3.20
Test your knowledge of this skill drill by filling in the correct words in the photo captions.

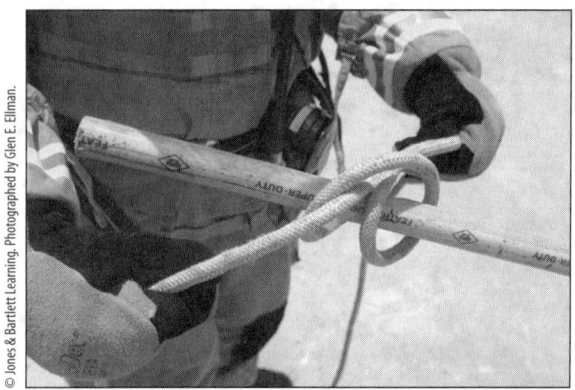

1. Place a _____ hitch over the bottom of the handle, and secure it close to the _____ of the handle. Leave enough length of rope below the clove hitch for a tag line while raising the pike pole.

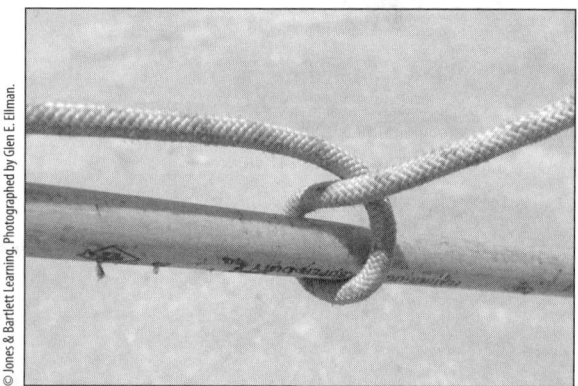

2. Place a half hitch around the _____ above the clove hitch to keep the rope parallel to the handle.

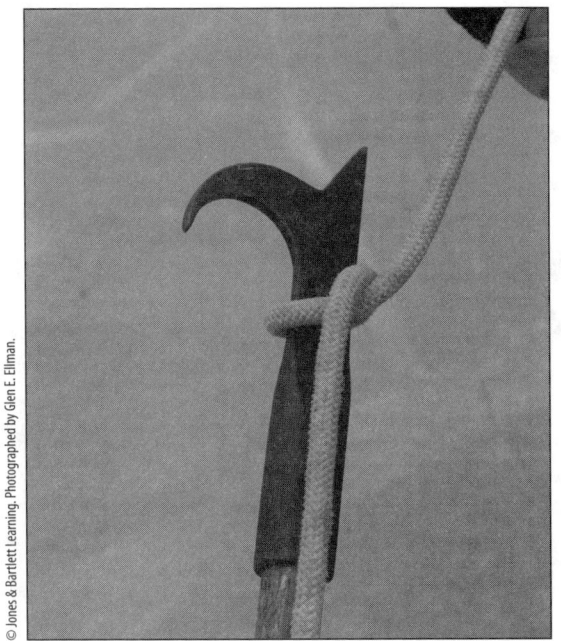

3. Slip a second _____ hitch over the handle, and secure it near the head of the pike pole.

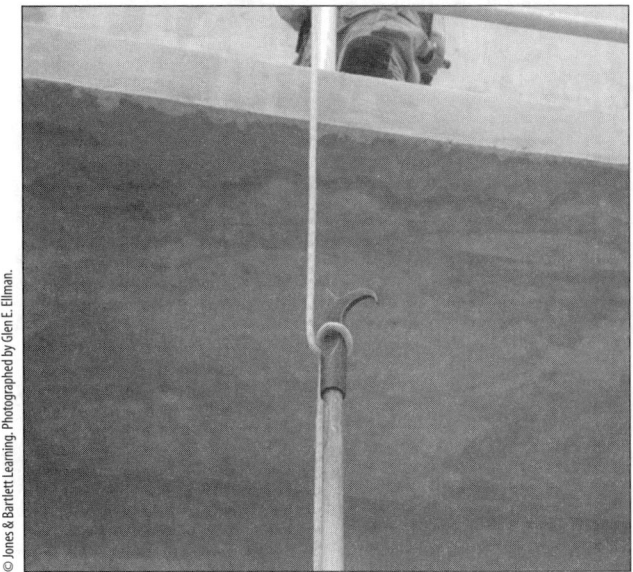

4. Communicate with the fire fighter above that the _____ is ready to raise.

Skill Drill 9-18: Hoisting a Ladder Fire Fighter I, NFPA 1001: 4.1.2, 4.3.20
Test your knowledge of this skill drill by placing the photos below in the correct order. Number the first step with a "1," the second step with a "2," and so on.

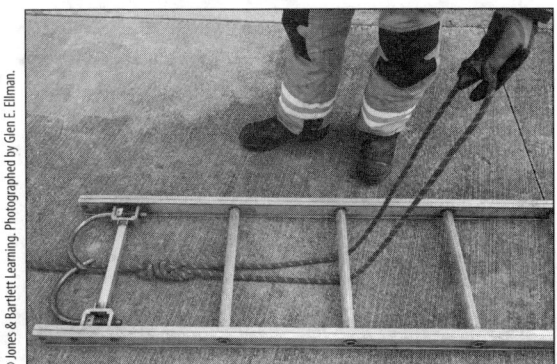

_____ Pass the rope between two beams of the ladder, three or four rungs from the top. Pull the end of the loop under the rungs and toward the tip at the top of the ladder.

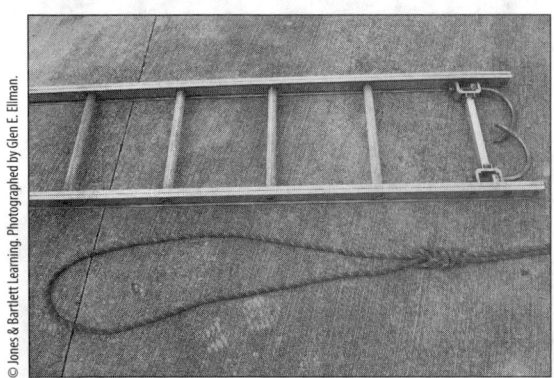

_____ The loop should be approximately 3 or 4 ft (1–1.3 m) in diameter and large enough to fit around both ladder beams.

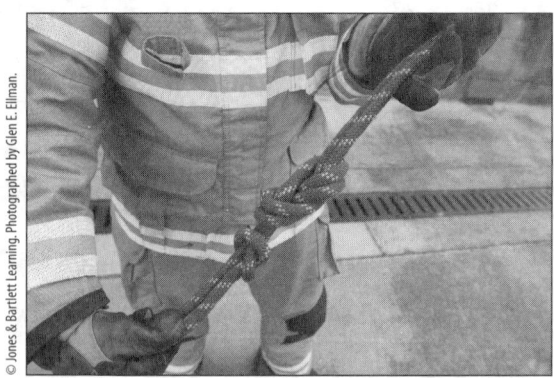

_____ Tie a figure eight on a bight to create a loop.

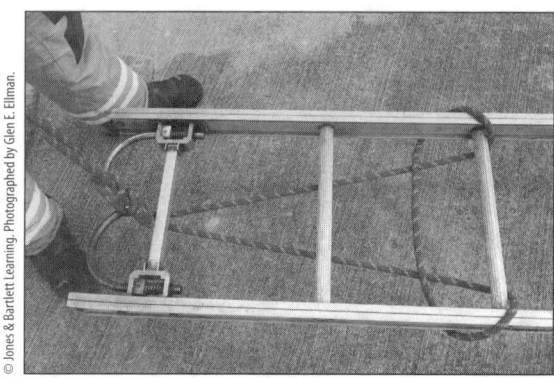

_____ Pull on the running end of the rope to remove the slack from the rope. Attach a tag line to the bottom rung of the ladder to stabilize it as it is being hoisted. Communicate with the fire fighter above that the ladder is ready to be raised. Hold on to the tag line to stabilize the bottom of the ladder as it is being hoisted.

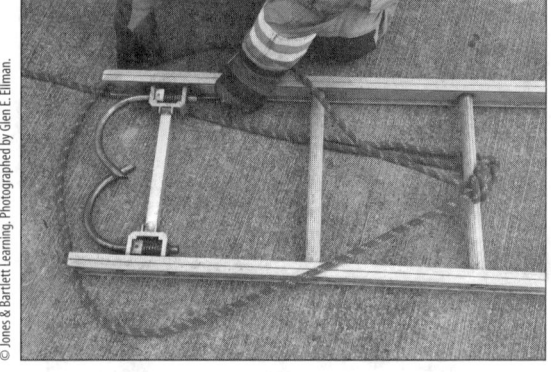

_____ Place the loop around the top tip of the ladder.

Skill Drill 9-21: Hoisting an Exhaust Fan or Power Tool Fire Fighter I, NFPA 1001: 4.1.2, 4.3.20
Test your knowledge of this skill drill by filling in the correct words in the photo captions.

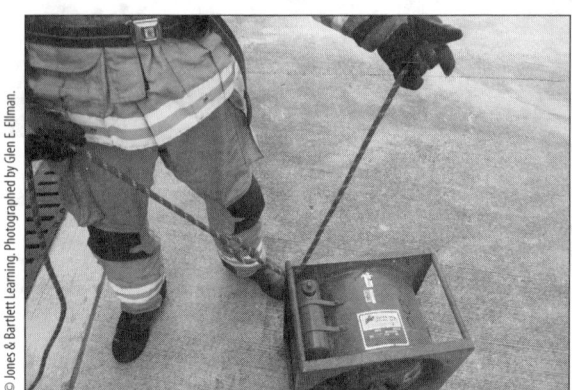

1. Tie a figure eight knot in the rope about 3 ft (1 m) from the _____ end of the rope.

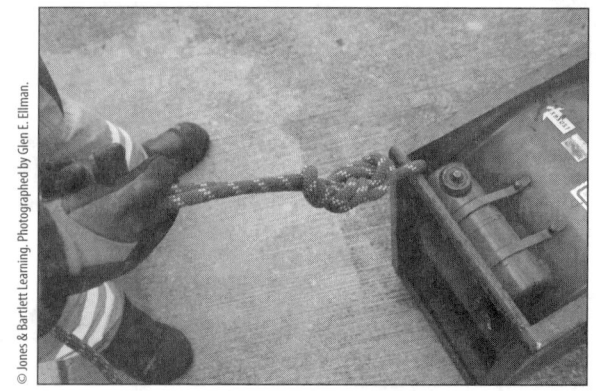

2. Loop the working end of the rope around the _____ and back to the figure eight knot.

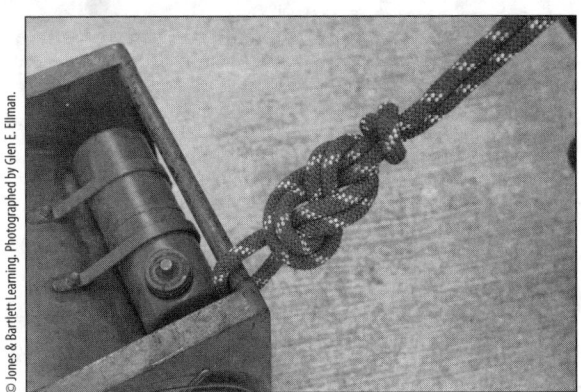

3. Secure the rope by tying a figure eight follow-through by threading the working end back through the first figure eight in the _____ direction.

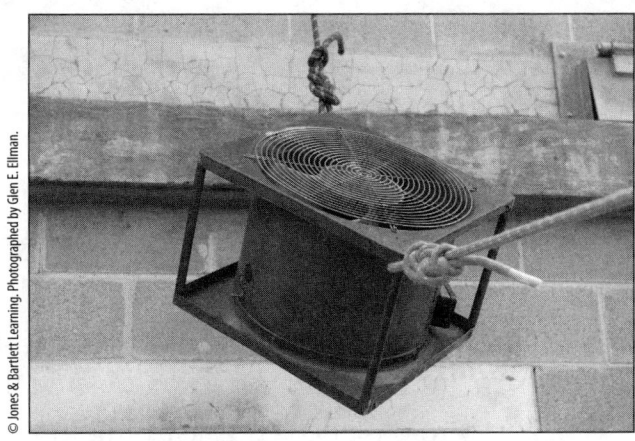

4. Attach a tag line to the _____ for better control. Communicate with the fire fighter above that the _____ is ready to hoist.

Forcible Entry

Workbook Activities

The following activities have been designed to help you. Your instructor may require you to complete some or all of these activities as a regular part of your fire fighter training program. You are encouraged to complete any activity your instructor does not assign to you, as a way to enhance your learning in the classroom.

Chapter Review

The following exercises provide an opportunity to refresh your knowledge of this chapter.

Matching

Match each of the terms in the left column to the appropriate definition in the right column.

_____ 1. Interior wall   A. A door design that consists of wood core blocks inside the door

_____ 2. Forcible entry   B. Usually the best point for forcing entry into a structure

_____ 3. Halligan   C. One part of the forcible entry tool "irons"

_____ 4. Latch   D. The U-shaped part of a padlock

_____ 5. Purchase point   E. A small opening made to enable better tool access in forcible entry

_____ 6. Solid-core   F. Gaining access to a structure when the normal means of entry are locked, secured, obstructed, blocked, or unable to be used

_____ 7. Rabbet   G. A cutting tool with a pry bar built into the cutting part of the tool

_____ 8. "A" tool   H. A type of door frame that has the stop for the door cut into the frame

_____ 9. Shackles   I. The part of the door lock that catches and holds the door frame

_____ 10. Door   J. A wall inside a building that divides a large space into smaller areas

Multiple Choice

Read each item carefully, and then select the best response.

_____ 1. Which type of tool is designed to cut into a lock cylinder and has a pry bar built into the cutting part of the tool?
  A. A tool
  B. K tool
  C. J tool
  D. Adz

_____ 2. Walls that support part of the weight of a structure are
  A. nonbearing.
  B. exterior walls.
  C. load bearing.
  D. partitions.

CHAPTER 10

_____ 3. The main part of a padlock that houses the locking mechanisms is the
   A. lock body.
   B. shackle.
   C. unlocking device.
   D. deadbolt.

_____ 4. Doors that have two sections and a double track where one side is fixed and the other slides are known as
   A. sliding doors.
   B. tempered doors.
   C. slab doors.
   D. honeycomb doors.

_____ 5. The two door locks that can be surface mounted on the interior of the door frame are rim locks and
   A. mortise locks.
   B. combination locks.
   C. key locks.
   D. deadbolts.

_____ 6. Gaining access to a structure when the normal means of entry are unable to be used is referred to as
   A. structure entry.
   B. forcible entry.
   C. operating access.
   D. forced access.

_____ 7. Vehicle windshields are most commonly made of
   A. tempered glass.
   B. laminated glass.
   C. plate glass.
   D. glazed glass.

_____ 8. The most common locks on the market today are
   A. mortise locks.
   B. cylindrical locks.
   C. padlocks.
   D. rim locks.

_____ 9. If you can see the hinges of a door, it is a(n)
   A. sliding door.
   B. inward-swinging door.
   C. outward-swinging door.
   D. overhead door.

_____ 10. The part of the door lock that catches and holds the door frame is called the
   A. latching device.
   B. operator lever.
   C. deadbolt.
   D. lock body.

_____ 11. Which types of tools are often used to force entry into buildings?
   A. Striking tools
   B. Cutting tools
   C. Prying tools
   D. Through-the-lock tools

_____ 12. Company officers usually select both the point of entry and the
   A. rate of entry.
   B. equipment to be used.
   C. method to be used.
   D. point of exit.

_____ 13. The slab door typically used for entrance doors because it is heavy and difficult to force open is a
   A. metal door.
   B. solid-core door.
   C. hollow-core door.
   D. glass door.

_____ 14. Another term for the doorknob is the
   A. latch.
   B. operator lever.
   C. deadbolt.
   D. lock body.

_____ 15. Which types of tools are used to generate a force directly on an object or another tool?
   A. Striking tools
   B. Cutting tools
   C. Prying tools
   D. Through-the-lock tools

_____ 16. Larger pieces or panes of glass are called
   A. annealed glass.
   B. tempered glass.
   C. laminated glass.
   D. plate glass.

_____ 17. The adz, the pick, and the claw are all incorporated into the
   A. hammer.
   B. Halligan tool.
   C. maul.
   D. pick axe.

_____ 18. The windows that are similar to sliding doors are called
   A. jalousie windows.
   B. casement windows.
   C. horizontal-sliding windows.
   D. projected windows.

_____ 19. Doors that have a wood frame inset with solid wood panels are called
   A. tempered doors.
   B. ledge doors.
   C. panel doors.
   D. slab doors.

_____ 20. Which type of circular saw blade can be used to cut through metal doors, locks, and gates?
   A. Steel blade
   B. Masonry-cutting blade
   C. Carbide-tipped blade
   D. Metal-cutting blade

Labeling

Label the following diagram with the correct terms.

1. Parts of a double-hung window

A. _____
B. _____
C. _____
D. _____
E. _____

2. Parts of a door lock

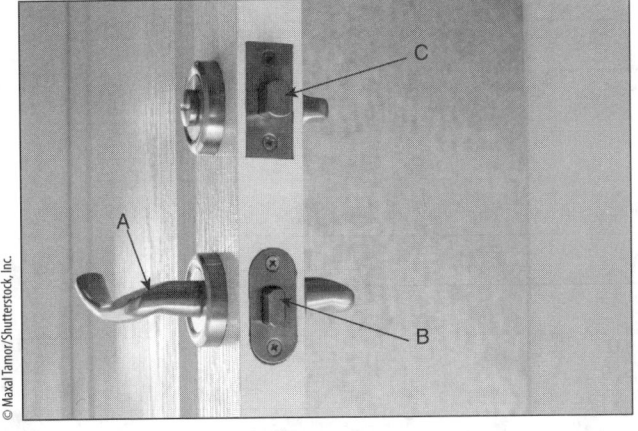

A. _____
B. _____
C. _____

Vocabulary

Define the following terms using the space provided.

1. Casement windows:
_____
_____
_____

Fundamentals of Fire Fighter Skills

2. Projected windows:
   _____
   _____
   _____

3. Lockbox:
   _____
   _____
   _____

4. Mortise locks:
   _____
   _____
   _____

5. Tempered glass:
   _____
   _____
   _____

6. K tool:
   _____
   _____
   _____

7. Jalousie windows:
   _____
   _____
   _____

8. Jamb:
   _____
   _____
   _____

Fill-In

Read each item carefully, then complete the statement by filling in the missing word(s).

1. _____ are used to cut metal components such as bolts, padlocks, and chains.

2. A(n) _____ is a three-piece hydraulic spreader operated by a hand-powered pump.

3. Forcible entry is usually required at emergency incidents where time is a(n) _____ factor.

4. _____ windows have two movable sashes that move freely up and down.

5. The quickest way to force entry through a(n) _____ roll-up door is to cut the door using a hinge cut.

6. _____ windows are similar in operation to jalousie windows, except that they usually have one large or two medium-sized glass panels instead of many small ones.

7. All tools should be kept in a(n) _____ state.

8. _____ provide air flow and light to the inside of the buildings, but can also provide emergency entrances.

9. _____-powered tools are portable and can be placed into operation quickly, but have limited power and operating times.

10. _____ doors are usually made of four glass panels with metal frames.

11. The circular saw blade that can stay sharp for long periods of time and can cut through hard surfaces or wood is the _____-tipped blade.

True/False

If you believe the statement to be more true than false, write the letter "T" in the space provided. If you believe the statement to be more false than true, write the letter "F."

1. _____ The best point from which to attempt forcible entry to a structure is the door or window.
2. _____ Interior walls are usually constructed of wood or metal studs and covered by plaster, gypsum, or sheetrock.
3. _____ Securing the premises after performing forcible entry is primarily the responsibility of the police department and the property owner, not the fire department.
4. _____ A rabbet tool is a three-piece hydraulic spreader operated by a hand-powered pump.
5. _____ A pry axe should be used only for cutting.
6. _____ The two most popular floor materials found in residences and commercial buildings are tile and steel.
7. _____ Outward-opening doors are most often used in residential occupancies.
8. _____ Double-pane glass is being used in many homes because it improves home insulation.
9. _____ Duck-billed lock breakers are cutting tools used to snip off the shackles of a lock.
10. _____ When breaking a window, always stand downwind.
11. _____ The locking mechanisms on sliding doors are not strong and can be pried open.

Short Answer

Complete this section with short written answers using the space provided.

1. Identify the four general carrying tips that apply to all tools.

   _____
   _____
   _____
   _____

2. List the four categories of forcible entry tools.

   _____
   _____
   _____
   _____

Fundamentals of Fire Fighter Skills

3. Identify the four general safety tips for using tools.

_____
_____
_____
_____

4. List the four basic components of a door.

_____
_____
_____
_____

Fire Alarms

The following real case scenarios will give you an opportunity to explore the concerns associated with forcible entry. Read each scenario, and then answer each question in detail.

1. It is 3:00 in the afternoon when your ladder truck company is dispatched to a residential structure fire. Upon arrival, your ladder truck is assigned to force entry through the overhead garage door on side D of the building. Your Lieutenant performs a size-up and tells you and your partner to gather the appropriate tools and force entry through the door. How do you proceed?

_____
_____
_____
_____
_____
_____

2. It is 1:30 in the morning when your engine company is dispatched to an alarm activation at an elementary school. Upon arrival, you find light smoke in the hallway and the alarm annunciator panel tells you that water is flowing. During his walk-around, your Captain finds a single sprinkler head that has activated in a classroom, and he reports that the fire has been contained. He directs your crew to force entry through the classroom doors and overhaul the fire. Upon size-up, you determine the entrance doors are glass, outward-opening doors with a steel frame. How should you proceed?

_____
_____
_____
_____
_____
_____

Skill Drills

Skill Drill 10-1: Forcing Entry into an Inward-Opening Door Fire Fighter I, NFPA 1001: 4.3.4
Test your knowledge of this skill drill by placing the photos below in the correct order. Number the first step with a "1," the second step with a "2," and so on.

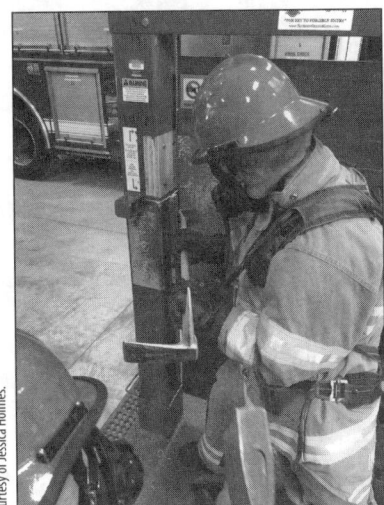

_____ Instruct a second fire fighter to drive the fork in forcefully with a flat-head axe. Keep constant pressure on the tool and move the tool away from the door as it is being driven in. The tool is set when the arch of the fork is even with the inside edge of the door/doorstop and is perpendicular to the door.

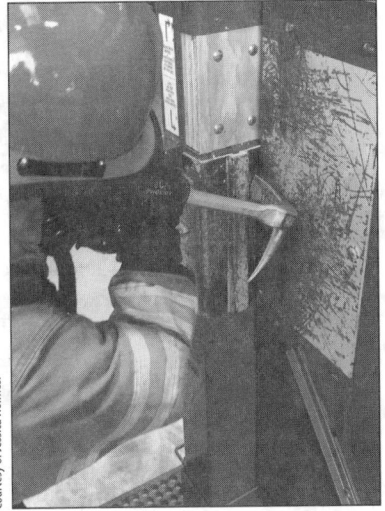

_____ Insert the adze end of a prying tool (such as a Halligan tool) into the space between the door and the door jamb about 6 in. (15 cm) above or below the door lock. Push up or down on the tool to rotate the adze and to create a gap (or crease) in the door. To capture your progress, insert a wedge or tool before removing the adze end of the tool from the door.

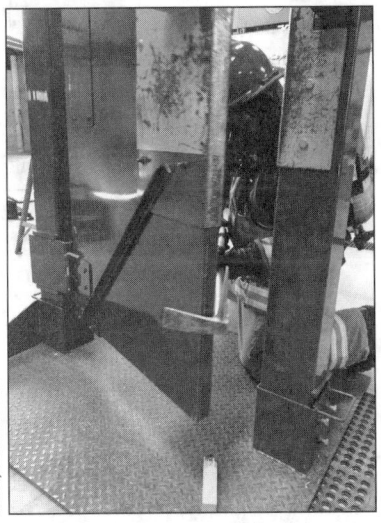

_____ Maintain control of the door when it opens by hooking the door with the adze end of the Halligan or by attaching a strap to the knob. Limit ventilation of the fire.

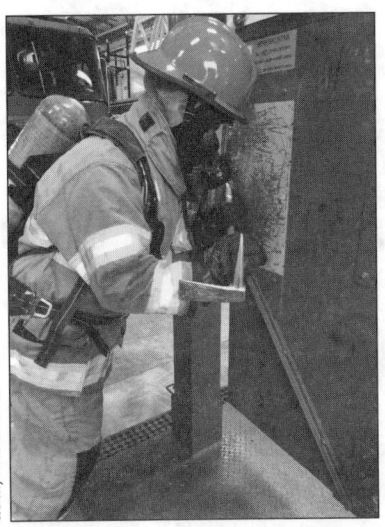

_____ When the Halligan tool is set, push the tool sharply inward toward the center of the door to create maximum force.

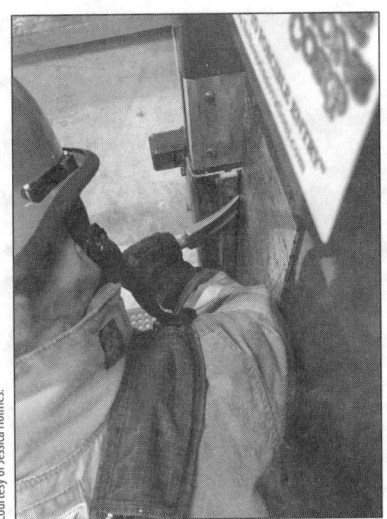

_____ Insert the fork end of the tool into the gap between the door and the door frame.

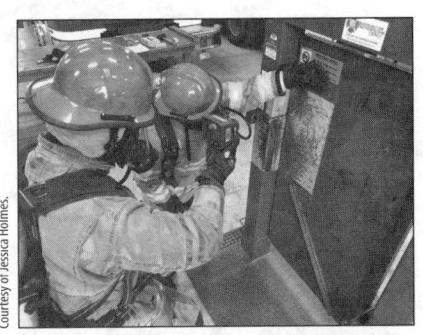

_____ Look for any safety hazards as you evaluate the door. Inspect the door for the location and number of locks and their mechanisms.

Skill Drill 10-2: Forcing Entry into an Outward-Opening Door Fire Fighter I, NFPA 1001: 4.3.4

Test your knowledge of the skill drill by filling in the correct words in the photo captions.

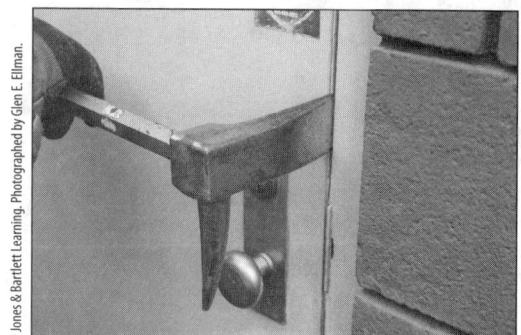

1. Size up the door, looking for any safety hazards. Determine the _____ and _____ of locks and the locking mechanism. Place the adze end of the Halligan tool in the space between the door and the door jamb. Gap the door by rocking the tool up and down to spread the door from the door jamb.

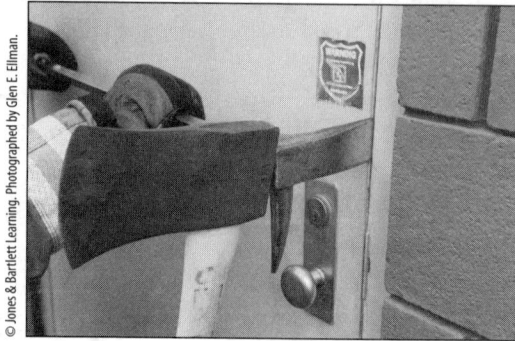

2. Set the tool, and pry the door out by pulling on the _____ tool so the _____ can be driven in past the door jamb. Be careful not to bury the tool in the door jamb. Strike the _____ tool to drive the adze end of the tool past the door jamb.

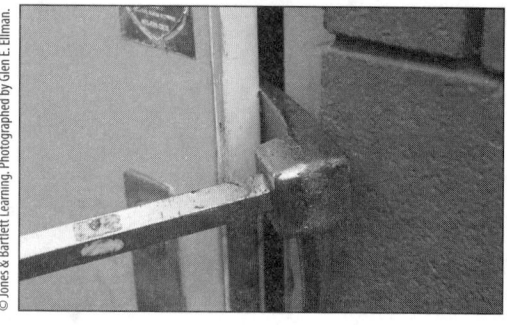

3. Force the door by pulling the _____ tool away from the door. Control the door to limit _____ of the fire and to prevent it from closing behind you.

Skill Drill 10-3: Opening an Overhead Garage Door Using the Triangle Method Fire Fighter I, NFPA 1001: 4.3.4

Test your knowledge of this skill drill by placing the photos below in the correct order. Number the first step with a "1," the second step with a "2," and so on.

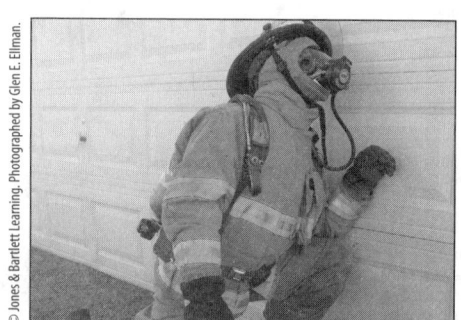

_____ Before cutting, check for any safety hazards during the size-up of the garage door. Select the appropriate tool to make the cut. (The best choice is a power saw with a metal-cutting blade.) Wearing full protective gear and eye protection, start the saw, and ensure it is in proper working order.

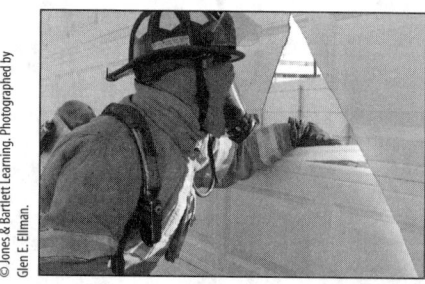

_____ Be aware of the environment behind the door. Check the outside of the door for heat. Try to lift the door to assure that it is not unlocked. If necessary, cut a small inspection hole, large enough to insert a hose nozzle.

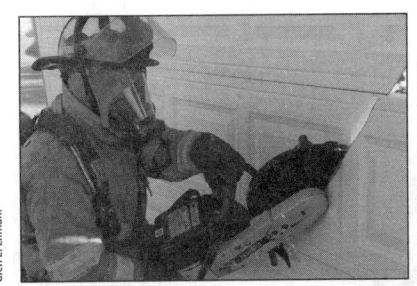 _____ Next to the same starting point, make a second diagonal cut to the left, down to the bottom of the door. Fold the door down to form a large triangle.

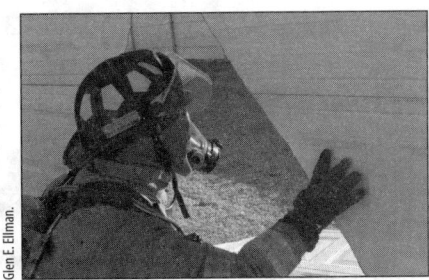 _____ If necessary, pad or protect the cut edges of the triangle and the bottom panel to prevent injuries as fire fighters enter or leave the premises. If you have time, you can remove the cut portion of the door and the bottom rail by raising the bottom rail with a prying tool and then cutting the bottom rail in two places.

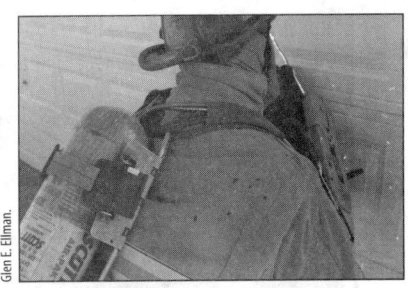 _____ Starting at a center high point in the door, make a diagonal cut to the right, down to the bottom of the door.

Skill Drill 10-4: Forcing Entry into an Outward-Opening Door Fire Fighter I, NFPA 1001: 4.3.4
Test your knowledge of this skill drill by filling in the correct words in the photo captions.

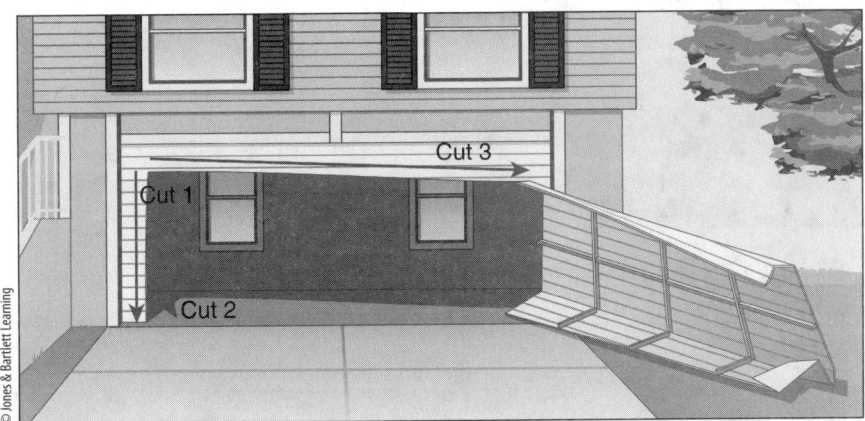

1. Before cutting, check for any safety hazards during the size-up of the garage door. Select the appropriate tool to make the _____. (The best choice is a power saw with a metal-cutting blade.) Wearing full protective gear and _____, start the saw, and ensure it is in proper working order.

2. Be aware of the environment behind the door. Check the outside of the door for _____. Try to lift the door to assure it is not unlocked. If necessary, cut a small inspection hole, large enough to insert a hose nozzle.

3. Make a vertical cut down the _____ side of the door starting as high as you can comfortably reach.

4. Make a diagonal cut about 18 in. (45 cm) from the bottom of the door starting at the first cut. Make a cut to the _____ of the door. This will make a small triangle. Kick or push in the triangle formed by these two cuts.

5. Insert the saw blade into the opening made by the _____ cuts at the bottom of the door. Cut through the angle iron, or L-shaped steel, at the bottom of the door.

6. Resting the saw on your shoulder, make a _____ cut the width of the door, starting at the top of the first cut. Continue cutting to the right side of the door. The uncut side of the door will act as the hinge.

7. Open the door flap _____. This will produce a large opening that can be opened and closed to control the flow of air to the fire. Secure the door in an open position anytime fire fighters are inside the building.

Skill Drill 10-6: Forcing Entry Through a Casement Window Fire Fighter I, NFPA 1001: 4.3.4
Test your knowledge of this skill drill by filling in the correct words in the photo captions.

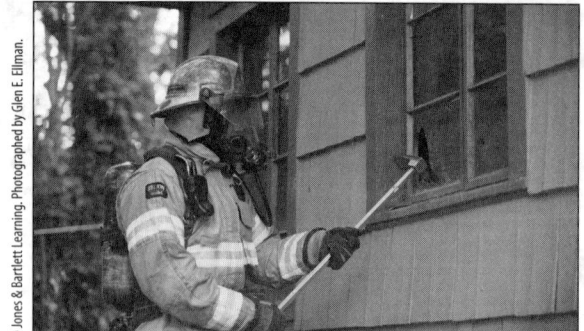

1. Size up the window to check for any safety hazards, and locate the _____. Select an appropriate tool to break out a windowpane. Stand to the windward side of the window, and break out the pane closest to the locking mechanism.

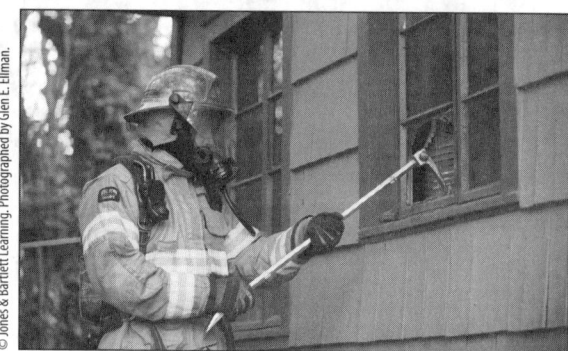

2. Remove all of the _____ in the pane to prevent injuries.

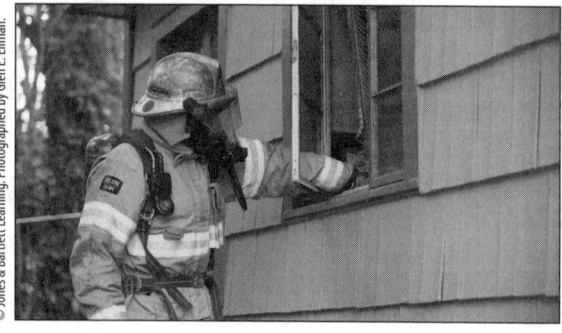

3. Reach in and unlock the window, then _____ operate the window crank to open the window.

Skill Drill 10-8: Forcing Entry Using a K Tool Fire Fighter I, NFPA 1001: 4.3.4
Test your knowledge of this skill drill by placing the photos below in the correct order. Number the first step with a "1," the second step with a "2," and so on.

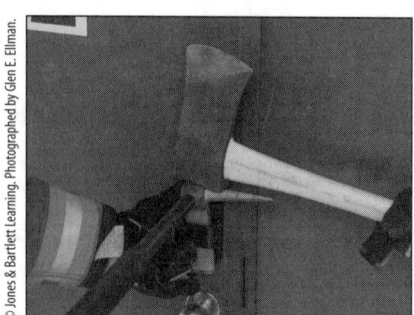

_____ Place the adze end of the Halligan tool or similar prying tool into the slot on the face of the K tool. Using a flat-head axe or similar striking tool, strike the end of the prying tool to drive the K tool farther onto the lock cylinder.

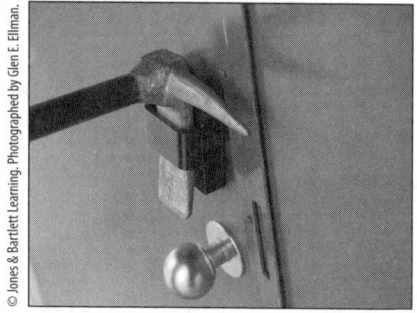

_____ Pry up on the tool to remove the lock cylinder and expose the locking mechanism. Using the small tools that come with the K tool, turn the locking mechanism to open the lock. The lock should release, allowing you to open the door.

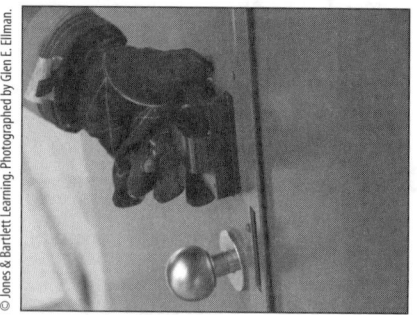

_____ Size up the door and lock area, checking for any safety hazards. Determine which type of lock is used, whether it is regular or heavy-duty construction, and whether the lock cylinder has a case-hardened collar, which may hamper proper cutting. Place the K tool over the face of the lock cylinder, noting the location of the keyway.

Skill Drill 10-9: Forcing Entry Using an A Tool Fire Fighter I, NFPA 1001: 4.3.4
Test your knowledge of this skill drill by filling in the correct words in the photo captions.

1. Size up the door and lock area, checking for any safety hazards. Determine which type of lock is used, whether it is regular or heavy-duty construction, and whether the lock cylinder has a _____, which may hamper proper cutting. Place the cutting edges of the A tool over the lock cylinder, between the lock cylinder and the door frame.

2. Using a _____-_____ axe or similar striking tool, drive the A tool onto the lock cylinder. Pry up on the _____ to remove the lock cylinder from the door. Insert a key tool into the hole to manipulate the locking mechanism and open the door.

Skill Drill 10-11: Breaching a Wall Frame Fire Fighter I, NFPA 1001: 4.3.4
Test your knowledge of this skill drill by filling in the correct words in the photo captions.

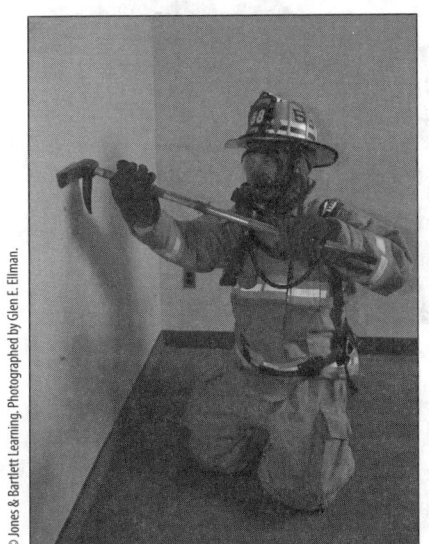

1. Size up the wall, checking for safety hazards such as electrical outlets, wall switches, or any signs of _____. Inspect the overall scene to ensure that the wall is not load bearing. Using a tool, sound the wall to locate any _____. Make a hole between the studs.

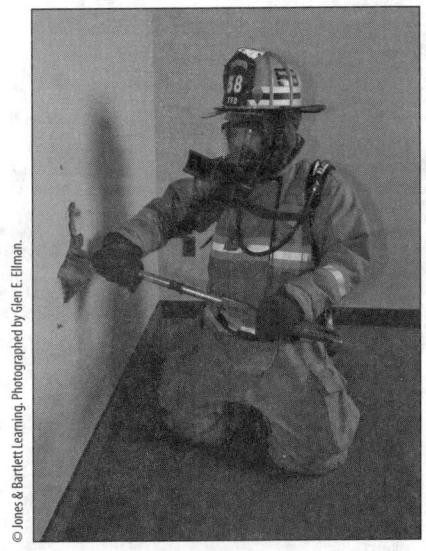

2. Cut the _____ as close to the studs as possible.

3. Enlarge the hole by extending it from _____ to _____ and as high as necessary.

Skill Drill 10-12: Breaching a Floor Fire Fighter I, NFPA 1001: 4.3.4

Test your knowledge of this skill drill by placing the photos below in the correct order. Number the first step with a "1," the second step with a "2," and so on.

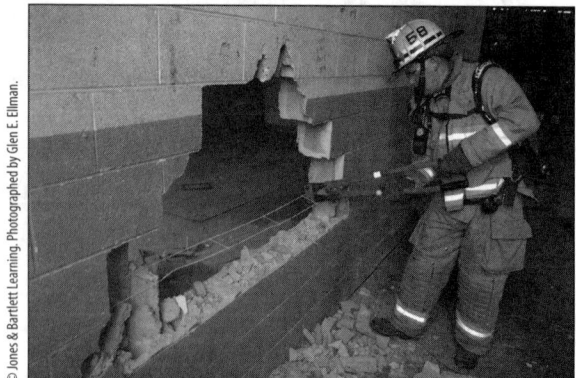

_____ Clear any reinforcing wire using bolt cutters, and enlarge the hole as needed.

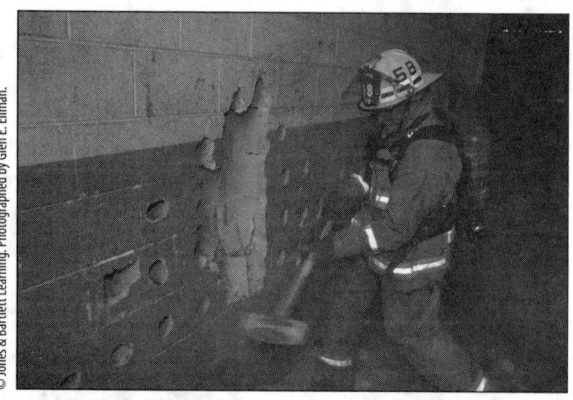

_____ Knock out the remaining portion of the masonry blocks by hitting the masonry blocks parallel to the wall rather than perpendicular to it.

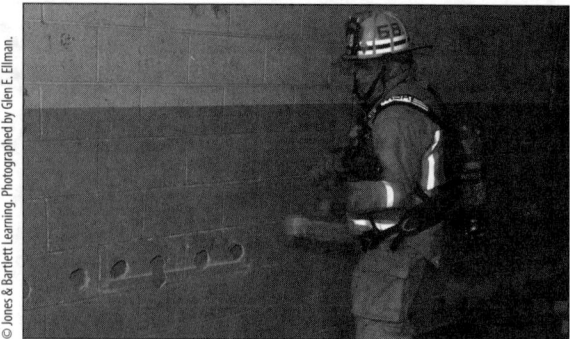

_____ Size up the wall, checking for any safety hazards such as electrical outlets, wall switches, and plumbing. Inspect the overall area to ensure that the wall is not load bearing. Select a row of five masonry blocks at 2 to 3 ft (61 to 91 cm) above the floor. Using a sledgehammer, knock two holes in each masonry block. Each hole should pierce into the hollow core of the masonry blocks.

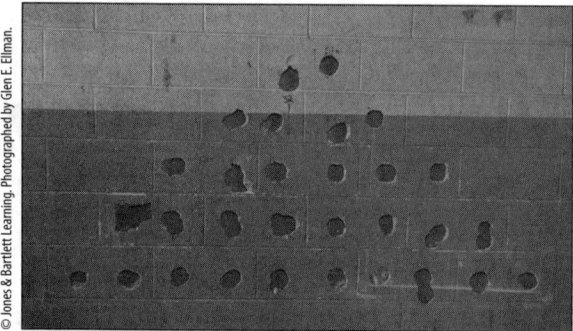

_____ Repeat the process on four masonry blocks above the first row. Repeat the process on three masonry blocks above the second row, on two masonry blocks above the third row, and on one masonry block above the fourth row. An inverted V-cut has now been created.

Skill Drill 10-14: Breaching a Masonry Wall Fire Fighter I, NFPA 1001: 4.3.4
Test your knowledge of this skill drill by placing the photos below in the correct order. Number the first step with a "1," the second step with a "2," and so on.

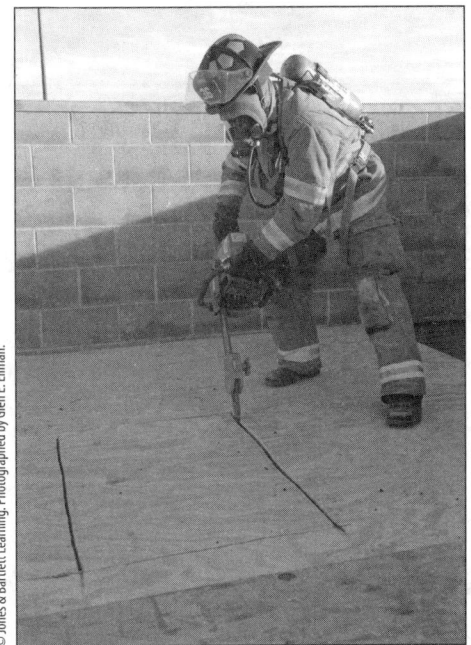

_____ Use an appropriate cutting tool to cut one side of the hole. Cut the opposite side. Make two additional cuts at right angles to the first cuts. This will form a rectangle. Avoid cutting into the floor joists.

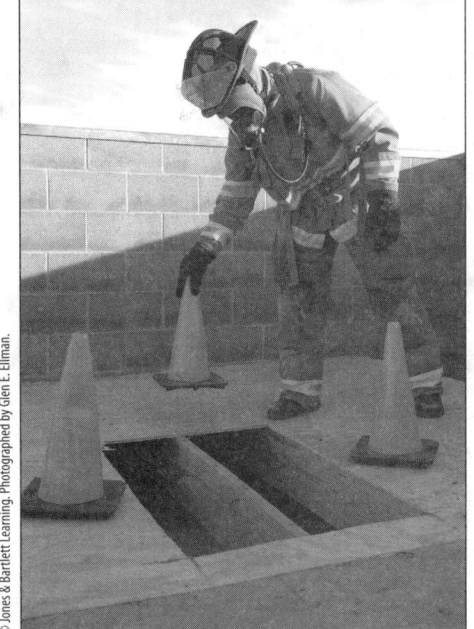

_____ Secure the area around the hole to prevent others working in the area from falling through the hole.

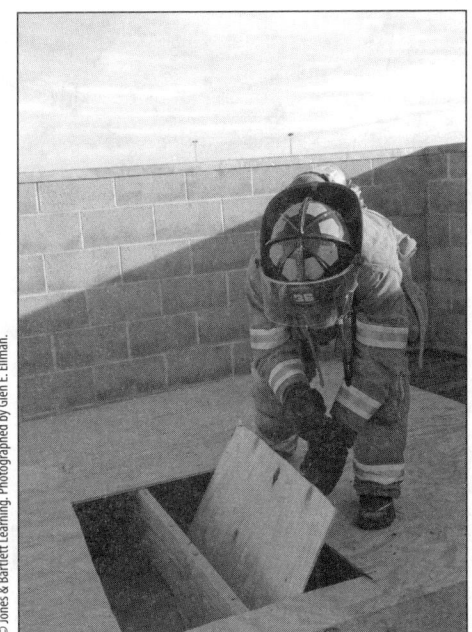

_____ Remove any flooring, such as carpet, tile, or floorboards that have been loosened. Cut a similar-size opening into the subfloor, until the proper-size hole is achieved.

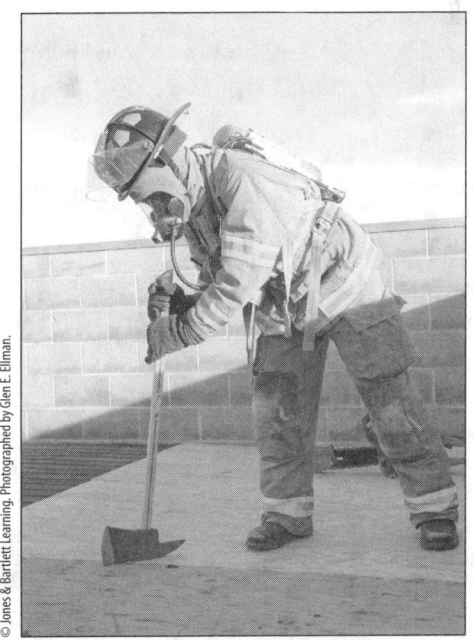

_____ Size up the floor area, checking for hazards in the area to be cut. Sound the floor with an axe or similar tool to locate the floor joists.

Ladders

Workbook Activities

The following activities have been designed to help you. Your instructor may require you to complete some or all of these activities as a regular part of your fire fighter training program. You are encouraged to complete any activity your instructor does not assign to you, as a way to enhance your learning in the classroom.

Chapter Review

The following exercises provide an opportunity to refresh your knowledge of this chapter.

Matching

Match each of the terms in the left column to the appropriate definition in the right column.

_____ 1. Stop   A. A piece of material that prevents the fly section(s) of a ladder from overextending and collapsing the ladder
_____ 2. Rung   B. A ladder crosspiece that provides a climbing step
_____ 3. Halyard   C. The end of the ladder that is placed against the ground when the ladder is raised
_____ 4. Staypoles   D. The very top of the ladder
_____ 5. Pawls   E. Part of a Bangor ladder
_____ 6. Tip   F. The ladder component that supports the rungs
_____ 7. Beam   G. The top and bottom surfaces of a trussed ladder
_____ 8. Guides   H. The rope or cable used to extend or hoist the fly section(s) of an extension ladder
_____ 9. Rail   I. Strips of metal or wood that guide a fly section of an extension ladder
_____ 10. Butt   J. A mechanical locking device used to secure the fly section(s) of a ladder

Multiple Choice

Read each item carefully, and then select the best response.

_____ 1. The rope or cable used to extend the fly section is the
   A. dog.
   B. guide.
   C. halyard.
   D. lift.

_____ 2. Ladders that are designed to allow access to attic scuttle holes and confined areas are
   A. folding ladders.
   B. pompier ladders.
   C. scaling ladders.
   D. combination ladders.

_____ **3.** When a fire fighter stands between the ladder and the structure, grasps the beams, and leans to pull the ladder into the structure, he or she is
   A. butting the ladder.
   B. guiding the ladder.
   C. heeling the ladder.
   D. dogging the ladder.

_____ **4.** The most important safety check is confirming the
   A. proximity to direct flames.
   B. location of overhead utility lines.
   C. identification of stable, level surfaces.
   D. size of the structure.

_____ **5.** Establishing verbal contact as quickly as possible is important when rescuing
   A. an unconscious patient.
   B. an infant.
   C. an elderly person.
   D. any person.

_____ **6.** A ladder that has no halyard, is generally short, and is designed for attic access is the
   A. pompier ladder.
   B. Bangor ladder.
   C. Fresno ladder.
   D. roof ladder.

_____ **7.** A ladder A-frame is used to access
   A. below-grade sites.
   B. above-grade sites.
   C. grade-level positions.
   D. interior above-grade sites.

_____ **8.** When climbing a ladder, the fire fighter's eyes should be looking
   A. forward, with an occasional glance upward.
   B. upward.
   C. downward.
   D. at the ladder's tip.

_____ **9.** The _____ is a small grooved wheel that is used to change the direction of the halyard pull.
   A. pulley
   B. foot
   C. heel
   D. stop

_____ **10.** Transferring the weight of the user to the beams is done through the
   A. halyards.
   B. rungs.
   C. butt spurs.
   D. tie rods.

_____ 11. Staypoles are required on ladders of
   A. 10 to 20 ft (3 to 6 m).
   B. 20 to 30 ft (6 to 9 m).
   C. 30 to 40 ft (9 to 12 m).
   D. 40 feet (12 m) or greater.

_____ 12. Most ladders are carried with the
   A. tip forward.
   B. fly-section forward.
   C. butt end forward.
   D. beam on top.

_____ 13. The horizontal-bending test evaluates the
   A. manufacturer's specifications.
   B. structural strength of the ladder.
   C. service testing of the ladder.
   D. extension hardware on the ladder.

_____ 14. The two common techniques for raising portable ladders are the
   A. team and self raises.
   B. beam and flat raises.
   C. beam and halyard raises.
   D. team and aerial raises.

_____ 15. Butt spurs prevent the ladder from
   A. losing contact with the exterior of the structure.
   B. damaging the structure.
   C. chaffing other surfaces.
   D. slipping out of position.

_____ 16. Ladders with staypoles or tormentors are typically referred to as
   A. aerial ladders.
   B. portable ladders.
   C. Bangor ladders.
   D. Fresno ladders.

_____ 17. What is the common rule of thumb when identifying the length of ladder to use on a structure?
   A. The tip of the ladder is in contact with the structure.
   B. The butt of the ladder is in contact with the structure.
   C. At least five ladder rungs should show above the roofline.
   D. The ladder must provide access to all possible incident outcomes.

_____ 18. The number of fire fighters required to raise a ladder depends on the
   A. length and width of the ladder.
   B. weight and target surface of the ladder.
   C. width and clearance of the ladder.
   D. length and weight of the ladder.

_____ 19. The proper climbing angle for maximum load capacity and strength is
   A. 30 degrees.
   B. 45 degrees.
   C. 60 degrees.
   D. 75 degrees.

_____ 20. A straight ladder equipped with retractable hooks to secure the tip of the ladder to a pitched roof is a
   A. roof ladder.
   B. Bangor ladder.
   C. combination ladder.
   D. Fresno ladder.

_____ 21. In most cases, a single fire fighter can safely carry a straight or roof ladder
   A. less than 18 ft (5.5 m) long.
   B. less than 24 ft (7 m) long.
   C. less than 4 ft (1.2 m) wide.
   D. less than 2 ft (0.6 m) wide.

_____ 22. Most portable ladders are designed to support a weight of
   A. 500 pounds (226.8 kg).
   B. 750 pounds (340.2 kg).
   C. 1000 pounds (453.6 kg).
   D. 1500 pounds (680.4 kg).

_____ 23. The rail is the
   A. top section of a solid beam.
   B. top section of a trussed beam.
   C. top or bottom section of a trussed beam.
   D. handrail at the tip of the ladder.

_____ 24. Pawls, ladder locks, or rung locks are also referred to as
   A. roof hooks.
   B. dogs.
   C. guides.
   D. truss locks.

_____ 25. Fire service ground ladders are limited to a maximum length of
   A. 25 ft (7.6 m).
   B. 50 ft (15.2 m).
   C. 75 ft (22.9 m).
   D. 100 ft (30.5 m).

_____ 26. The part of an extension ladder that is raised or extended from the bed section is the
   A. fly section.
   B. elevating section.
   C. lift section.
   D. aerial section.

_____ 27. The metal bar that runs from one beam of the ladder to the other and keeps the beams from separating is the
   A. butt spur.
   B. rung.
   C. rail.
   D. tie rod.

_____ 28. A truss block is a piece that connects the two
   A. rails of a trussed beam.
   B. rungs of a trussed beam.
   C. pulleys of an I-beam.
   D. rungs of an I-beam.

120 FUNDAMENTALS OF FIRE FIGHTER SKILLS

Labeling
Label the following diagram with the correct terms.

1. Basic components of an extension ladder.

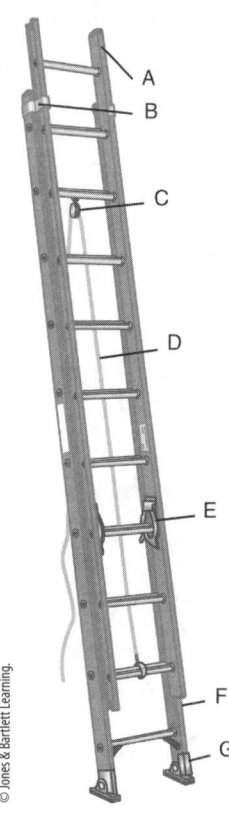

A. _____

B. _____

C. _____

D. _____

E. _____

F. _____

G. _____

Vocabulary
Define the following terms using the space provided.

1. Guides:

_____

_____

_____

2. Ladder belt:

_____
_____
_____

3. Heat sensor label:

_____
_____
_____

4. Tie rod:

_____
_____
_____

5. Roof hooks:

_____
_____
_____

6. Protection plates:

_____
_____
_____

7. Pawls:

_____
_____
_____

8. Bed section:

_____
_____
_____

9. Halyard:

_____
_____
_____

10. Pulley:
_____
_____
_____

Fill-In

Read each item carefully, and then complete the statement by filling in the missing word(s).

1. A(n) _____ ladder is an assembly of two or more ladder sections that can be extended or retracted to adjust the length.

2. Fire fighters who are working from a ladder should use a ladder belt or a(n) _____ to secure themselves to the ladder.

3. A(n) _____ ladder can be converted from a straight ladder to a stepladder configuration.

4. When dismounting a ladder, the fire fighter should try to maintain contact with the ladder at _____ points.

5. The _____ ladder is one of the most functional, versatile, and rapidly deployable tools used by fire fighters.

6. A rope, a rope-hose tool, or _____ can be used to secure a ladder in place.

7. A(n) _____ ladder is a single-section, fixed-length ladder.

8. The _____ serve as the steps of a ladder.

9. _____ ladders are permanently mounted, power-operated ladders with a working length of at least 50 feet (15.2 meters).

10. Ladders can be used as _____ to assist in moving equipment during emergencies.

11. Ladders should always be inspected and maintained in accordance with the _____ recommendations.

True/False

If you believe the statement to be more true than false, write the letter "T" in the space provided. If you believe the statement to be more false than true, write the letter "F."

1. _____ Ladders consist of two rungs connected by a series of parallel beams.

2. _____ The butt and the heel of a ladder are at opposite ends of a portable ladder.

3. _____ Pulling on the halyard extends the bed sections of a combination ladder.

4. _____ The ladder is one of the fire fighter's basic tools.

5. _____ In general, ladder manufacturers recommend that the fly sections of metal ground ladders be placed toward the structure.

6. _____ A fire fighter working from a ladder is in a less stable position than a fire fighter working on the ground.

7. _____ During a three-fire-fighter shoulder carry, the middle fire fighter should be on the opposite side of the other two.

8. _____ When roof ladders are properly attached, they will not support the weight of the ladder and a fire fighter.

9. _____ When using an extension ladder, never wrap the halyard around your hand.

10. _____ A ladder can be deployed across a small opening to create a bridge.

11. _____ Self-contained breathing apparatus (SCBA) is not required when working on the roof at a chimney fire.

12. _____ There are two tips on a portable ladder.

Short Answer

Complete this section with short written answers using the space provided.

1. Identify five basic considerations when lifting a ground ladder.

   _____
   _____
   _____
   _____

2. Identify five basic safety considerations when descending a ground ladder.

   _____
   _____
   _____
   _____

3. Describe the three basic types of beam construction.

   _____
   _____
   _____
   _____

4. Identify five fundamental ladder maintenance tasks.

   _____
   _____
   _____
   _____

Fire Alarms

The following real case scenarios will give you an opportunity to explore the concerns associated with ladders. Read each scenario, and then answer each question in detail.

1. It is 10:45 in the morning when your company is dispatched to an older two-story apartment complex. The fire is located in two units on the second floor. Upon arrival, the incident commander assigns you to Division C. Your Captain receives instructions to deploy a roof ladder utilizing the extension ladder already in place on side C of the structure. The Captain tells you and your partner to remove the roof ladder from the apparatus and place it on the roof. How should you proceed?

   _____
   _____
   _____
   _____
   _____

2. It is 11:30 in the evening when your engine company is dispatched to a two-story residential building for a structure fire with a life threat. As you exit your engine, you can hear cries for help. When you look toward the structure, you see a middle-aged woman straddling a second-floor window with smoke pouring out from behind her. The adjacent window is engulfed with fire. Your Lieutenant tells you to ladder the window for a rescue. How should you proceed?

_____
_____
_____
_____
_____

Skill Drills

Skill Drill 11-1: Inspect, Clean, and Maintain a Ladder Fire Fighter I, NFPA 1001: 4.5.1

Test your knowledge of this skill drill by filling in the correct words in the photo captions.

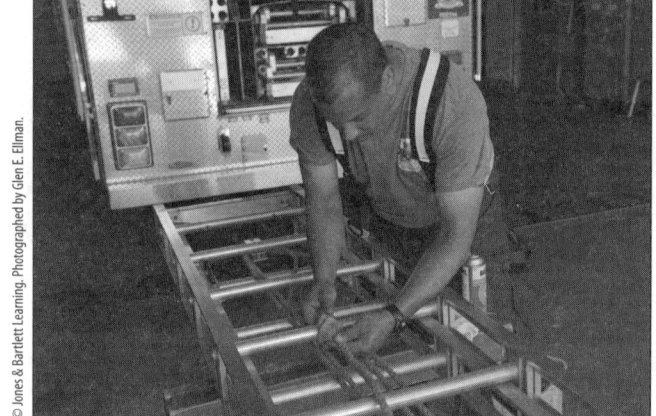

1. Clean all components, following _____ and _____ standards. Visually inspect the ladder for wear and damage.

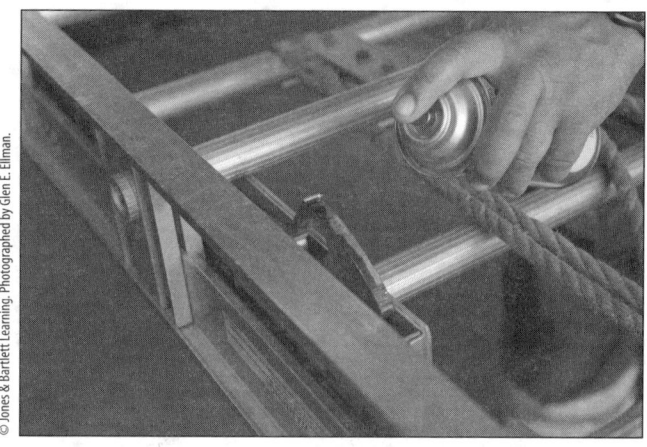

2. _____ the ladder pawls, guides, and pulleys using the recommended material.

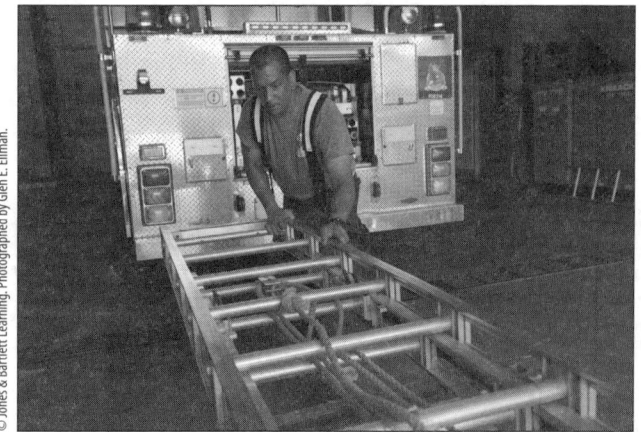

3. Perform a _____ of all components.

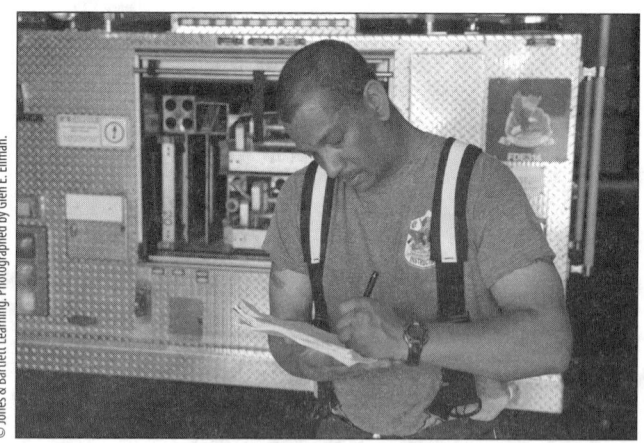

4. Complete the _____ record for the ladder. Tag and remove the ladder from service if deficiencies are found. Return the ladder to the apparatus or storage area.

Skill Drill 11-2: One-Fire Fighter Shoulder Carry Fire Fighter I, NFPA 1001: 4.3.6
Test your knowledge of this skill drill by filling in the correct words in the photo captions.

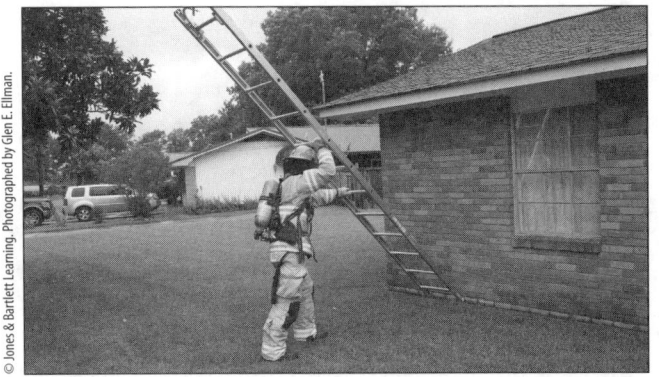

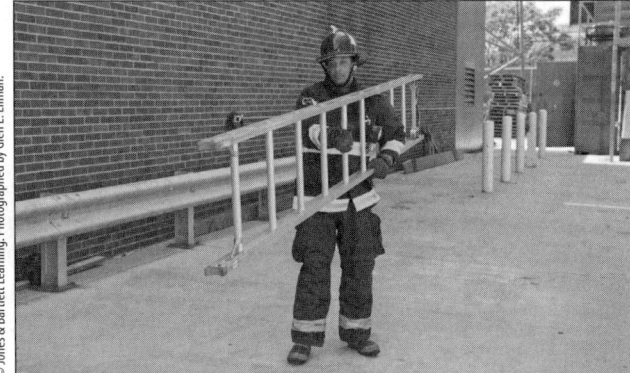

1. Start with the ladder mounted in a _____ or standing on one _____. Locate the center of the ladder. Grasp the two rungs on either side of the middle rung.

2. Lift the ladder and rest it on your _____.

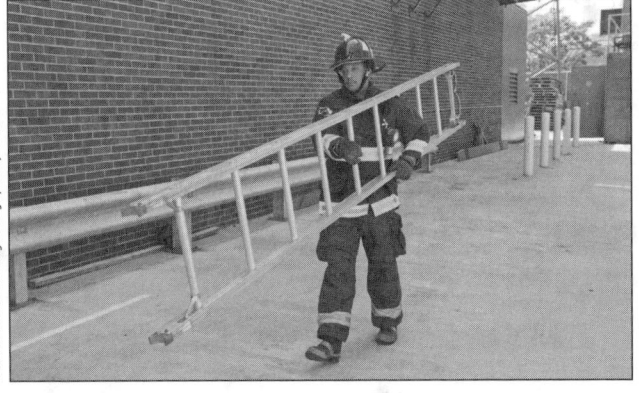

3. Walk carefully with the butt end first and pointed slightly _____.

Skill Drill 11-3: Two-Fire Fighter Shoulder Carry Fire Fighter I, NFPA 1001: 4.3.6
Test your knowledge of this skill drill by filling in the correct words in the photo captions.

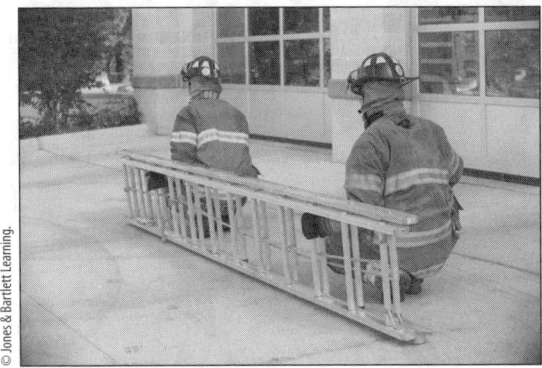

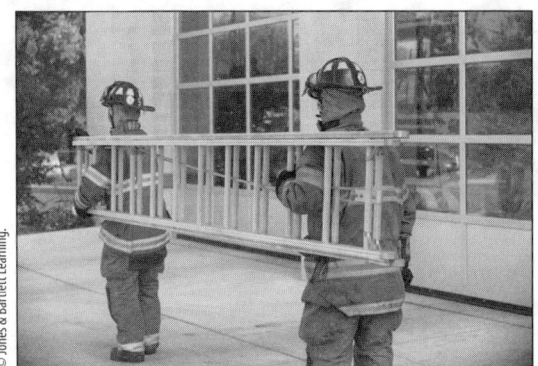

1. Start with the ladder mounted in a bracket or standing on one beam. Both fire fighters are positioned on the same side of the ladder. Facing the _____ end of the ladder, one fire fighter is positioned near the butt end of the ladder, and a second fire fighter is positioned near the _____ of the ladder.

2. Both fire fighters place one arm between two _____ and, on the leader's command, lift the ladder onto their shoulders. The ladder is carried butt end first.

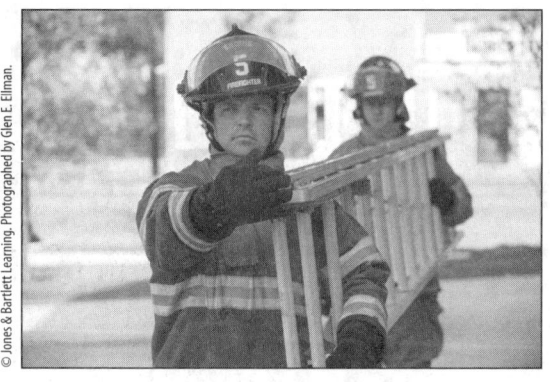

3. The fire fighter closest to the butt end covers the sharp butt _____ with a gloved hand to prevent injury to other fire fighters.

Skill Drill 11-8: Four-Fire Fighter Flat Carry Fire Fighter I, NFPA 1001: 4.3.6
Test your knowledge of this skill drill by placing the photos below in the correct order. Number the first step with a "1," the second step with a "2," and so on.

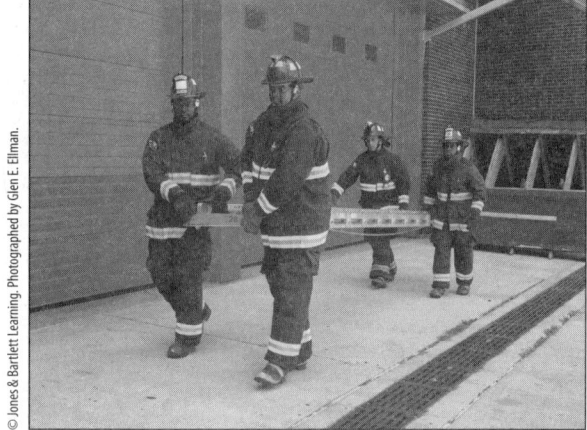

_____ The fire fighters closest to the butt end cover the sharp butt spurs with gloved hands to prevent injury to other fire fighters.

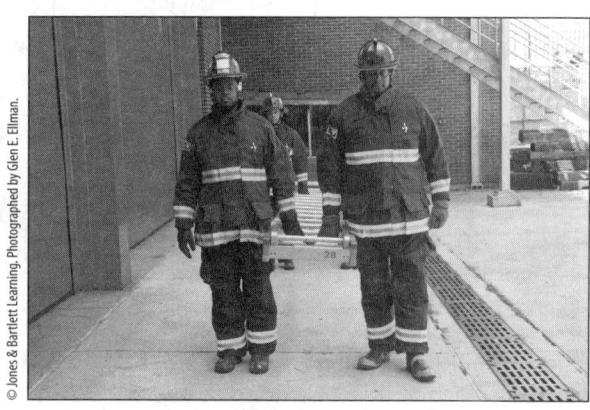

_____ On the leader's command, all four fire fighters pick up the ladder and carry it butt end forward.

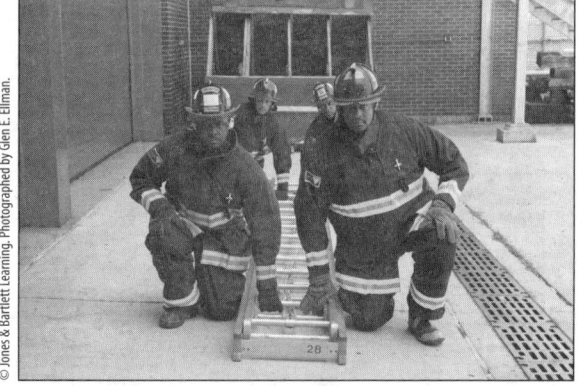

_____ On the leader's command, all four fire fighters kneel down and grasp the closer beam at arm's length.

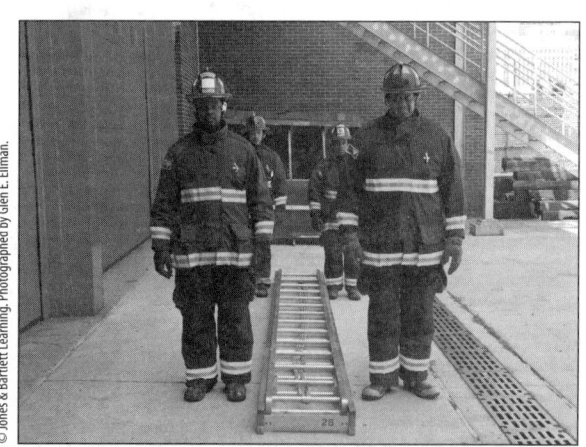

_____ The carry begins with the bed section of the ladder flat on the ground. Two fire fighters stand on each side of the ladder. All four fire fighters face the butt end of the ladder. One fire fighter is positioned at each corner of the ladder, with two fire fighters at the butt end of the ladder and two fire fighters at the tip end of the ladder.

Skill Drill 11-10: Four-Fire Fighter Flat Shoulder Carry Fire Fighter I, NFPA 1001: 4.3.6
Test your knowledge of this skill drill by placing the photos below in the correct order. Number the first step with a "1," the second step with a "2," and so on.

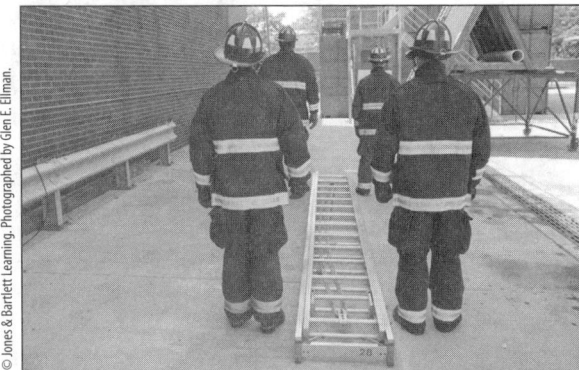

_____ The carry begins with the bed section of the ladder flat on the ground. Two fire fighters are positioned on each side of the ladder. All four fire fighters face the tip end of the ladder. One fire fighter is positioned at each corner of the ladder, with two fire fighters at the butt end and two fire fighters at the tip end of the ladder.

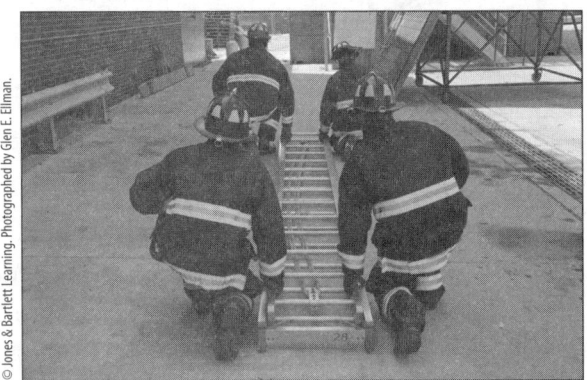

_____ On the leader's command, all four fire fighters kneel and grasp the closer beam.

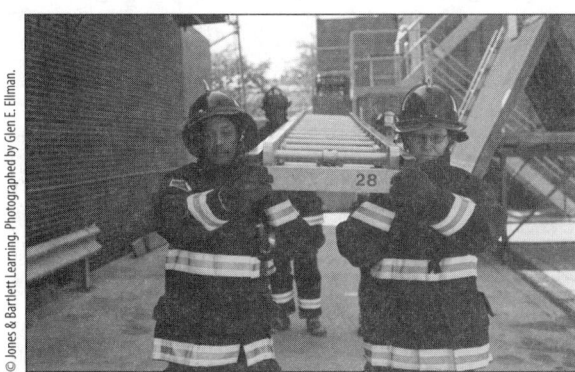

_____ The fire fighters place the beam of the ladder on their shoulders. All four fire fighters face the butt of the ladder. The ladder is carried in this position, with the butt moving forward. The fire fighters closest to the butt end cover the sharp butt spurs with gloved hands to prevent injury to other fire fighters.

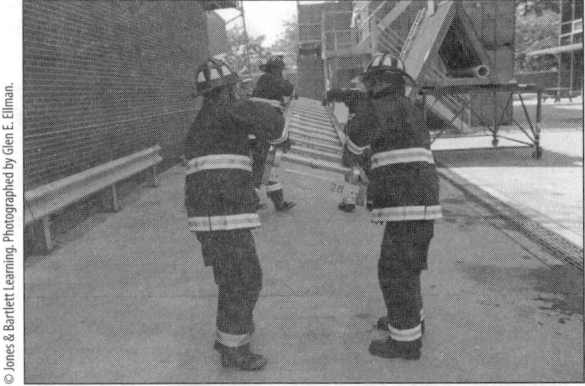

_____ On the leader's command, the fire fighters stand, raising the ladder.

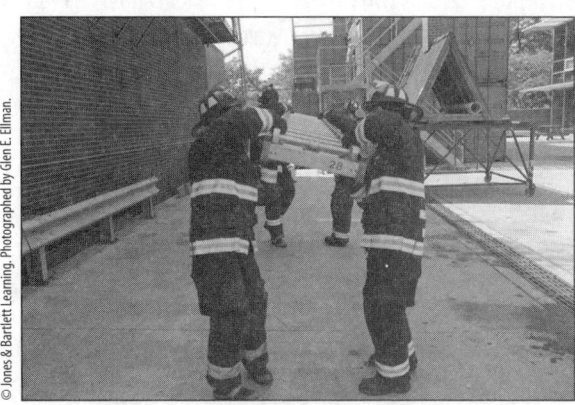

_____ As the ladder approaches chest height, the fire fighters all pivot toward the ladder.

Skill Drill 11-11: One-Fire Fighter Flat Raise for Ladders Less Than 14 Feet Long Fire Fighter I, NFPA 1001: 4.3.6

Test your knowledge of this skill drill by filling in the correct words in the photo captions.

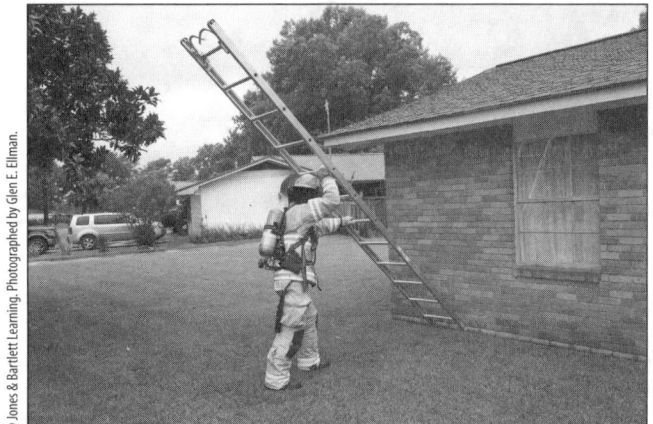

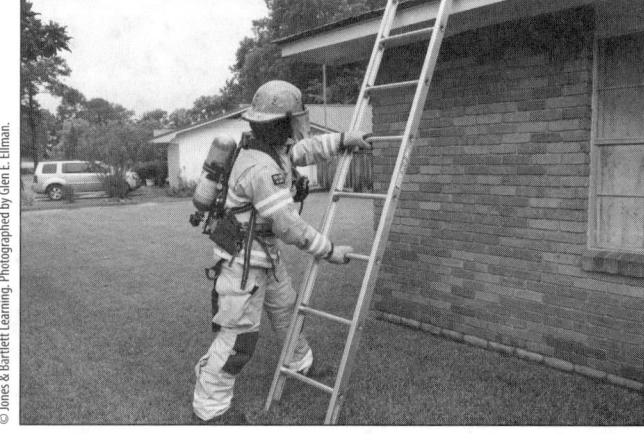

1. Place the butt of the ladder on the ground directly against the structure so that both butt spurs contact the _____ and the _____. Lay the ladder on the ground. If the ladder is an extension ladder, place the bed (base) section on the ground. Stand at the tip of the ladder, and check for overhead hazards. Take hold of a rung near the tip, bring that end of the ladder to chest height, and then step beneath the ladder. Raise the ladder using a _____ - _____ - _____ motion as you walk toward the structure until the ladder is vertical and against the structure. If an extension ladder is being used, hold the ladder vertical against the structure, and extend the _____ by pulling the halyard smoothly, with a hand-over-hand motion, until the desired height is reached and the pawls are locked.

2. Pull the butt of the ladder out from the structure to create a _____ - _____ climbing angle. To move the butt away from the structure, grip a lower _____, and lift slightly while pulling outward. At the same time, apply pressure to an upper rung to keep the tip of the ladder against the structure. If the ladder is an extension ladder, it will be necessary to rotate the ladder so the fly section is out. The _____ should be tied as described in the "Tying the Halyard" skill drill. Check the tip and the butt of the ladder to ensure safety before climbing.

Skill Drill 11-12: One-Fire Fighter Flat Raise for Ladders More Than 14 Feet Long Fire Fighter I, NFPA 1001: 4.3.6

Test your knowledge of this skill drill by placing the photos below in the correct order. Number the first step with a "1," the second step with a "2," and so on.

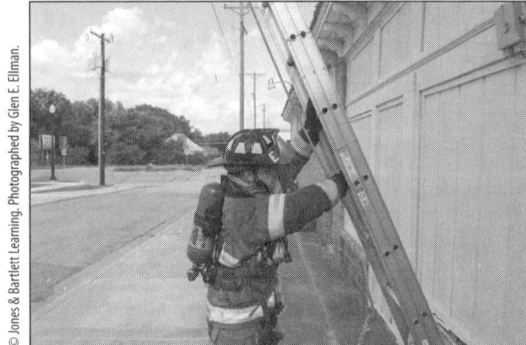

_____ Raise the ladder using a hand-over-hand motion as you walk toward the structure until the ladder is vertical and against the structure.

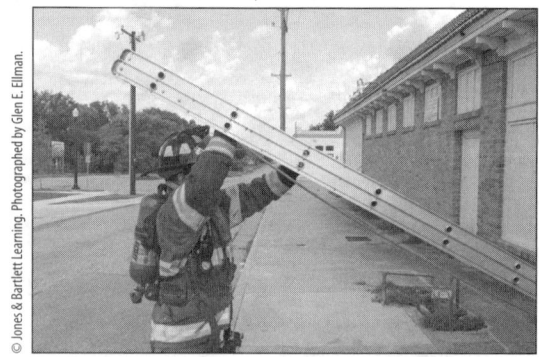

_____ Take hold of a rung near the tip, bring that end of the ladder to chest height, and then step beneath the ladder.

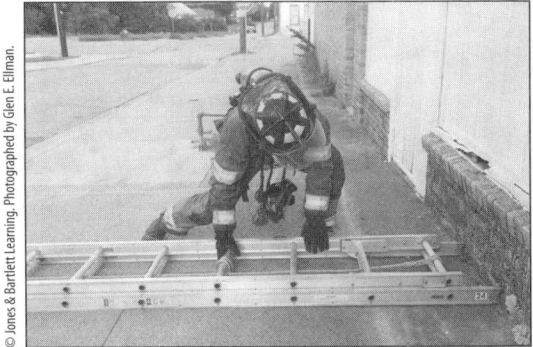

_____ Place the butt of the ladder on the ground directly against the structure so that both spurs contact the ground and the structure. Lay the ladder on the ground. If the ladder is an extension ladder, place the base section on the ground. Stand at the tip of the ladder and check for overhead hazards.

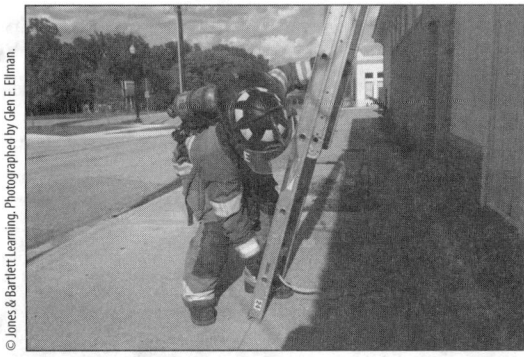

_____ Pull the butt of the ladder out from the structure to create a 75-degree climbing angle. To move the butt away from the structure, grip a lower rung, and lift slightly while pulling outward. At the same time, apply pressure to an upper rung to keep the tip of the ladder against the structure.

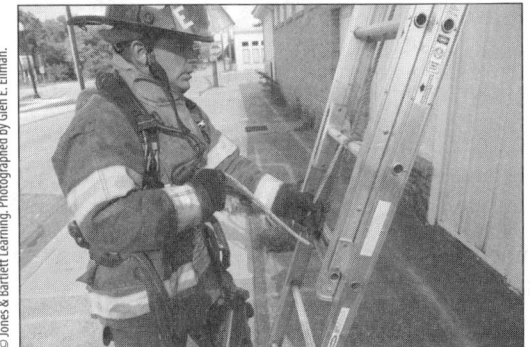

_____ If the ladder is an extension ladder, it will be necessary to rotate the ladder so the fly section is out. The halyard should be tied as described in the Tying the Halyard skill drill. Check the tip and the butt of the ladder to ensure safety before climbing.

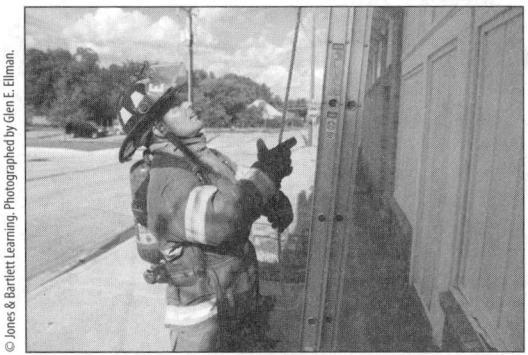

_____ If an extension ladder is being used, hold the ladder vertical against the structure, and extend the fly section by pulling the halyard smoothly, with a hand-over-hand motion, until the desired height is reached and the pawls are locked.

Skill Drill 11-14: Two-Fire Fighter Beam Raise Fire Fighter I, NFPA 1001: 4.3.6

Test your knowledge of this skill drill by placing the photos below in the correct order. Number the first step with a "1," the second step with a "2," and so on.

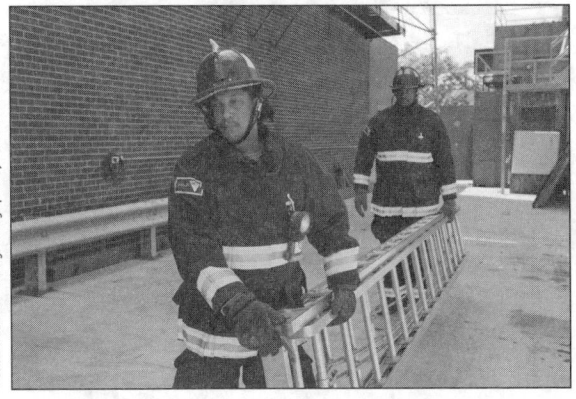

_____ The two-fire fighter beam raise begins with a shoulder or suitcase carry. One fire fighter stands near the butt end of the ladder, and the other fire fighter stands near the tip.

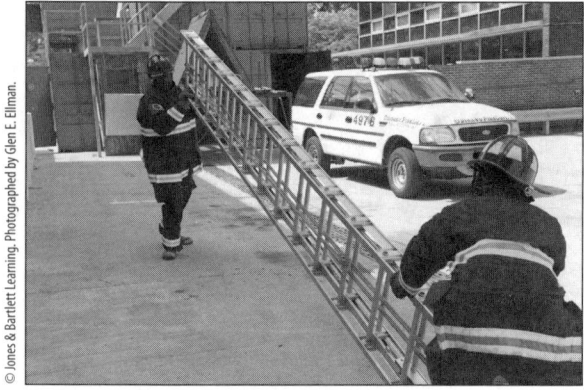
_____ The fire fighter at the butt of the ladder places that end of the ladder on the ground, while the fire fighter at the tip of the ladder holds that end.

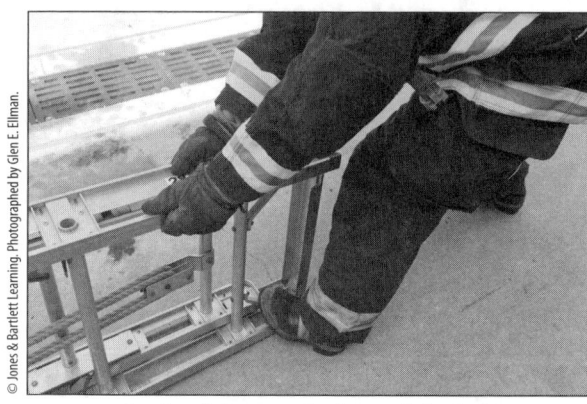
_____ The fire fighter at the butt of the ladder places a foot on the butt of the beam that is in contact with the ground and grasps the upper beam.

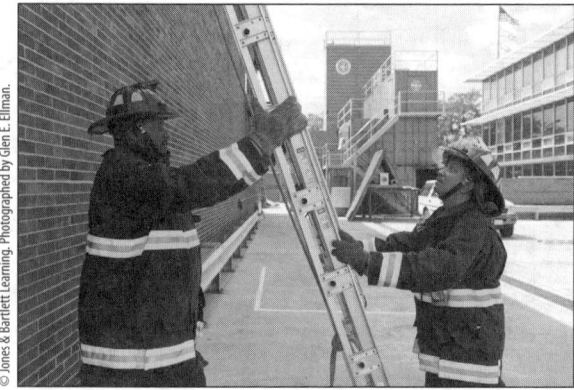
_____ The fire fighter facing the structure places one foot against one beam of the ladder, and then both fire fighters lean the ladder into place. The halyard is tied. The fire fighters check the ladder for a 75-degree climbing angle and check for stability at the tip and at the butt end of the ladder.

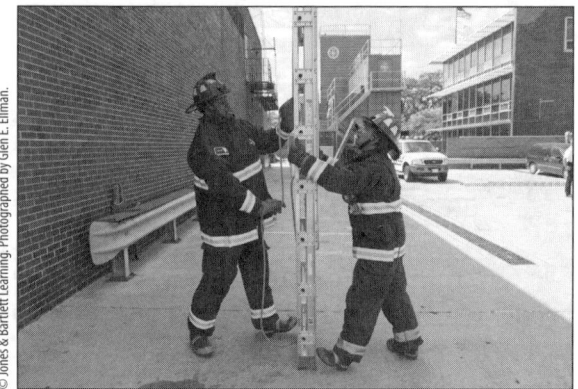
_____ One fire fighter extends the fly section by pulling the halyard smoothly with a hand-over-hand motion until the fly section is at the height desired and the pawls are locked. The other fire fighter stabilizes the ladder by holding the outside of the base section beams so that if the fly comes down suddenly it will not strike the fire fighter's hands.

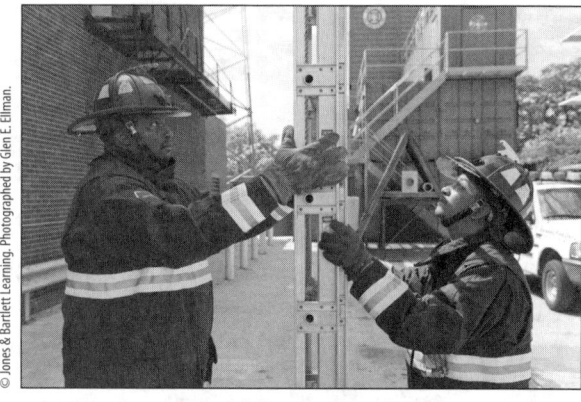
_____ The two fire fighters pivot the ladder into position as necessary.

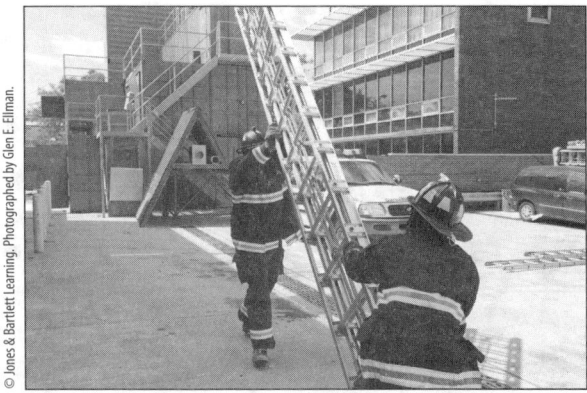

_____ The fire fighter at the tip of the ladder checks for overhead hazards and then begins to walk toward the butt, while raising the lower beam in a hand-over-hand fashion until the ladder is vertical.

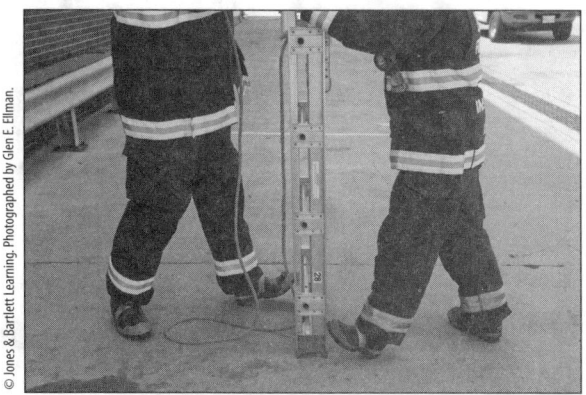

_____ The fire fighters face each other, one on each side of the ladder, and heel the ladder by each placing the toe or instep of one boot against the opposing beams of the ladder.

Skill Drill 11-17: Four-Fire Fighter Flat Raise Fire Fighter I, NFPA 1001: 4.3.6
Test your knowledge of this skill drill by filling in the correct words in the photo captions.

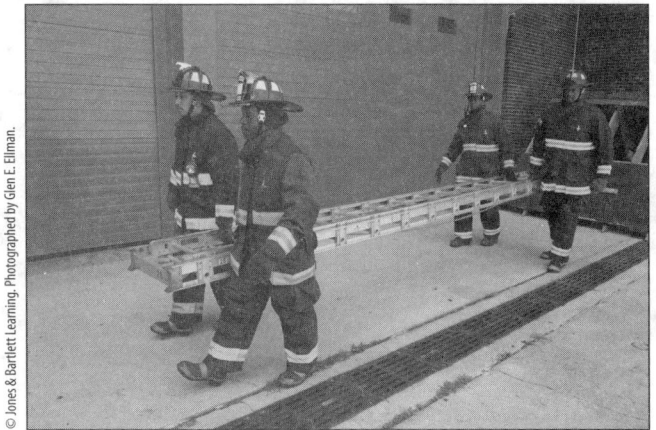

1. The raise begins with a four-fire fighter flat carry. Two fire fighters are at the _____ of the ladder, and two fire fighters are at the _____.

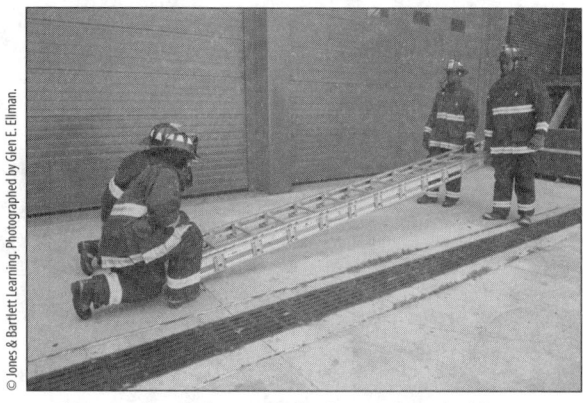

2. The two fire fighters at the butt of the ladder place the butt end of the ladder on the _____, while the two fire fighters at the tip _____ that end.

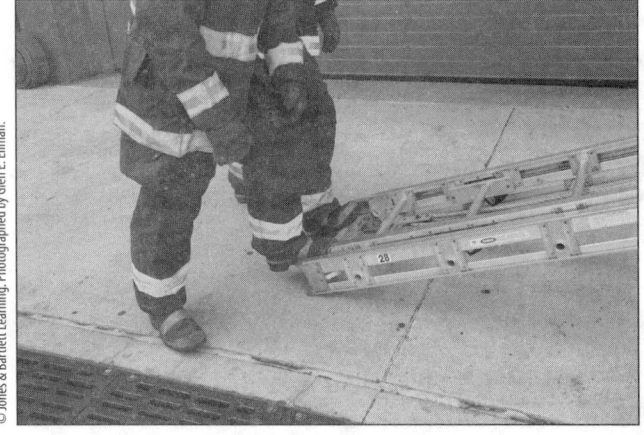

3. The two fire fighters at the butt of the ladder stand side by side, _____ the ladder. Each fire fighter places the inside foot on the bottom rung and the other foot on the ground outside the beam. Both crouch down, grab a rung and the beam, and lean backward.

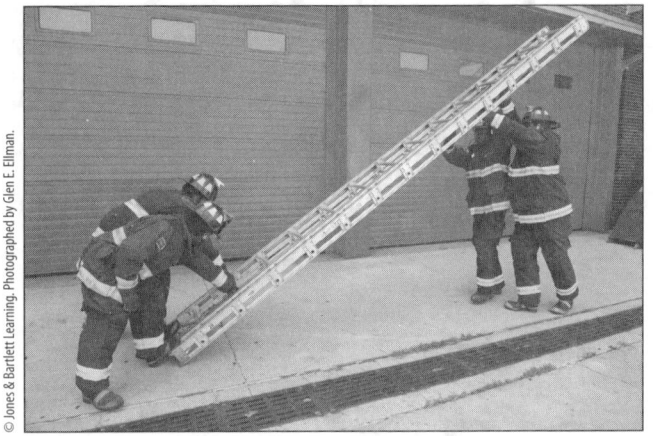

4. The two fire fighters at the tip of the ladder check for overhead hazards and then begin to walk toward the butt of the ladder, advancing down the rungs in a _____ - _____ - _____ fashion until the ladder is vertical.

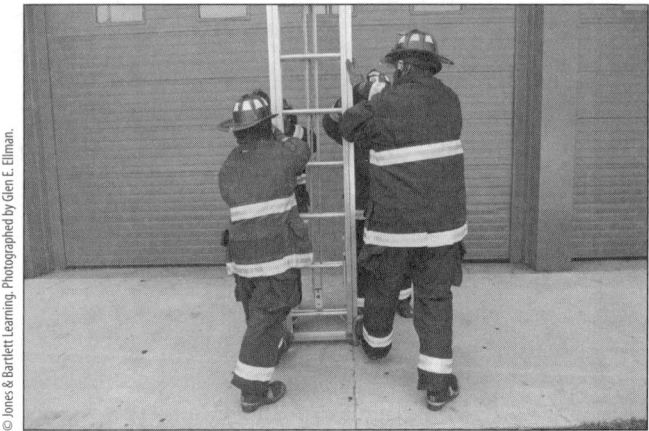

5. The fire fighters _____ the ladder into position, as necessary.

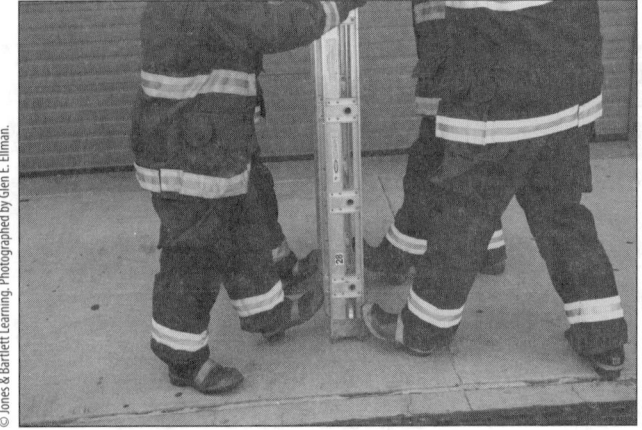

6. Two fire fighters heel the ladder by placing a boot against each _____. Each fire fighter places the toe or instep of one boot against one of the beams. The third fire fighter stabilizes the ladder by holding it on the outside of the rails.

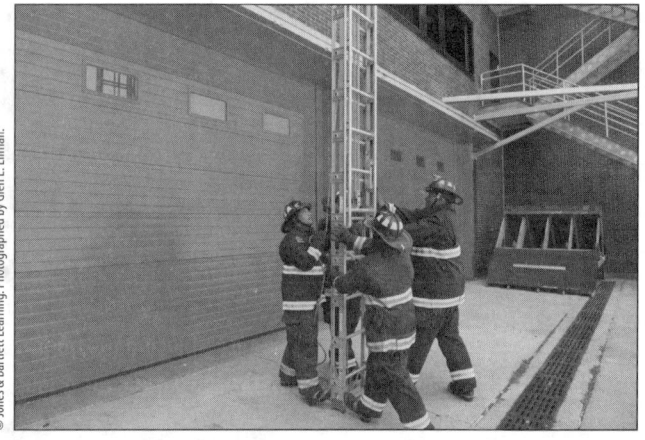

7. The fourth fire fighter extends the fly section by pulling the halyard smoothly with a hand-over-hand motion until the tip reaches the desired height and the _____ are locked.

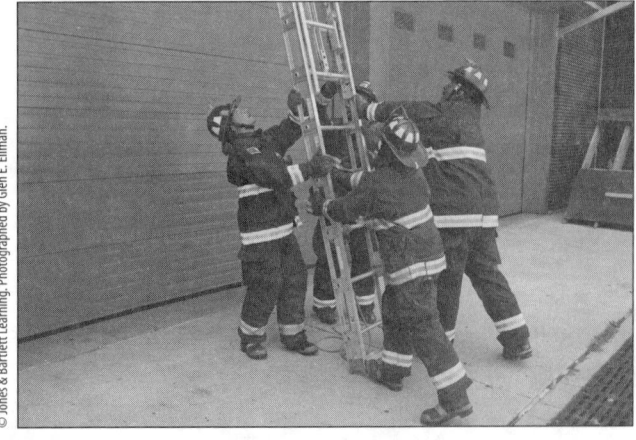

8. The two fire fighters facing the structure each place one foot against one beam of the ladder while the other two fire fighters lower the ladder into place. The _____ is tied. The fire fighters check the ladder for a _____ - _____ climbing angle and for security at the tip and at the butt end of the ladder.

Skill Drill 11-20: Deploying a Roof Ladder Fire Fighter I, NFPA 1001: 4.3.12

Test your knowledge of this skill drill by placing the photos below in the correct order. Number the first step with a "1," the second step with a "2," and so on.

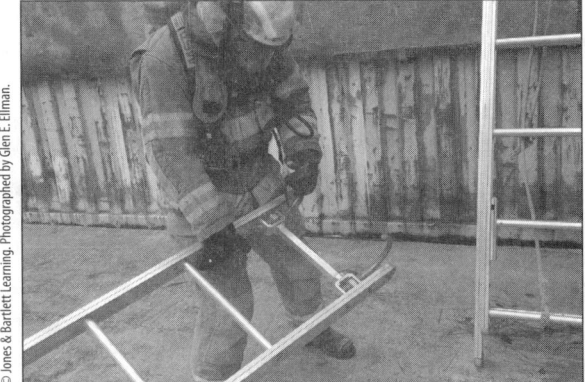

_____ Place the butt end of the roof ladder on the ground, and rotate the hooks of the roof ladder to the open position.

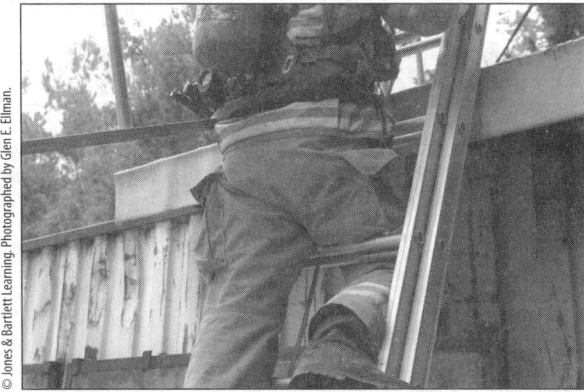

_____ Climb to the roofline of the structure, carrying the roof ladder on one shoulder. Secure yourself to the ladder.

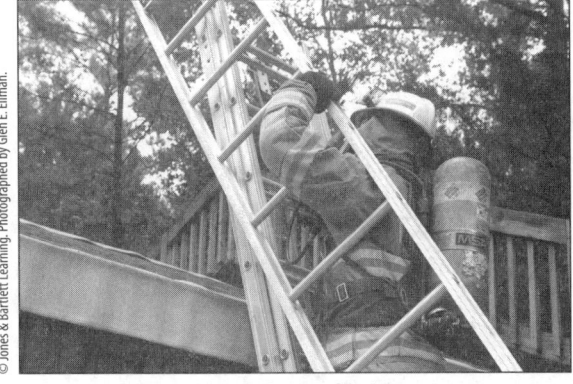

_____ Raise and lean the roof ladder against one beam of the other ladder with the hooks oriented outward, away from you. Climb the lower climbing ladder until you reach the midpoint of the roof ladder that is positioned next to you, and then slip one shoulder between two rungs of the roof ladder, and shoulder the roof ladder.

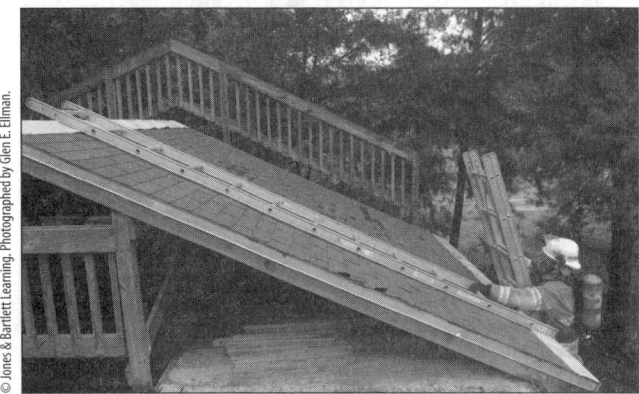

_____ Once the hooks have passed the peak, pull back on the roof ladder to set the hooks, and check that they are secure. To remove a roof ladder from the roof, reverse the process just described. After releasing the hooks from the peak, it may be necessary to turn the ladder on one of its beams or turn it so the hooks are pointing up to slide the ladder down the roof without catching the hooks on the roofing material. Carrying a roof ladder in this manner requires strength and practice.

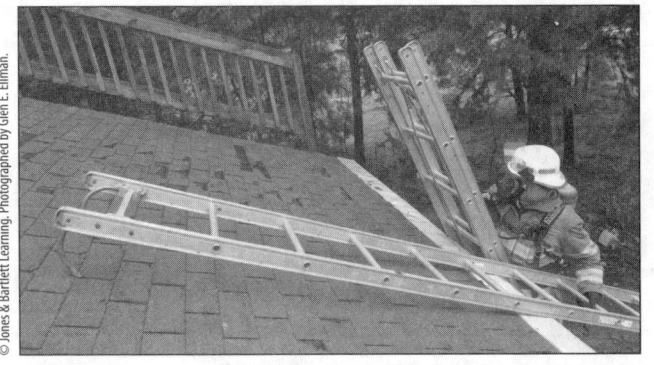

_____ Place the roof ladder on the roof surface with hooks down. Push the ladder up toward the peak of the roof with a hand-over-hand motion.

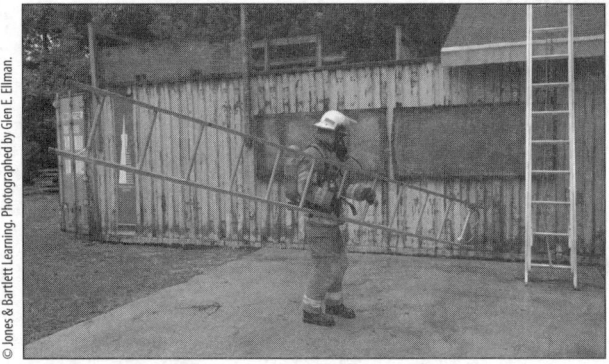

_____ Carry the roof ladder to the base of the climbing ladder that is already in place to provide access to the roofline.

Search and Rescue

Workbook Activities

The following activities have been designed to help you. Your instructor may require you to complete some or all of these activities as a regular part of your fire fighter training program. You are encouraged to complete any activity your instructor does not assign to you, as a way to enhance your learning in the classroom.

Chapter Review

The following exercises provide an opportunity to refresh your knowledge of this chapter.

Matching

Match each of the terms in the left column to the appropriate definition in the right column.

_____ 1. Secondary search   A. A return to flaming combustion after apparent but incomplete extinguishment

_____ 2. Primary search   B. An offensive fire attack initiated by an exterior, indirect handline operation into the fire compartment to initiate cooling while transitioning into an interior attack

_____ 3. Search and rescue   C. The process of looking for living victims who are in danger

_____ 4. Search   D. Assists, drags, and carries

_____ 5. Rescue techniques   E. Similar to a video camera except that it captures heat display images instead of visible light images

_____ 6. Transitional attack   F. The removal of a person from danger

_____ 7. Rescue   G. A more thorough search undertaken after the fire is under control

_____ 8. Rekindle   H. May be performed by any fire company or unit

_____ 9. Thermal imager   I. Quick initial search for victims

_____ 10. Search rope   J. A guide rope that allows fire fighters to maintain contact with a fixed point

Multiple Choice

Read each item carefully, and then select the best response.

_____ 1. Search ropes should be used to
   A. help fire fighters maintain their orientation.
   B. keep search teams connected.
   C. search wide open spaces.
   D. both A and C.

_____ 2. If a victim is capable of walking, rescuers may only need to use the
   A. one-person walking assist.
   B. two-person seat carry.
   C. cradle-in-arms carry.
   D. three-person walking assist.

CHAPTER 12

_____ 3. To rescue a victim through a window, raise the ladder and secure it in the rescue position with the tip
   A. above the windowsill.
   B. in the open window.
   C. just below the windowsill.
   D. upwind from the window.

_____ 4. When rescuing a heavy adult using a ladder, the rescuer should
   A. get more help—three rescuers at a minimum.
   B. use two ladders.
   C. place two ladders side by side.
   D. All of the above.

_____ 5. A webbing sling provides a secure grip around
   A. the victim's upper body.
   B. the victim's waist.
   C. the victim's arms.
   D. the victim's legs and feet.

_____ 6. When rescuing an unconscious victim on a ladder, the fire fighter on the ladder should
   A. maintain continuous eye contact with the victim.
   B. maintain eye contact with the second fire fighter.
   C. face the victim.
   D. remain on the ladder until a rescue team can assist the descent.

_____ 7. After the fire is under control, fire fighters should begin a
   A. primary search.
   B. secondary search.
   C. rescue.
   D. safety search.

_____ 8. When a ladder rescue involves a conscious victim, the fire fighter should
   A. establish verbal contact.
   B. urge the victim to jump.
   C. have the victim climb down facing the fire fighter.
   D. have the victim exit head first.

_____ 9. After the area immediately around the fire is searched in an apartment building, the next priority is to search the
   A. area directly above the fire.
   B. area directly below the fire.
   C. highest floors in the building.
   D. hallways and exits.

_____ 10. A search begins with the areas in which
   A. the greatest number of hazards exist.
   B. the building experiences the greatest traffic.
   C. occupants are expected.
   D. victims are at the greatest risk.

_____ 11. When conducting a search, a rapid rise in the amount of heat or flame may indicate the potential for a(n)
   A. collapse.
   B. flashover.
   C. backdraft.
   D. smoke explosion.

_____ 12. Assisting someone down a ladder carries a considerable risk to
   A. the victim.
   B. the fire fighters.
   C. the safety officer.
   D. both A and B.

_____ 13. Status and results from search operations needs to be communicated to the
   A. secondary search team.
   B. incident commander.
   C. safety officer.
   D. rapid intervention company/crew.

_____ 14. Adults that have tried to escape from a structure on their own are often found
   A. in a bathtub or shower.
   B. inside the garage.
   C. in closets.
   D. near doors or windows.

_____ 15. When a building is occupied, fire fighters should first rescue the occupants who are
   A. in the most immediate danger.
   B. in the least danger.
   C. the most easily accessed.
   D. closest to the exits.

_____ 16. When using the standard search method, fire fighters should
   A. search individually.
   B. carry no radios.
   C. enter the fire room at the same time.
   D. keep the hallway door open for egress.

_____ 17. The three most important senses during a search are
   A. sight, sound, and taste.
   B. touch, sight, and taste.
   C. sight, sound, and touch.
   D. sound, taste, and touch.

_____ 18. The two-person seat carry is used when the victim
   A. is very large.
   B. must be carried up or down stairs.
   C. is a child.
   D. is disabled or paralyzed.

_____ 19. The fire fighter drag utilizes the victim's
   A. clothing as a handle.
   B. tied wrists.
   C. weight to assist the movement.
   D. ability to assist moving.

_____ 20. The clothes drag is used to move a victim who is on the floor and
   A. is too heavy for one rescuer.
   B. must be carried up or down stairs.
   C. is disabled or paralyzed.
   D. is difficult to reach.

Vocabulary

Define the following terms using the space provided.

1. Exit assist:

   _____
   _____
   _____

2. Shelter-in-place:

   _____
   _____
   _____

3. Two-in/two-out rule:

   _____
   _____
   _____

4. Primary search:

   _____
   _____
   _____

5. Transitional attack:

   _____
   _____
   _____

Fill-In

Read each item carefully, and then complete the statement by filling in the missing word(s).

1. Saving _____ has the highest priority at a fire scene.

2. Search team members may have to _____ to stay below layers of hot gases and smoke.

3. Occupants who are asleep are at a(n) _____ risk than occupants who are awake.

4. The incident commander is responsible for managing the level of _____ during emergency operations.

5. Search teams must have a(n) _____ escape route in case fire conditions change.

6. Searched rooms should be _____ so other searchers will know they have been searched.

7. In a structure, searching the area directly above the fire and the rest of that floor represents the _____ priority.

8. _____ _____ to determine whether they are stable is a dangerous practice and should be discouraged.

9. Searchers need to be aware of the _____ _____ _____ in a building and avoid actions that could place them in a dangerous position.

10. The _____ _____ is the most commonly taught search method used by fire fighters.

True/False
If you believe the statement to be more true than false, write the letter "T" in the space provided. If you believe the statement to be more false than true, write the letter "F."

1. _____ Although search and rescue is a top priority, it is rarely the only action taken by first-arriving fire fighters.
2. _____ It is justifiable to risk the safety of fire fighters only if there is a potential to save lives.
3. _____ In some situations, the best option is to shelter occupants in place.
4. _____ Some of the most accurate information can be obtained from people who have just escaped from a burning building.
5. _____ Most people who realize they are in danger will attempt to escape on their own.
6. _____ The overall plan for a fire incident must focus on the life-safety priority as long as search and rescue operations are still underway.
7. _____ Any search operation conducted in the flow path increases the risks posed to fire fighters.
8. _____ Observations of the size and arrangement of the building can provide valuable information when trying to determine a search plan.
9. _____ The two-in/two-out rule can be broken if there is an imminent life-threatening situation.
10. _____ The standard search is conducted with a search team of two or more members.

Short Answer
Complete this section with short written answers using the space provided.

1. Describe three benefits of thermal imagers.

   _____
   _____
   _____
   _____

2. List six pieces of search and rescue equipment.

   _____
   _____
   _____
   _____

3. Identify the six guidelines fire fighters need to remember during search and rescue operations.

   _____
   _____
   _____
   _____

4. Identify five pieces of valuable information a preincident plan can provide for search and rescue operations.

   _____
   _____
   _____
   _____

5. Identify the four simple carries that can be used to move a victim who is conscious and responsive, but incapable of standing or walking.

   _____
   _____
   _____
   _____

6. Identify four considerations for search and rescue size-up.

   _____
   _____
   _____
   _____

Fire Alarms

The following real case scenarios will give you an opportunity to explore the concerns associated with search and rescue. Read each scenario, and then answer each question in detail.

1. You are the leader of a search and rescue team about to enter a carpet warehouse. Two employees are missing and thought to be located in the fire building. The warehouse has sprinklers, and the fire is confined. Your officer warns that the inside floor plan is complex owing to the numerous remodels. To make matters worse, the smoke is thick and black because of the burning carpet, and it is cold and hugging the floor because of the activation of the sprinkler system. Knowing that this is a very dangerous task, you want to ensure the safety of yourself and your crew. How should you proceed?

   _____
   _____
   _____
   _____
   _____
   _____

2. It is 1:00 in the morning when you are dispatched to an old three-story apartment complex. The main stairway is located in the center of the building. The fire is located on the first floor. A suppression crew has been sent to the seat of the fire. There are mixed reports on whether the building has been evacuated. Your engine company has been assigned to the third floor for search and rescue. How should you proceed?

_____

_____

_____

_____

_____

_____

_____

_____

Skill Drills

Skill Drill 12-1: Conducting a Primary Search Using the Standard Search Method Fire Fighter I, NFPA 1001: 4.3.9

Test your knowledge of this skill drill by filling in the correct words in the photo captions.

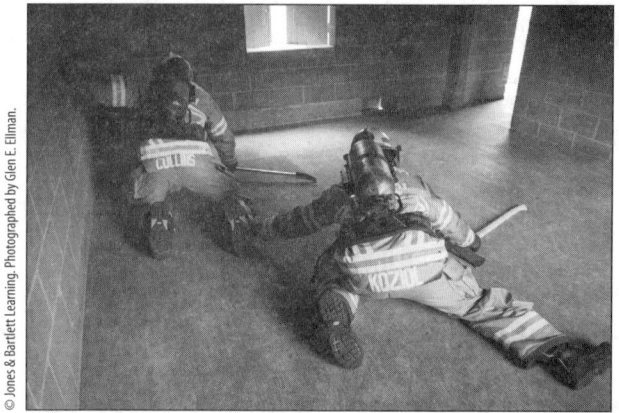

1. _____ your personal protective equipment (PPE), including SCBA, and enter the personnel accountability system. Bring hand tools, a hand light, a radio, a thermal imaging device, and search ropes if indicated. Notify command that the search is starting and indicate the area to be searched and the direction of the search. Use hand tools or ground ladders if needed to gain access to the site. Conduct a quick and systematic search by staying on an outside wall and searching from room to room. Maintain contact with an outside wall.

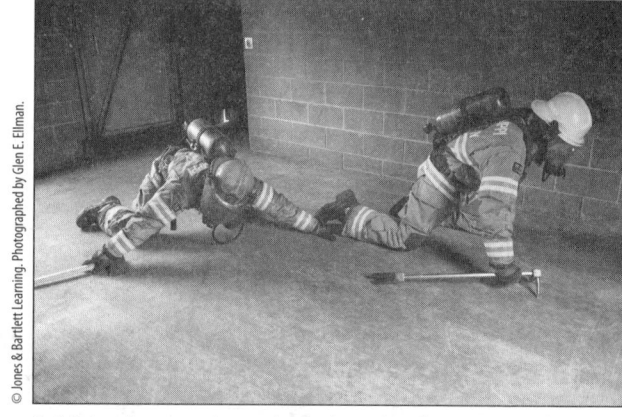

2. Maintain team integrity using visual, voice, or direct contact. Use the most efficient movement based on the hazard encountered: duck walk, crawl, stand only when you can see your feet and it is not hot. Use tools to extend your reach if recommended by your department. Clear each room _____ or by _____, and then close the door. Search the area, including stairs up to the landing on the next floor.

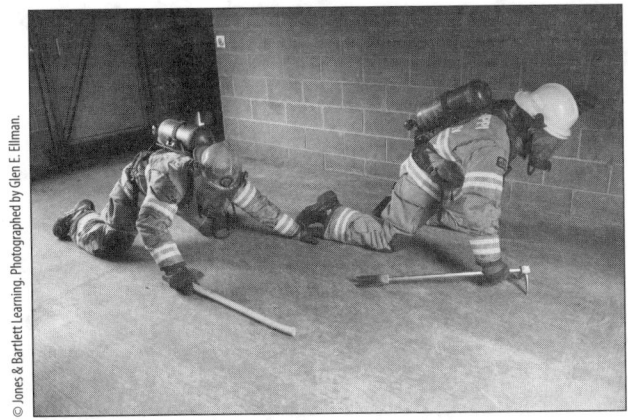

3. Periodically listen for _____ and _____ of fire. Communicate the locations of doors, windows, and inside corners to other team members. Observe fire, smoke, and heat conditions; update command on this information. Locate and remove victims; notify the IC. When the search is complete, conduct a personnel accountability report. Report the results of the search to your officer.

Skill Drill 12-2: Conducting a Primary Search Using the Oriented Search Method Fire Fighter I, NFPA 1001: 4.3.9
Test your knowledge of this skill drill by placing the photos below in the correct order. Number the first step with a "1," the second step with a "2," and so on.

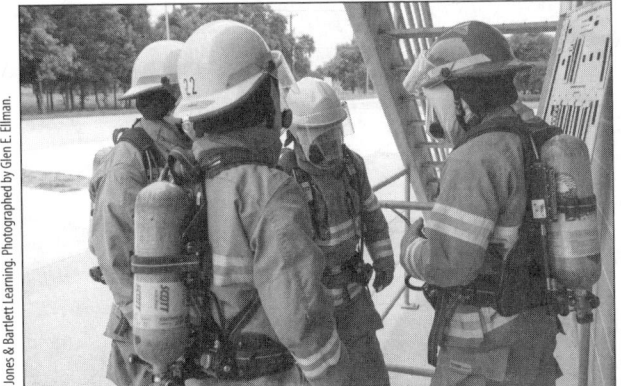

_____ A search team consisting of one officer or team leader and one to three searchers is assembled.

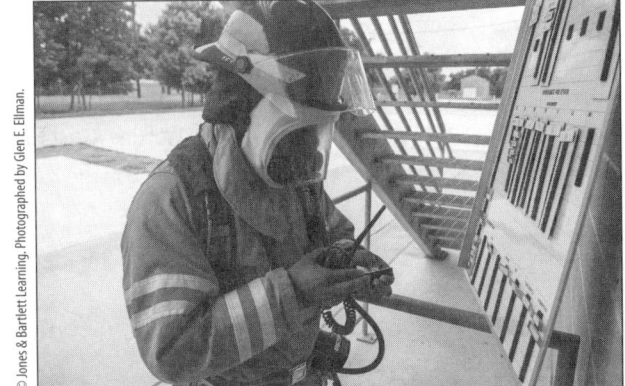

_____ Searchers don their personal protective equipment (PPE), including SCBA and hand tools, and enter the personnel accountability system.

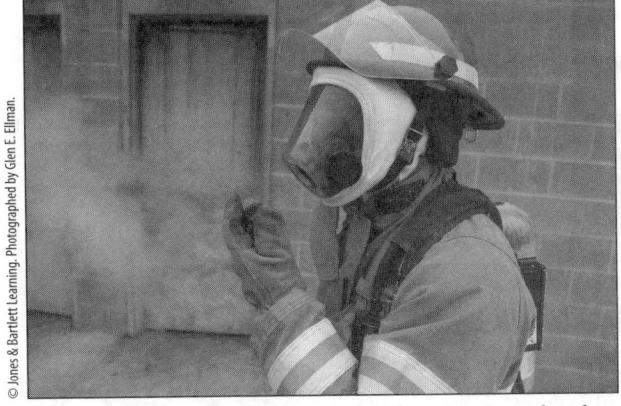

_____ The officer notifies the incident commander that search is starting and directs the searchers to the area to be searched.

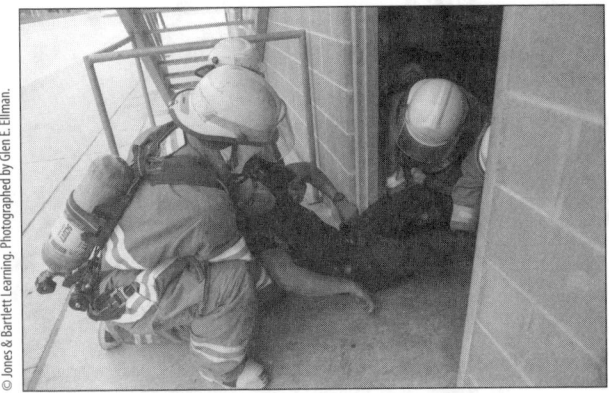

_____ Searchers use a left-handed or a right-handed search pattern and perform two to three side crawls as necessary to extend the search toward the center of the room. Upon completion of the search of each room, the officer directs searchers to the next rooms to be searched and closes the door. If a victim is found, the officer notifies the incident commander and requests a second team to help remove the victim. The search team moves the victim toward the exit and turns over the care and removal of the victim to the second team.

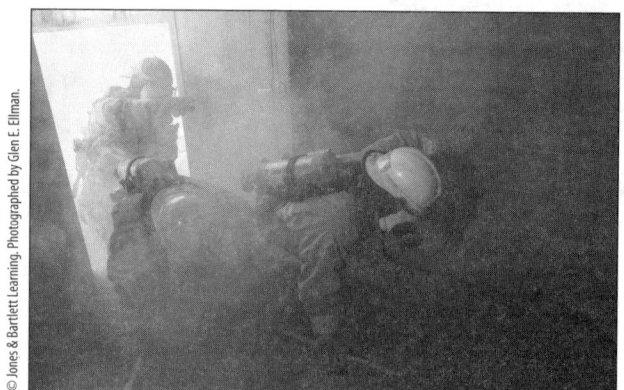

_____ The officer remains outside the rooms to be searched to monitor safety conditions, air supplies, and the status of the fire. The officer maintains a systematic search pattern and coordinates activities with the incident commander.

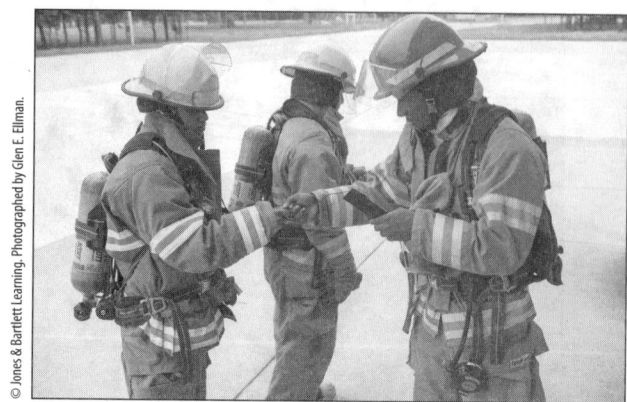

_____ The search team then returns to the last location searched and continues the systematic search of the building. When the search is complete, the officer conducts a personnel accountability report. The officer reports the results of the search and the personnel accountability report to the incident commander.

Skill Drill 12-5: Performing a Two-Person Walking Assist Fire Fighter I, NFPA 1001: 4.3.9
Test your knowledge of the skill drill by filling in the correct words in the photo captions.

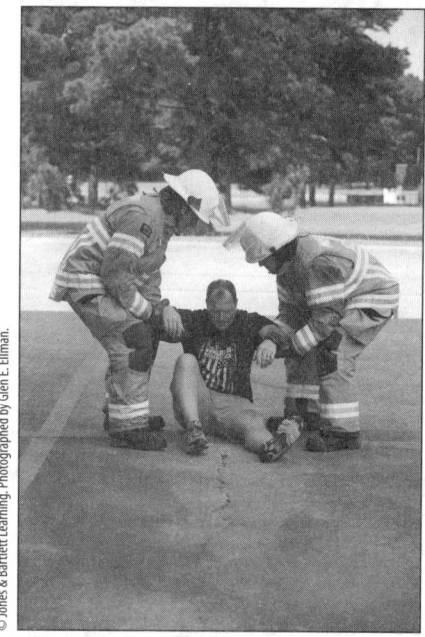

1. Two fire fighters stand facing the victim, one on each side of the victim. Both fire fighters assist the victim to a _____ position.

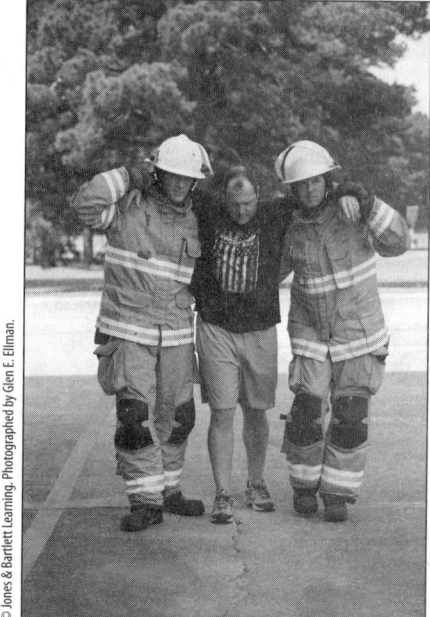

2. Once the victim is fully upright, place the victim's right arm around the neck of the fire fighter on the right side. Place the victim's left arm around the neck of the fire fighter on the left side. The victim's arms should drape over the fire fighter's _____. The fire fighters hold the victim's _____ in one hand.

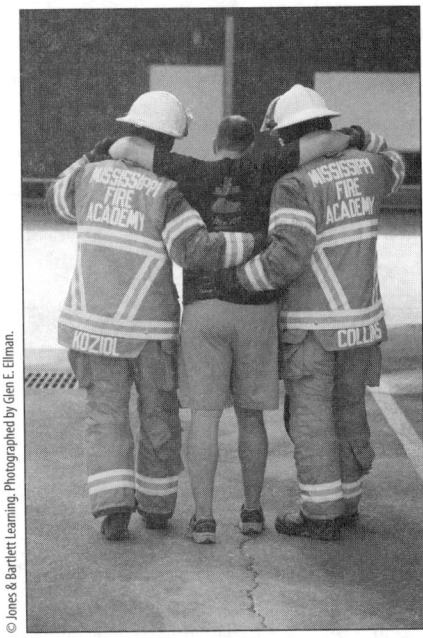

3. Both fire fighters put their free arms around the victim's _____ for added support and slowly assist the victim to walk. Fire fighters must coordinate their movements and move slowly.

Skill Drill 12-6: Performing a Two-Person Extremity Carry Fire Fighter I, NFPA 1001: 4.3.9

Test your knowledge of this skill drill by placing the photos below in the correct order. Number the first step with a "1," the second step with a "2," and so on.

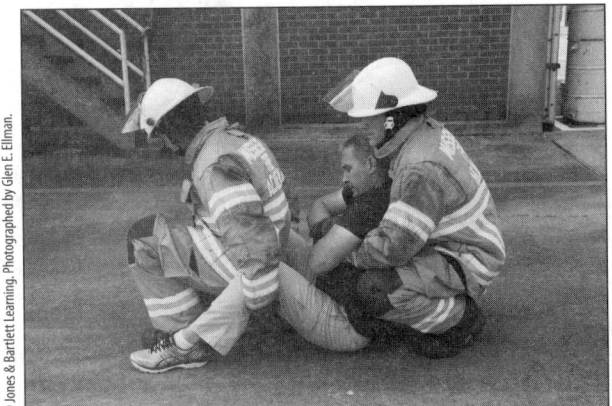

_____ The second fire fighter backs in between the victim's legs, reaches around, and grasps the victim behind the knees.

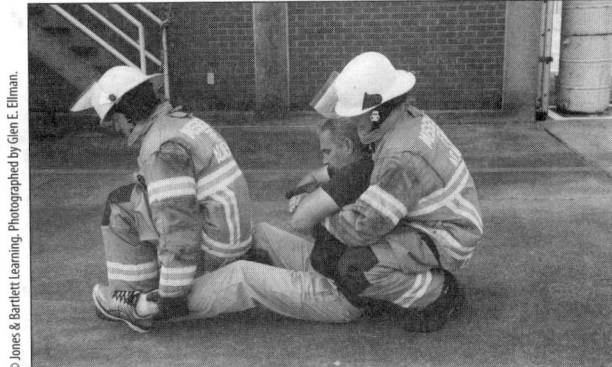

_____ The first fire fighter kneels behind the victim, reaches under the victim's arms, and grasps the victim's wrists.

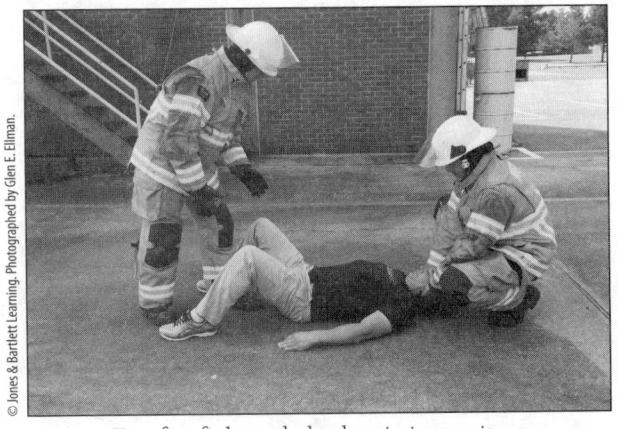

_____ Two fire fighters help the victim to sit up.

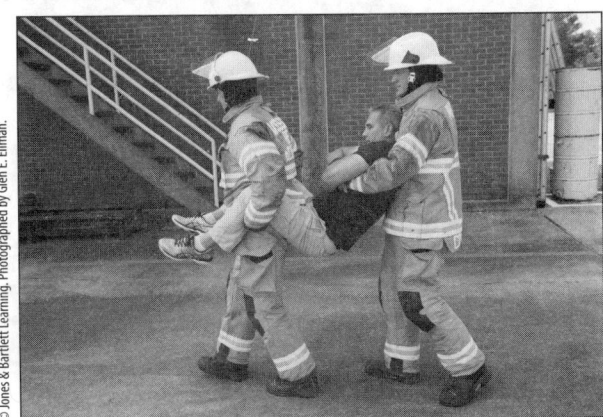

_____ The first fire fighter gives the command to stand and carry the victim away, walking straight ahead. Both fire fighters must coordinate their movements.

Skill Drill 12-8: Performing a Two-Person Chair Carry Fire Fighter I, NFPA 1001: 4.3.9

Test your knowledge of this skill drill by filling in the correct words in the photo captions.

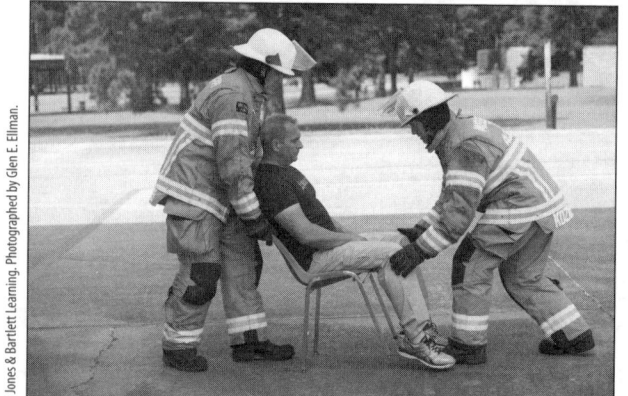

1. Tie the victim's hands together, or have the victim grasp his or her hands together. This prevents the victim from reaching for a _____ object while you are moving him or her. One fire fighter stands behind the seated victim, reaches down, and grasps the back of the chair.

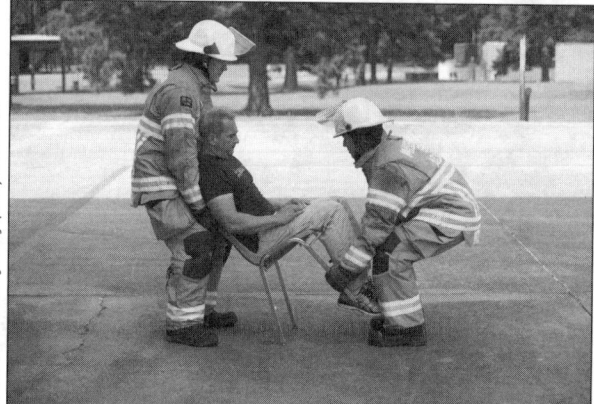

2. The fire fighter tilts the chair slightly _____ on its rear legs so that the second fire fighter can step back between the legs of the chair and grasp the tips of the chair's front legs. The victim's legs should be between the legs of the chair.

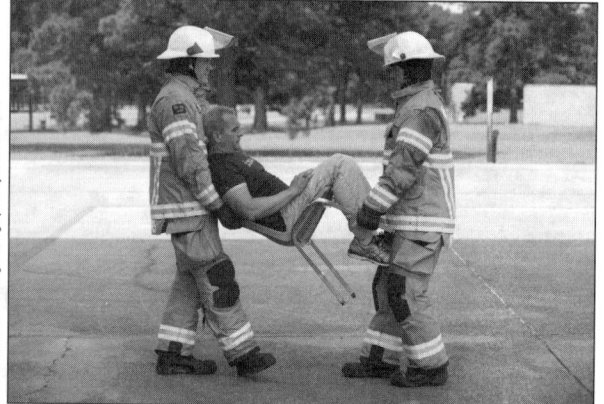

3. When both fire fighters are correctly positioned, the fire fighter behind the chair gives the command to _____ and walk away. Because the chair carry may force the victim's head forward, watch the victim for _____ problems.

Skill Drill 12-12: Performing a Standing Drag Fire Fighter I, NFPA 1001: 4.3.9

Test your knowledge of this skill drill by placing the photos below in the correct order. Number the first step with a "1," the second step with a "2," and so on.

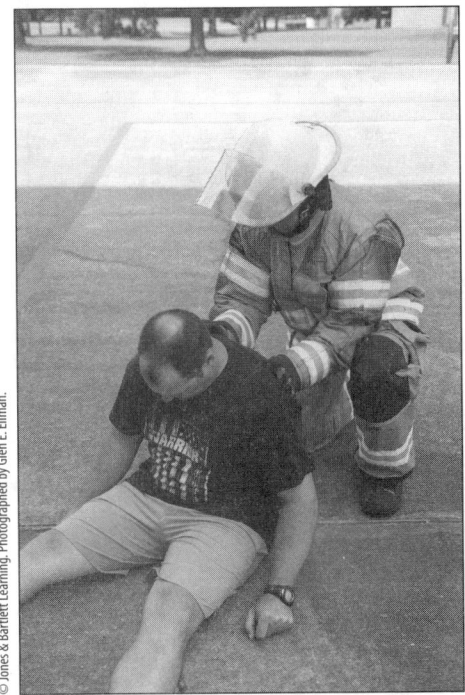

_____ Raise the victim's head and torso by 90 degrees so that the victim is leaning against you.

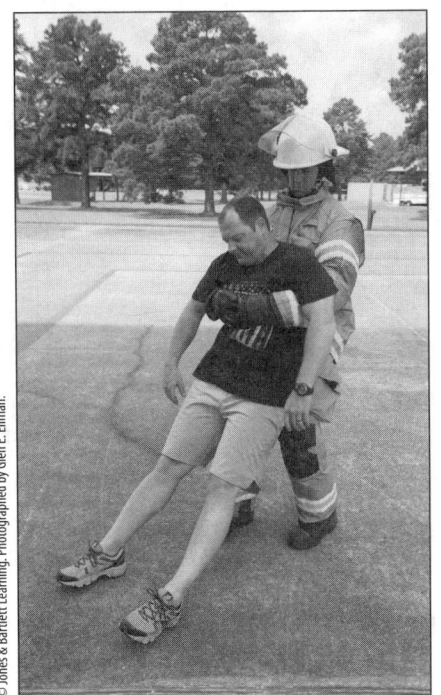

_____ Stand straight up using your legs. Drag the victim out.

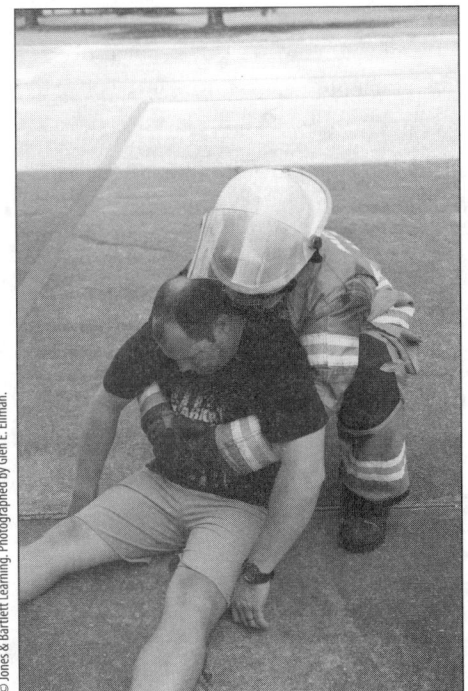

_____ Reach under the victim's arms, wrap your arms around the victim's chest, and lock your arms.

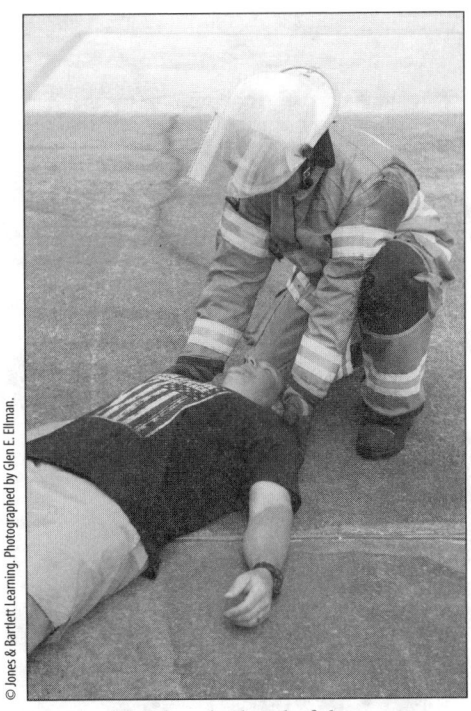

_____ Kneel at the head of the supine victim.

Skill Drill 12-16: Rescuing a Conscious Victim from a Window Fire Fighter I, NFPA 1001: 4.3.9
Test your knowledge of this skill drill by filling in the correct words in the photo captions.

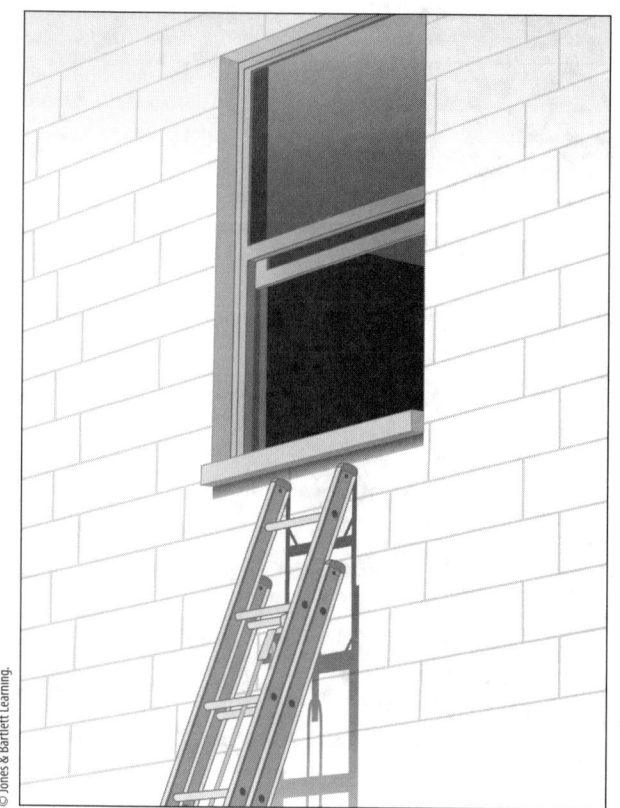

1. The rescue team places the ladder in the rescue position, with the tip of the ladder just below the _____, and secures the ladder in place.

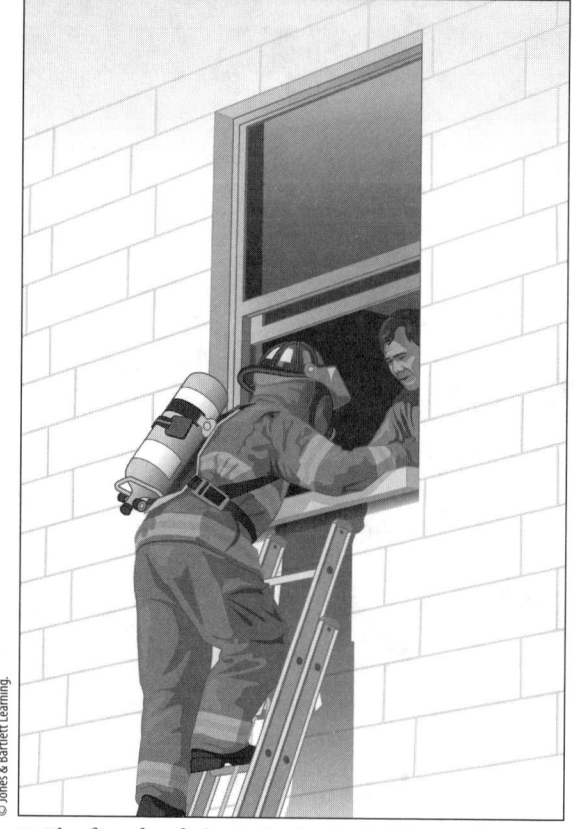

2. The first fire fighter climbs the ladder, makes _____ with the victim, and climbs inside the window to assist the victim. The fire fighter should make contact as soon as possible to calm the victim and encourage the victim to stay at the window until the rescue can be performed.

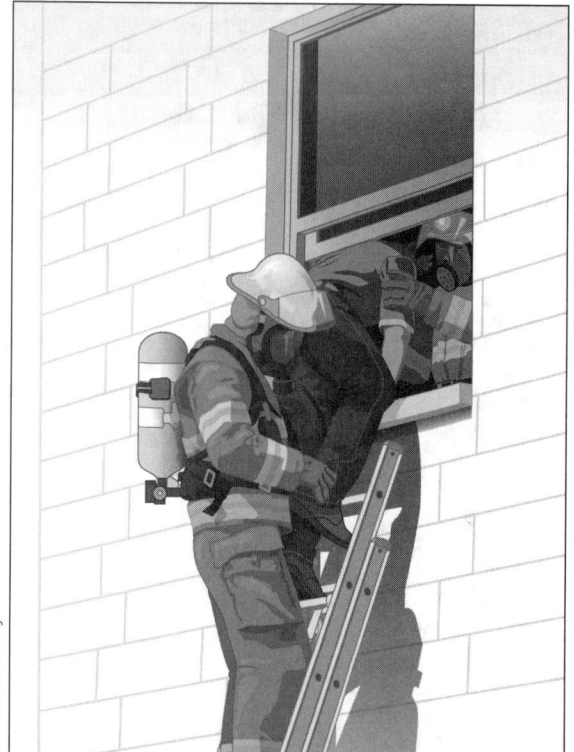

3. The second fire fighter climbs up to the window, leaving at least one _____ available for the victim. When ready, the fire fighter advises the victim to slowly come out onto the ladder, feet _____ and facing the ladder.

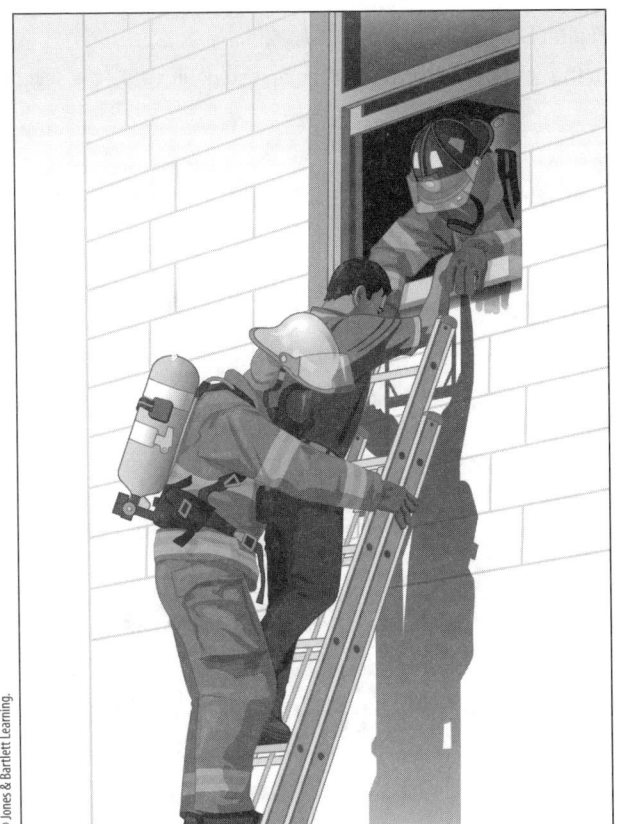

4. The second fire fighter forms a

_____-_____

around the victim, with both hands on the beams of the ladder.

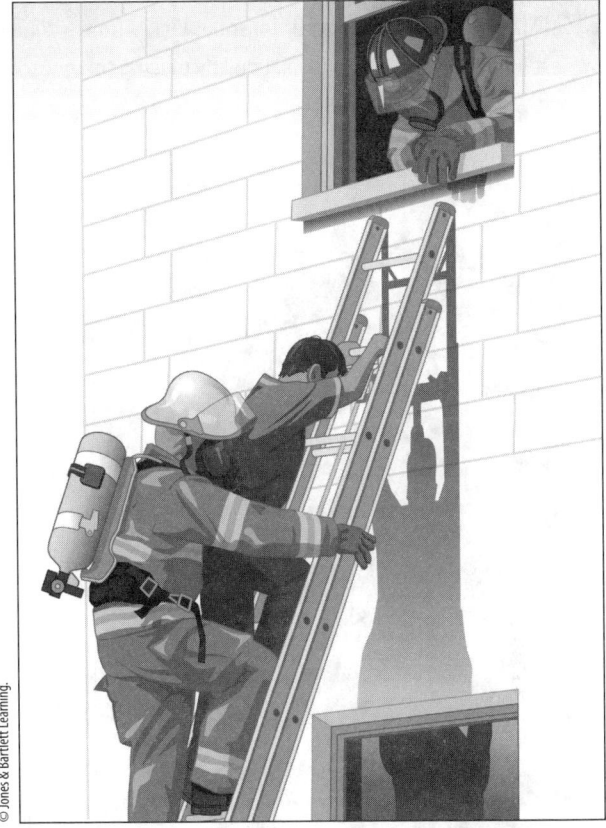

5. The second fire fighter and victim proceed slowly down the ladder, one rung at a time, with the fire fighter always staying one rung below the victim. If the victim slips or loses his or her footing, the fire fighter's _____ should keep the victim from falling. The fire fighter can take control of the victim at any time by leaning in toward the ladder and squeezing the victim against the ladder. The fire fighter should _____ each step and talk to the person being rescued to help reassure and calm him or her and encourage the person to keep his or her gaze forward.

Skill Drill 12-17: Rescuing an Unconscious Victim from a Window Fire Fighter I, NFPA 1001: 4.3.9

Test your knowledge of this skill drill by placing the photos below in the correct order. Number the first step with a "1," the second step with a "2," and so on.

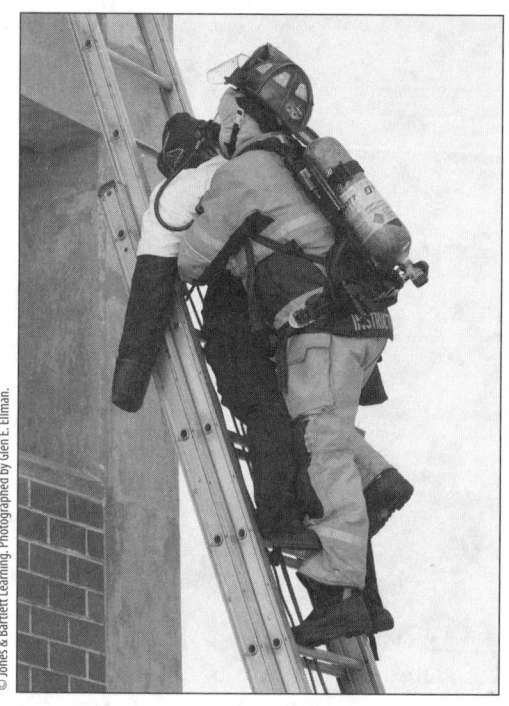

_____ The victim is lowered so that he or she straddles the second fire fighter's leg. The fire fighter's arms should be positioned under the victim's arms, holding on to the rungs. The fire fighter keeps the balls of both feet on the rungs of the ladder to make it easier to move his or her feet. The fire fighter climbs down the ladder slowly, one rung at a time, transferring the victim's weight from one leg to the other. The victim's arms can also be secured around the fire fighter's neck.

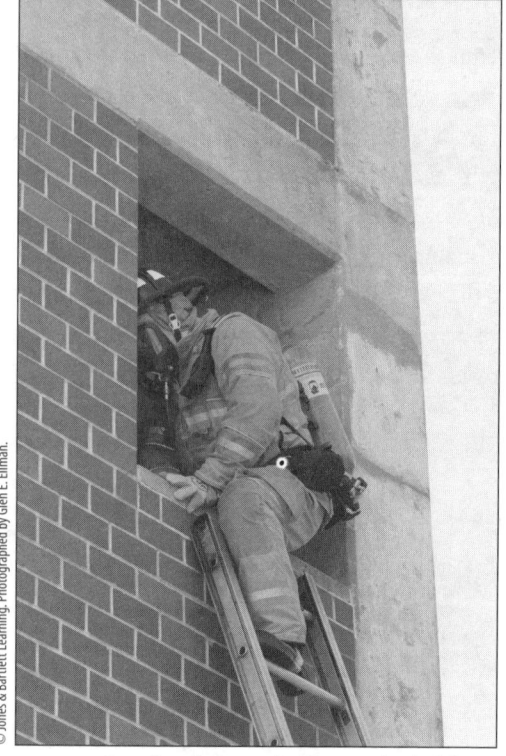

_____ One fire fighter climbs up the ladder and enters the window to rescue the victim. The second fire fighter climbs up to the window opening and waits for the victim.

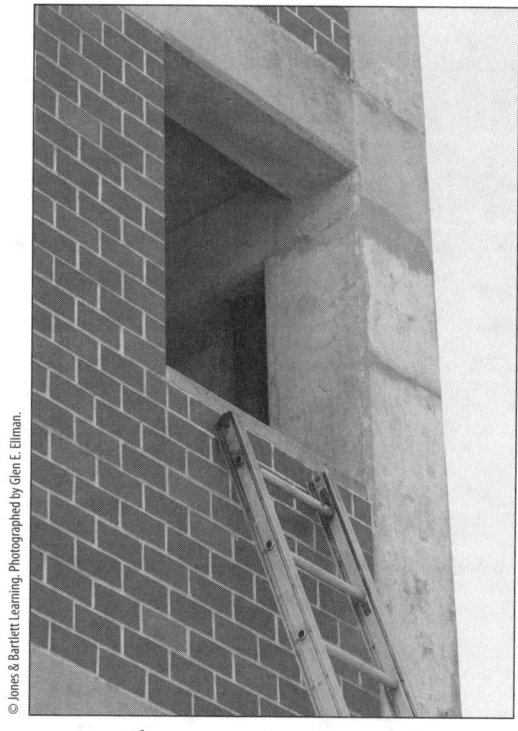

_____ The rescue team sets up and secures the ladder in rescue position with the tip of the ladder just below the windowsill.

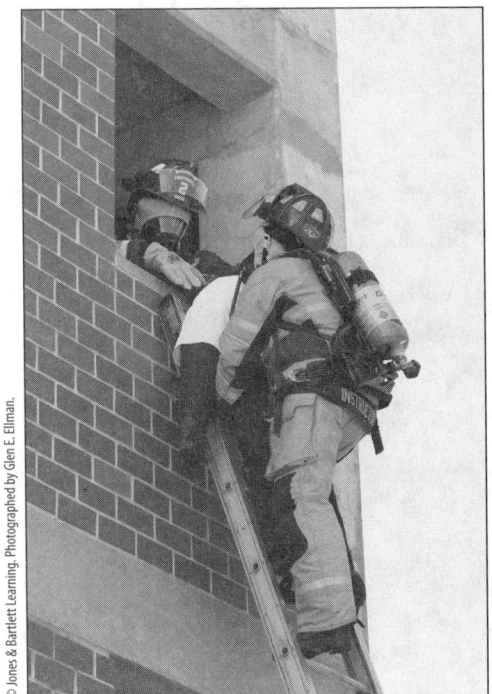

_____ The second fire fighter places both hands on the rungs of the ladder, with one leg straight and the other horizontal to the ground with the knee at an angle of 90 degrees. The foot of the straight leg should be one rung below the foot of the bent leg. When both fire fighters are ready, the first fire fighter passes the victim out through the window and onto the ladder, keeping the victim's back toward the ladder.

Skill Drill 12-18: Rescuing an Unconscious Child or a Small Adult from a Window Fire Fighter I, NFPA 1001: 4.3.9
Test your knowledge of this skill drill by filling in the correct words in the photo captions.

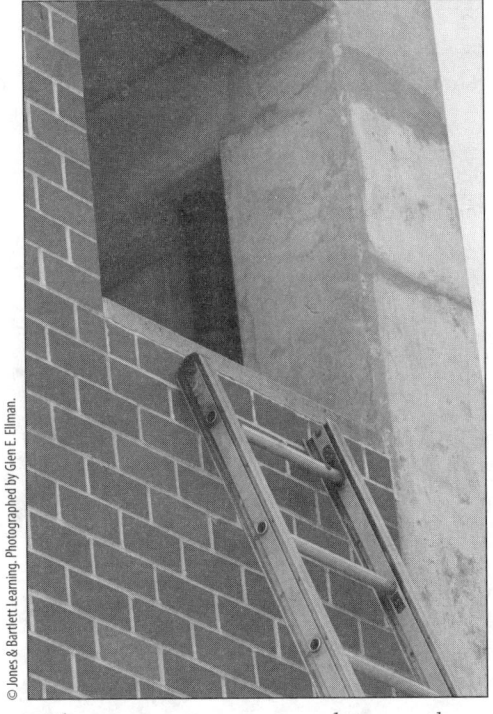

1. The rescue team sets up and secures the ladder in _____ position, with the tip below the windowsill.

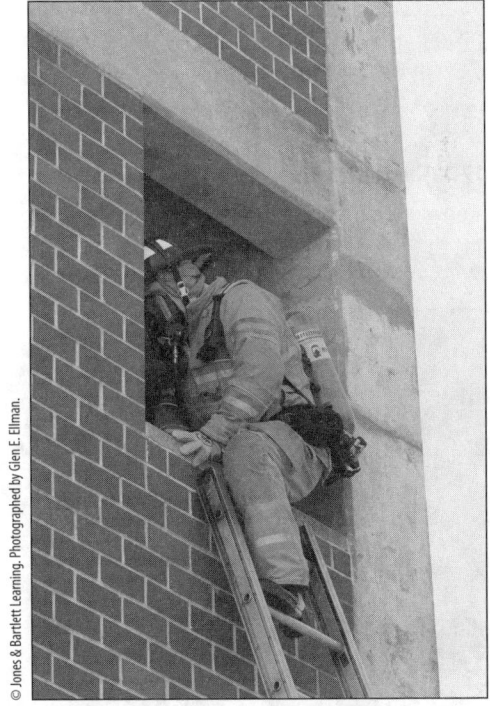

2. The first fire fighter climbs the ladder and enters the window to assist the victim. The second fire fighter climbs the ladder to the window opening and waits to receive the victim. Both of the second fire fighter's _____ should be level with his or her hands on the beams.

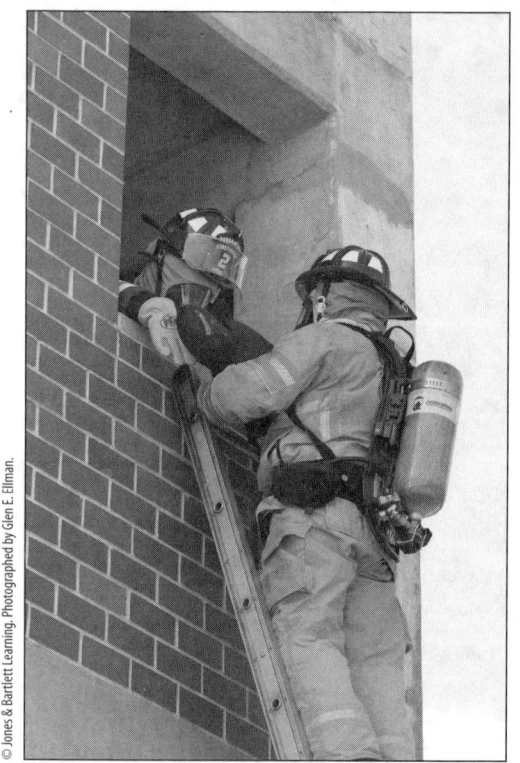

3. When ready, the first fire fighter passes the victim to the second fire fighter so the victim is _____ across the second fire fighter's arms.

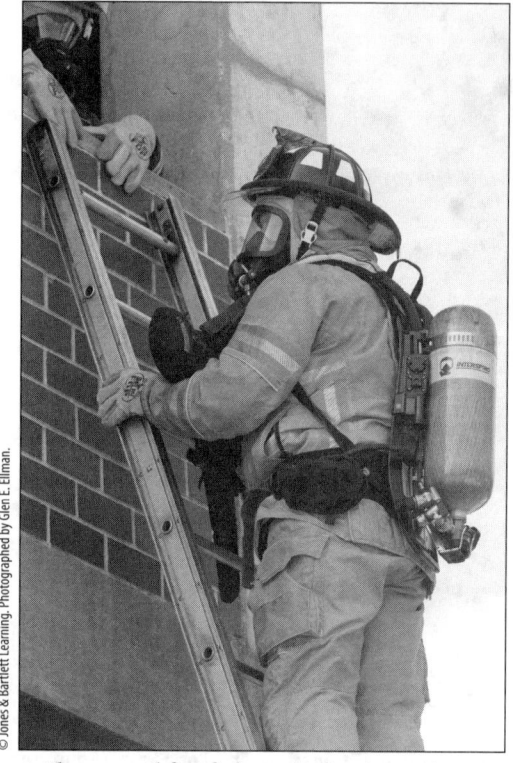

4. The second fire fighter climbs down the ladder slowly, with the victim being held in his or her arms. The fire fighter's arms should stay _____, and his or her hands should slide down the beams.

Skill Drill 12-19: Rescuing a Large Adult from a Window Fire Fighter I, NFPA 1001:4.3.9

Test your knowledge of this skill drill by placing the photos below in the correct order. Number the first step with a "1," the second step with a "2," and so on.

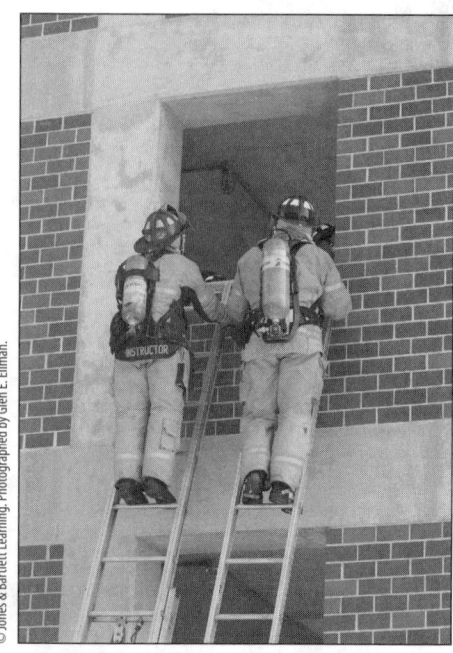

_____ The rescue team places and secures two ladders, side by side, in the rescue position. The tips of the two ladders should be just below the windowsill.

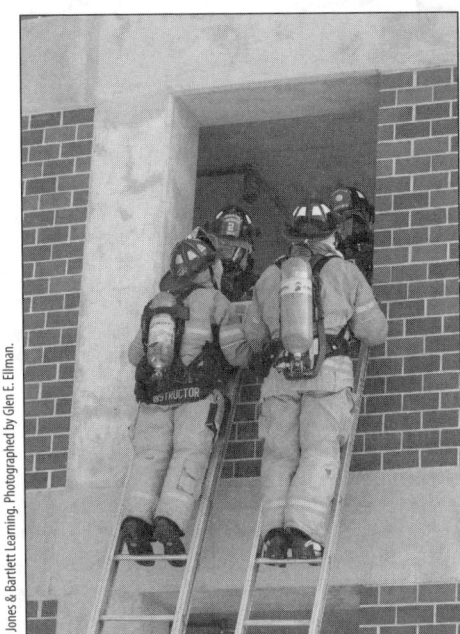

_____ Multiple fire fighters may be required to enter the window to assist from the inside.

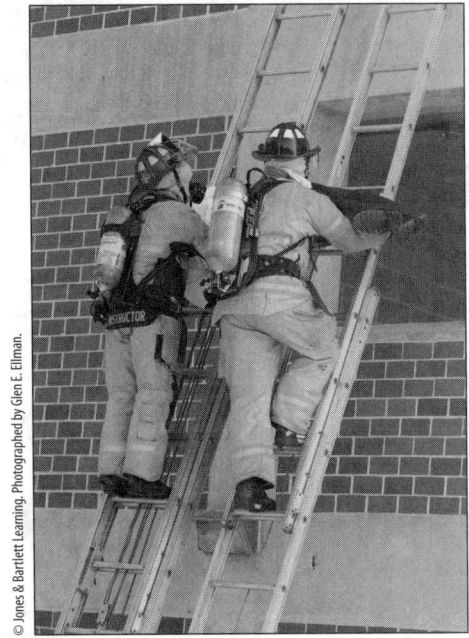

_____ When ready, the victim is lowered down across the arms of the fire fighters, with one fire fighter supporting the victim's legs and the other supporting the victim's arms. Once in place, the fire fighters can slowly descend the ladder, using both hands to hold on to the ladder rungs.

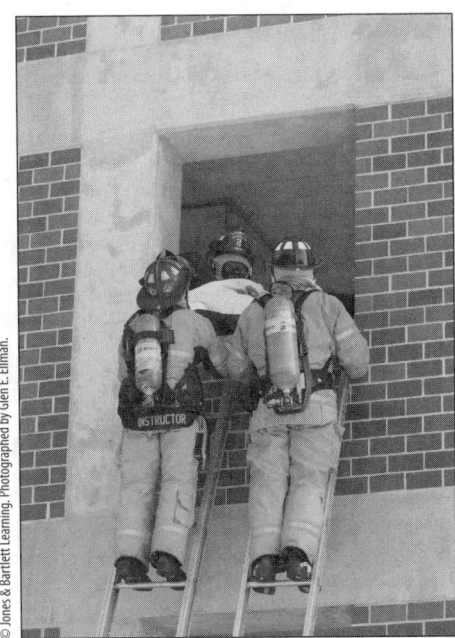

_____ Two fire fighters, one on each ladder, climb up to the window opening and wait to receive the victim.

Ventilation

Workbook Activities

The following activities have been designed to help you. Your instructor may require you to complete some or all of these activities as a regular part of your fire fighter training program. You are encouraged to complete any activity your instructor does not assign to you, as a way to enhance your learning in the classroom.

Chapter Review

The following exercises provide an opportunity to refresh your knowledge of this chapter.

Matching

Match each of the terms in the left column to the appropriate definition in the right column.

_____ 1. Pitched roofs
_____ 2. Roof decking
_____ 3. Neutral plane
_____ 4. Laths
_____ 5. Rafters
_____ 6. Flashover
_____ 7. Smoke ejectors
_____ 8. Cockloft
_____ 9. Parapet walls
_____ 10. Transitional attack

A. The open space between the top-floor ceiling and the roof of a building
B. The transition from a fire that is growing to a fire where all of the exposed surfaces have ignited
C. Thin parallel strips of wood used to make the supporting structure for roof tiles
D. An offensive fire attack initiated by a quick, indirect, exterior attack into the fire compartment
E. Electric or gasoline fans used in negative-pressure ventilation
F. The rigid roof component made of wooden boards, plywood sheets, or metal panels
G. Solid structural components that support a roof
H. The interface at a ventilation opening such as a doorway or a window
I. Have a visible slope that provides for rain, ice, and snow runoff
J. Freestanding walls on a flat roof that extend above the roofline

Multiple Choice

Read each item carefully, and then select the best response.

_____ 1. Negative-pressure ventilation fans are called
   A. ventilators.
   B. conductors.
   C. smoke ejectors.
   D. HVAC systems.

_____ 2. Which type of ventilation occurs when fans are used to force clean air into a space to displace smoke?
   A. Positive-pressure ventilation
   B. Natural ventilation
   C. Hydraulic ventilation
   D. Negative-pressure ventilation

CHAPTER 13

_____ 3. A cut that works well on metal roofing because it prevents the decking from rolling away is a
   A. kerf cut.
   B. rectangular cut.
   C. louver cut.
   D. triangular cut.

_____ 4. Ventilation openings should never be
   A. opened directly into the atmosphere.
   B. between the fire fighters and the escape route.
   C. created without incident commander (IC) direction.
   D. opened before proper sounding.

_____ 5. A triangular examination hole created with three small cuts is a
   A. kerf cut.
   B. rectangular cut.
   C. louver cut.
   D. triangular cut.

_____ 6. What should fire fighters do before opening a door, taking out a window, or putting a hole in a roof at a structure fire?
   A. Why am I ventilating?
   B. Where do I want to accomplish the ventilation?
   C. When do I want to perform the ventilation?
   D. A, B, and C

_____ 7. A cut that can create a large opening quickly and is particularly suitable for flat or sloping roofs with plywood decking is a
   A. kerf cut.
   B. rectangular cut.
   C. louver cut.
   D. triangular cut.

_____ 8. When fire fighters need quick or immediate ventilation, they often use
   A. natural ventilation.
   B. mechanical ventilation.
   C. hydraulic ventilation.
   D. vertical ventilation.

_____ 9. Trusses are connected with heavy-duty staples or by
   A. triangular plates.
   B. gusset plates.
   C. plate locks.
   D. truss plates.

_____ 10. The firefighting operation of controlled and coordinated removal of heat and smoke from a structure is called
   A. ventilation.
   B. convection.
   C. conduction.
   D. smoke inversion.

_____ 11. All roofs have three major components
    A. a support structure, roof decking, and roof covering.
    B. beams, rafters, and decking.
    C. a support structure, truss system, and roof covering.
    D. a platform, assembly method, and roofing.

_____ 12. A bearing wall is used
    A. as an exterior wall.
    B. to support the weight of a floor or roof.
    C. as an interior wall.
    D. to extend the firewall.

_____ 13. The act of closing the front door of a structure after forcible entry will
    A. create a strong downdraft.
    B. create a strong updraft.
    C. limit air supply and slow fire growth.
    D. create greater resistance to air movement.

_____ 14. A type of building construction in which all of the structural components are made of noncombustible materials is known as
    A. Type I.
    B. Type II.
    C. Type III.
    D. Type IV.

_____ 15. Hydraulic ventilation is most useful for clearing smoke and heat out of a room because it creates
    A. a low-pressure area behind the nozzle.
    B. a high-pressure area behind the nozzle.
    C. a mist that traps smoke particles and heat.
    D. water vapor.

_____ 16. _____ fans are powered by internal combustion engines and can increase carbon monoxide levels if they run for significant periods of time after the fire is extinguished.
    A. Negative-pressure
    B. Horizontal
    C. Mechanical
    D. Positive-pressure

_____ 17. When breaking glass for ventilation purposes, the fire fighter should always use a(n)
    A. "all clear" call.
    B. hand tool.
    C. hose line.
    D. safety break before splintering.

_____ 18. Ventilating directly over the fire will
    A. produce the fastest impact on the fire's behavior.
    B. exhaust the greatest amount of combustion products.
    C. cause stack effect.
    D. A and B

_____ 19. Horizontal ventilation is most effective when the opening goes directly
    A. to another space within the structure.
    B. into a stairwell.
    C. into the space where the fire is located.
    D. past the attack team.

_____ 20. The neutral plane is the interface at a vent between the hot gas flowing out of a compartment and
    A. water flowing into the compartment.
    B. cool air flowing into the compartment.
    C. hot smoke flowing out of the compartment.
    D. particulate flowing out of the compartment.

_____ 21. Which type of ventilation occurs when fans are used to pull smoke through openings?
   A. Positive-pressure ventilation
   B. Natural ventilation
   C. Hydraulic ventilation
   D. Negative-pressure ventilation

_____ 22. The easiest place to horizontally ventilate is usually
   A. the door.
   B. a skylight.
   C. a roof.
   D. windows.

_____ 23. A backdraft occurs when smoke, heat, and gases accumulate with a rich supply of partially burned fuels and are suddenly introduced to
   A. a flame.
   B. increased temperature.
   C. clean air.
   D. open fuels.

_____ 24. Which type of roof has a visible slope for rain or snow runoff?
   A. Bowstring roof
   B. Arched roof
   C. Flat roof
   D. Pitched roof

Vocabulary

Define the following terms using the space provided.

1. Smoke inversion:

   _____
   _____
   _____

2. Ventilation:

   _____
   _____
   _____

3. Ordinary construction:

   _____
   _____
   _____

4. Fire-resistive construction:

   _____
   _____
   _____

FUNDAMENTALS OF FIRE FIGHTER SKILLS

5. Gusset plates:
_____
_____
_____

6. Vertical ventilation:
_____
_____
_____

7. Stack effect:
_____
_____
_____

8. Horizontal ventilation:
_____
_____
_____

9. Flow path:
_____
_____
_____

10. Ventilation limited fire:
_____
_____
_____

Fill-In

Read each item carefully, and then complete the statement by filling in the missing word(s).

1. The most obvious risk to fire fighters performing vertical ventilation is _____ _____.

2. _____ _____ ventilation creates a large opening ahead of the fire, removing a section of fuel for the fire to spread and increasing smoke and gas flow out of a building.

3. _____ ventilation is most useful after a fire is under control.

4. Heavy timber construction features exterior walls made of _____ and interior walls made of wood.

5. A _____ fire attack reduces the chance of a backdraft or flashover.

6. _____ ventilation takes advantage of the doors and windows on the same level as the fire, as well as any other horizontal openings that are available.

7. Fire fighters should be _____ from the ventilation openings so the wind will push the heat and smoke away.

8. The collapse of a(n) _____ truss roof is usually very sudden. For this reason, the presence of such a roof must be noted during preincident planning.

9. Positive-pressure fans operate at _____ velocity and can be very noisy.

10. _____ is a powerful force that can rapidly change the direction and speed of a fire and its flow path.

True/False

If you believe the statement to be more true than false, write the letter "T" in the space provided. If you believe the statement to be more false than true, write the letter "F."

1. _____ Examination holes allow the team members to evaluate conditions under the roof and to verify the proper location for a ventilation opening.

2. _____ Smoke can be cooled with automatic sprinkler systems.

3. _____ HVAC or other building systems can cause fire to spread through vertical fire extension.

4. _____ A backdraft can occur when a building is charged with hot gases and oxygen is at the normal percentage in the building.

5. _____ Horizontal ventilation operations often involve opening or breaking a window.

6. _____ Ventilation should occur as close to the seat of the fire as possible.

7. _____ A strong concern that arises when structures have metal roofs is the release of flammable vapors, which can be the result of leaking roof coverings.

8. _____ During ventilation, cutting several smaller holes is better than making one large hole.

9. _____ Creating roof ventilation openings requires the use of many different tools and techniques, depending on the type of construction and roof decking.

10. _____ When attacking basement fires, the use of interior stairs for ventilation should not be considered a safe option because of the danger of fire fighters being in the exhaust flow path of hot gases from the fire.

Short Answer

Complete this section with short written answers using the space provided.

1. Describe the impact that door control can have on fire growth.

_____
_____
_____
_____

2. What is the objective of any roof ventilation operation?

_____
_____
_____
_____

3. List five indicators that it is time for immediate retreat from the roof of a structure.

___

4. Explain the "Three W's of Ventilation."

___

Fire Alarms
The following real case scenarios will give you an opportunity to explore the concerns associated with ventilation. Read each scenario, and then answer each question in detail.

1. It is 12:30 in the afternoon when your engine is dispatched to a two-story apartment building. Dispatch reports that the fire is located on the second floor. The interior attack teams are fighting the fire as you arrive. The attack team reports that the fire is knocked down on the second floor but there is fire in the attic. The IC tells your Lieutenant to ladder the building and perform vertical ventilation. Your Lieutenant tells two members of your crew to ladder the building and instructs you and your partner to grab the chainsaw and complete a louver cut over the seat of the fire. How should you proceed?

___

2. It is 2:00 in the morning when your engine is dispatched to a residential structure fire. You are on the second engine to arrive on scene. The interior attack team is met with smoke and high heat at the front door. The attack team notifies the IC that ventilation is needed prior to entering the structure. The IC assigns you and your partner to coordinate positive-pressure ventilation with the attack team. How should you proceed?

___

Skill Drills

Skill Drill 13-1: Breaking Glass with a Hand Tool Fire Fighter I, NFPA 1001: 4.3.11
Test your knowledge of this skill drill by filling in the correct words in the photo captions.

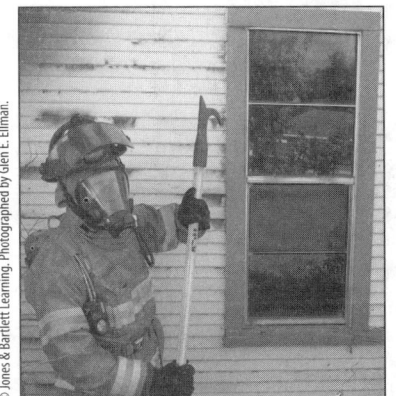 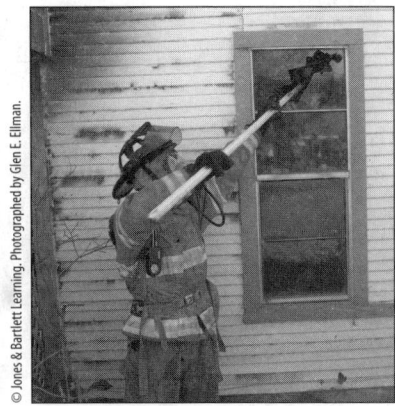 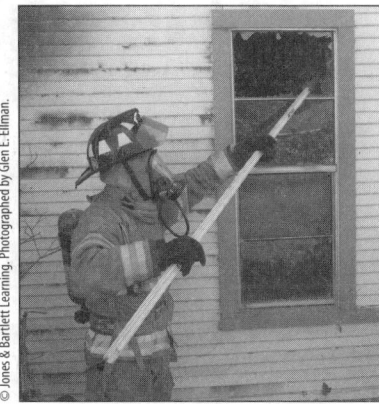

1. Wear full personal protective equipment (PPE), including eye protection and self-contained breathing apparatus (SCBA). Select a hand tool and position yourself to the _____ of the window.

2. With your back _____ the wall, swing backward forcefully with the tip of the tool striking the top _____-_____ of the glass.

3. Clear the remaining _____ from the opening with the hand tool.

Skill Drill 13-2: Breaking Windows with a Ladder Fire Fighter I, NFPA 1001: 4.3.11
Test your knowledge of this skill drill by placing the photos below in the correct order. Number the first step with a "1," the second step with a "2," and so on.

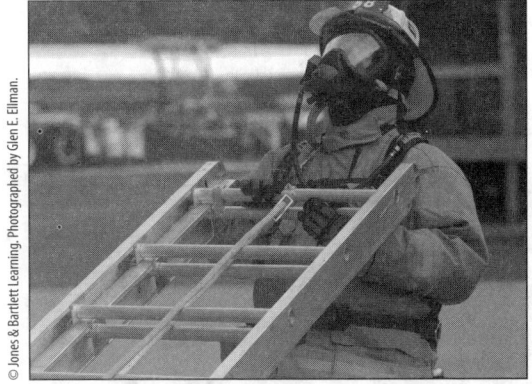 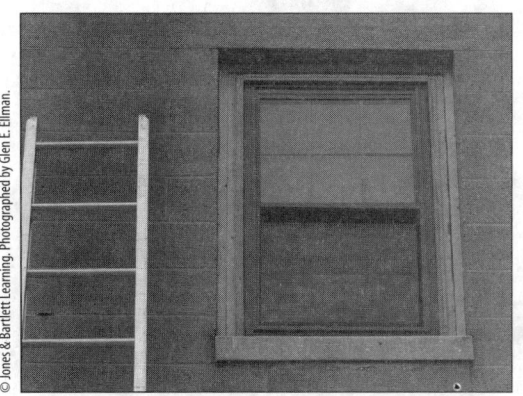

_____ Wear full PPE, including eye protection. Select the proper size ladder for the job. Check for overhead lines. Use standard procedures for performing a ladder raise.

_____ Raise the ladder next to the window. Extend the tip so that it is even with the top third of the window. If a roof ladder is used, extend the hooks toward the window.

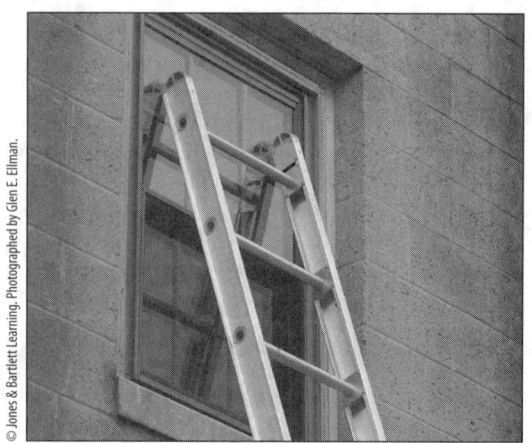

_____ Coordinate operations with the incident's tactical objectives. Position the ladder in front of the window.

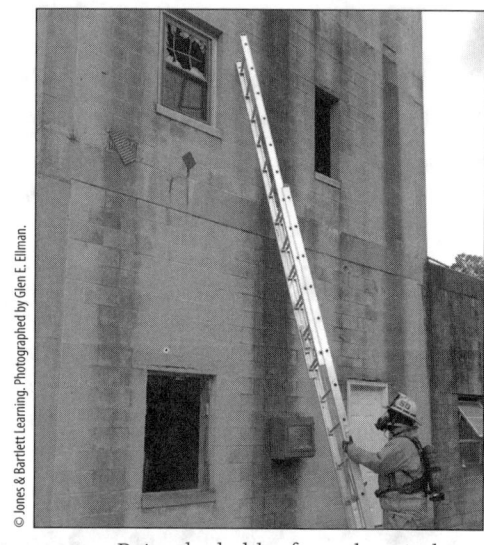

_____ Raise the ladder from the window, and move it to the next window to be ventilated. Either carry the ladder vertically or pivot the ladder on its feet.

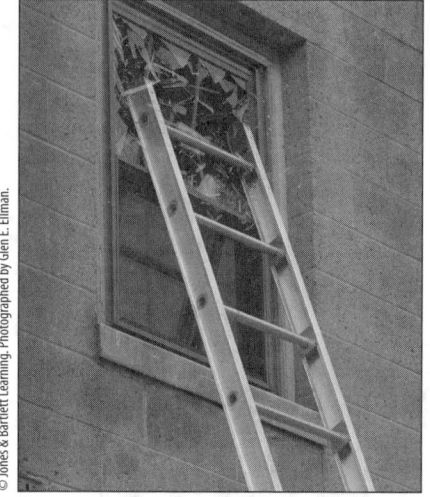

_____ Forcibly drop the ladder into the window. Exercise caution—falling glass can cause serious injury.

Skill Drill 13-4: Delivering Positive-Pressure Ventilation Fire Fighter I, NFPA 1001: 4.3.12
Test your knowledge of this skill drill by filling in the correct words in the photo captions.

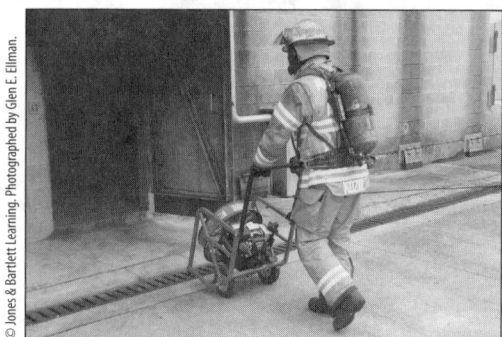

1. Place the fan in front of the opening to be used for the fire attack. The exact position depends on the size of the opening, the size of the fan, and the _____ of the wind.

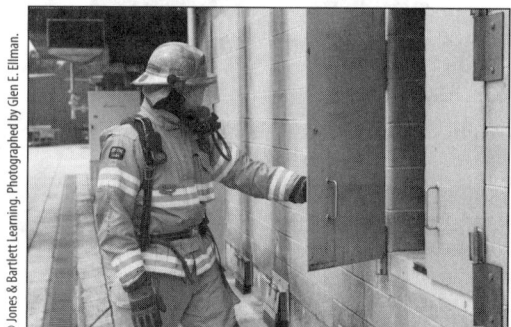

2. Provide an exhaust opening in the fire room. This opening can be made either _____ the fan is started or when the fan is started.

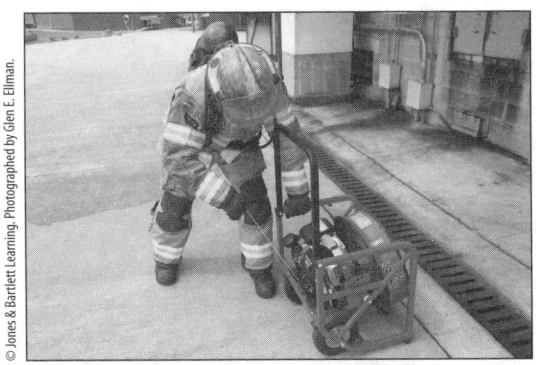

3. Start the _____.

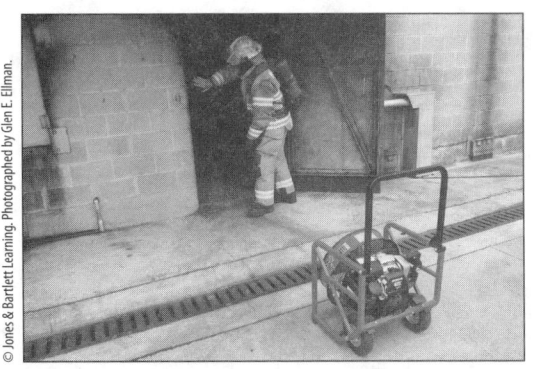

4. Check the cone of air produced; it should completely cover the opening. This can be checked by running a hand around the door frame to feel the direction of air currents. Monitor the exhaust opening to ensure there is a _____ flow. Allow the smoke to clear.

Skill Drill 13-5: Delivering Hydraulic Ventilation Fire Fighter I, NFPA 1001: 4.3.12
Test your knowledge of this skill drill by filling in the correct words in the photo captions.

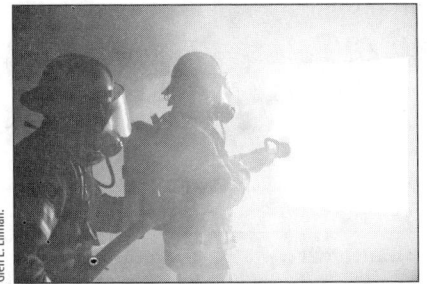

1. Enter the room and remain close to the _____ opening. Place the nozzle through the opening, and open the nozzle to a narrow _____ or broken-pattern spray.

2. Keep directing the stream _____ and back into the room until the stream almost fills the opening. The nozzle should be 2 to 4 ft (0.6 to 1.2 m) inside the opening.

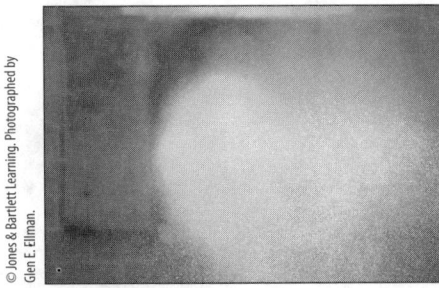

3. Stay _____, out of the heat and smoke, or to one side to keep from partially obstructing the opening.

Skill Drill 13-8: Making a Seven, Nine, Eight (7, 9, 8) Rectangular Cut Fire Fighter I, NFPA 1001: 4.3.12

Test your knowledge of this skill drill by placing the photos below in the correct order. Number the first step with a "1," the second step with a "2," and so on.

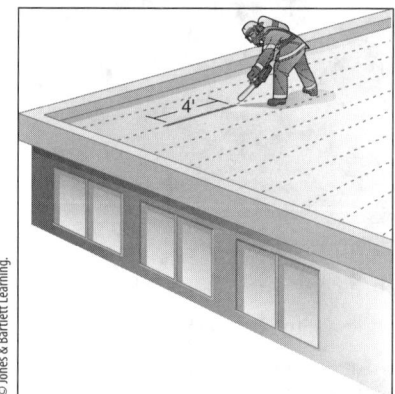

_____ Locate the roof supports by sounding. Make the first cut parallel to the roof supports. The cut should be 3.5 to 4 ft (1 to 1.2 m) long.

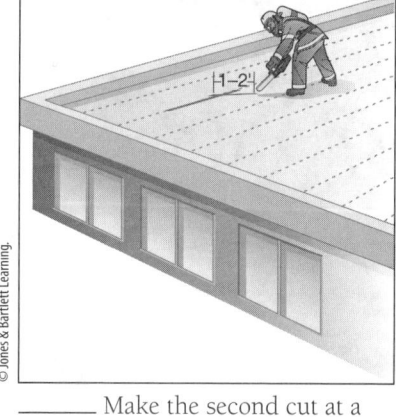

_____ Make the second cut at a 45-degree angle to the first cut. The length of this knock-out cut should be 1 to 2 ft (0.3 to 0.6 m) in length.

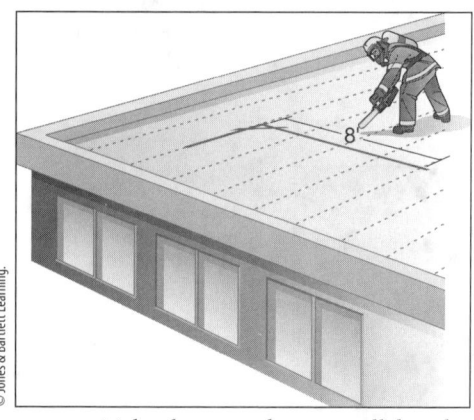

_____ Make the seventh cut parallel to the first cut and the fifth cut. Start on the side of the sixth cut, and cut toward the side of the third cut, until the cuts are connected. These seven cuts should produce the shape of the number "8."

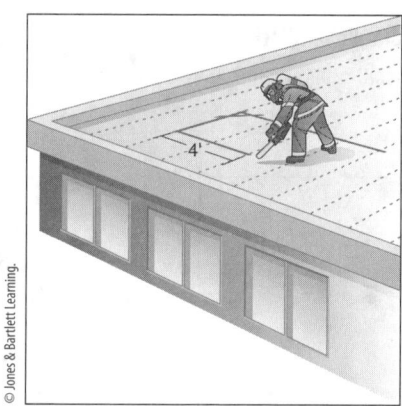

_____ Make the fourth cut perpendicular to the first cut on the opposite side of the knock-out cut (the second cut). The cut should be about 4 ft (1.2 m) long.

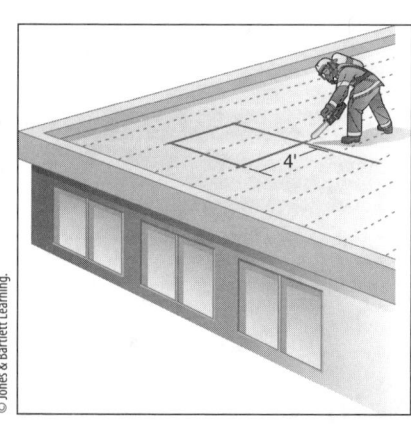

_____ Make the sixth cut perpendicular to the first cut. Extend the fourth cut approximately 4 ft (1.2 m) until it is even with the third cut.

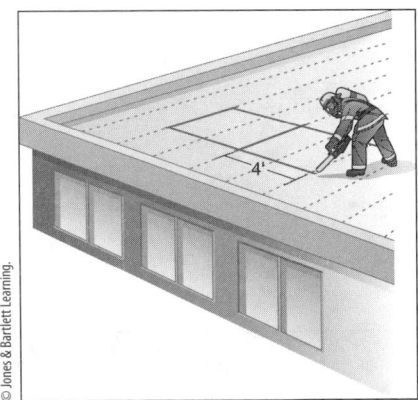

_____ Make the fifth cut parallel to the first cut. Starting on the thirdcut side of the hole, make a cut that connects with the fourth-cut side of the hole. These five cuts should produce the shape of the number "9."

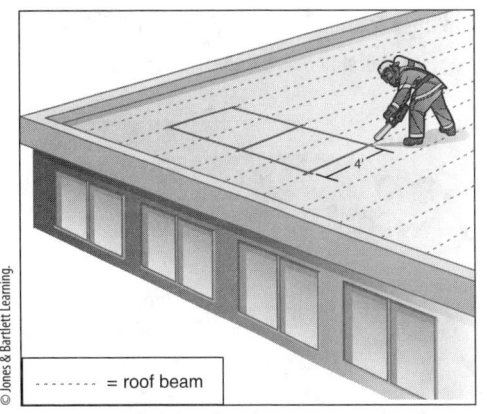

= roof beam

_____ Make the third cut perpendicular to the first cut from the corner where the knock-out cut was made. This cut should be about 8 ft (2.4 m) long. The three cuts should produce the shape of the number "7".

Skill Drill 13-9: Making a Louver Cut Fire Fighter I, NFPA 1001:4.3.12
Test your knowledge of this skill drill by filling in the correct words in the photo captions.

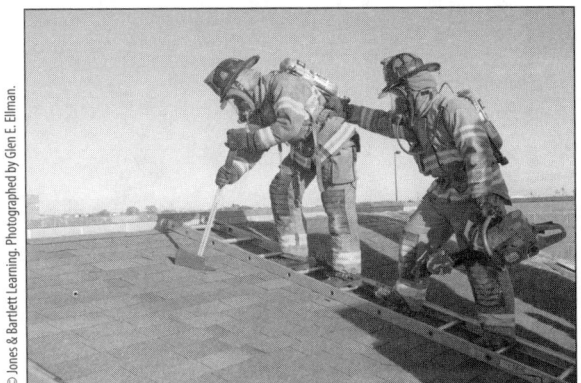

1. Locate the roof supports by _____.

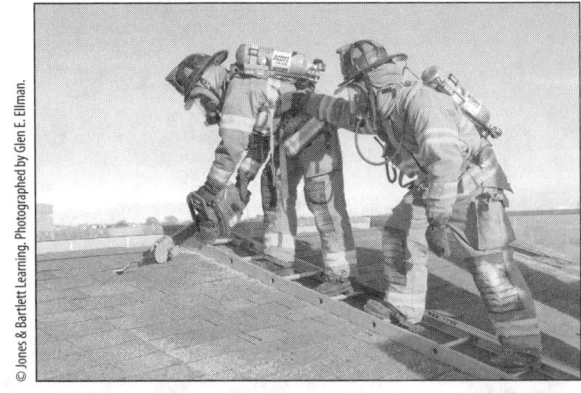

2. Make two _____ cuts perpendicular to the roof supports.

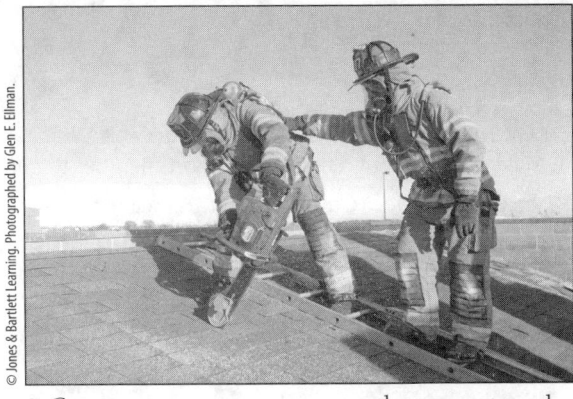

3. Cut _____ to the supports and between pairs of supports in a rectangular pattern.

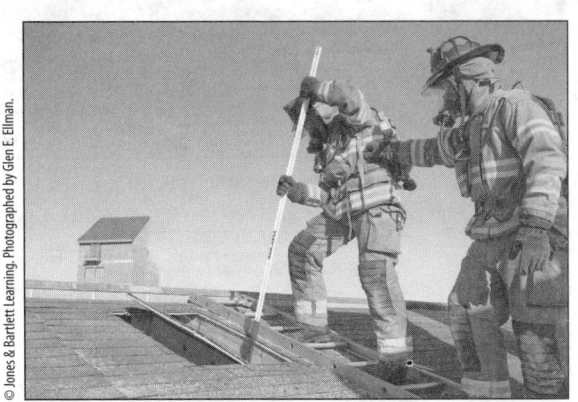

4. Tilt the panel to a _____ position. Open the interior ceiling area below the opening by using the butt end of a _____ _____. This hole should be the same size as the opening made in the roof decking.

Skill Drill 13-10: Making a Triangular Cut Fire Fighter I, NFPA 1001: 4.3.12
Test your knowledge of this skill drill by filling in the correct words in the photo captions.

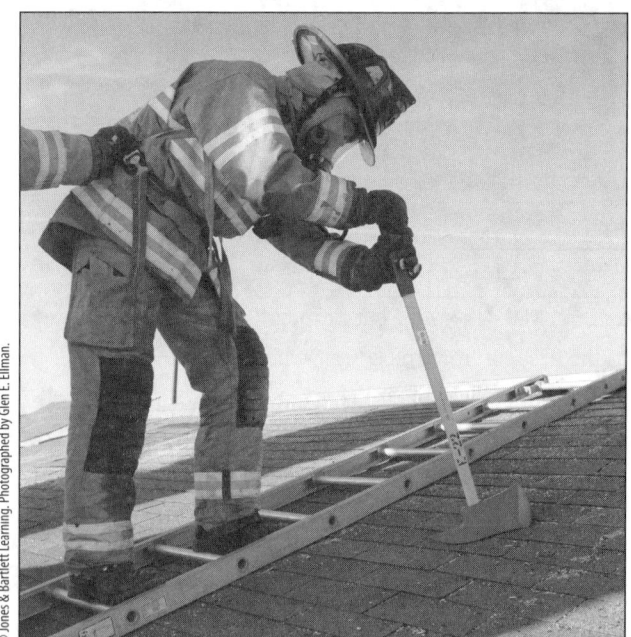

1. Locate the roof _____.

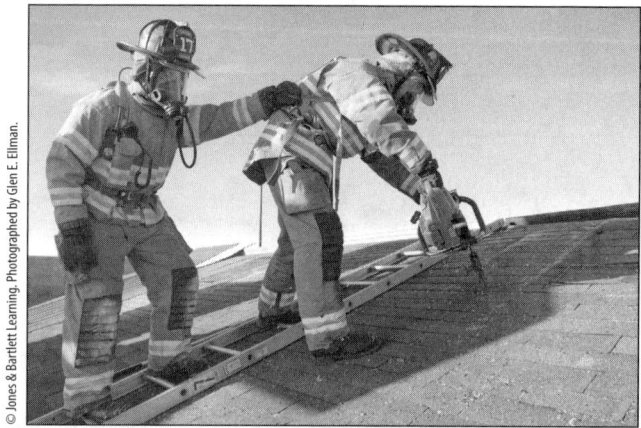

2. Make the first cut from just inside a support member in a _____ direction toward the next support member.

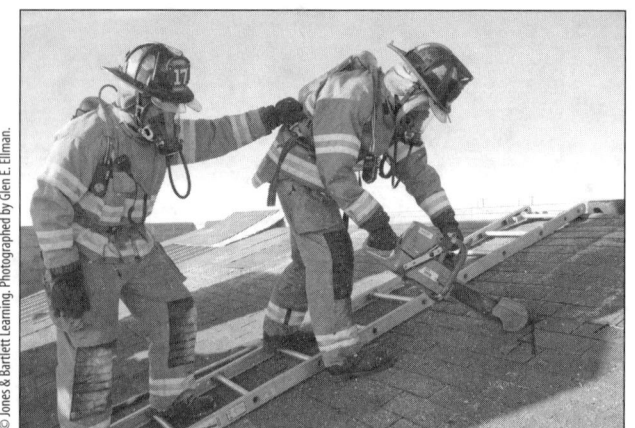

3. Begin the second cut at the same location as the first, and make it in the _____ diagonal direction, forming a _____ shape.

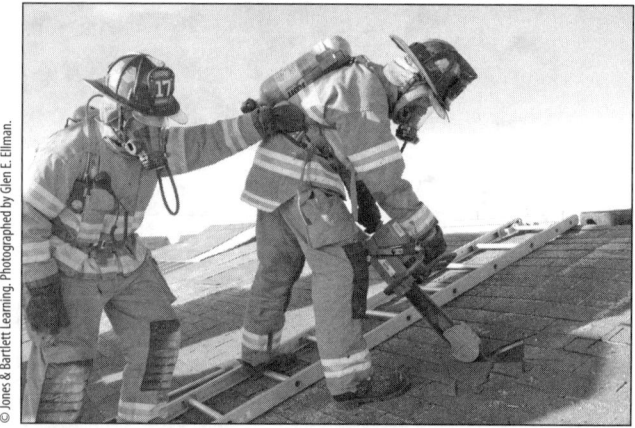

4. Make the final cut along the support member to connect the first two cuts. Cutting from this location allows fire fighters the full support of the member directly below them while performing _____.

Skill Drill 13-11: Making a Peak Cut Fire Fighter I, NFPA 1001: 4.3.12
Test your knowledge of this skill drill by placing the photos below in the correct order. Number the first step with a "1," the second step with a "2," and so on.

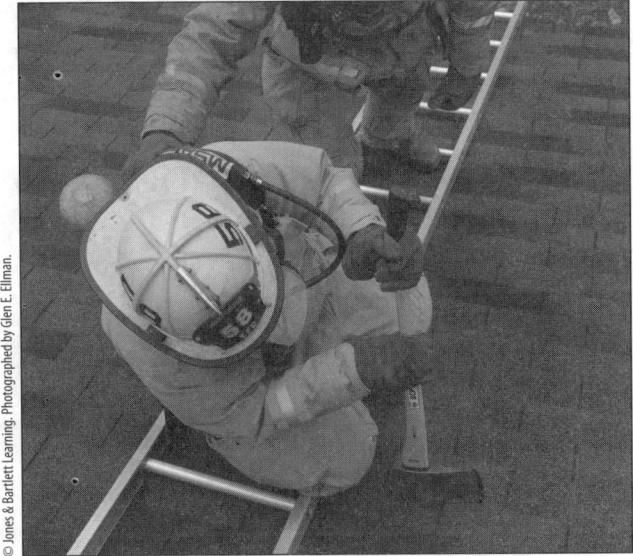

_____ Clear the roofing materials away from the roof peak.

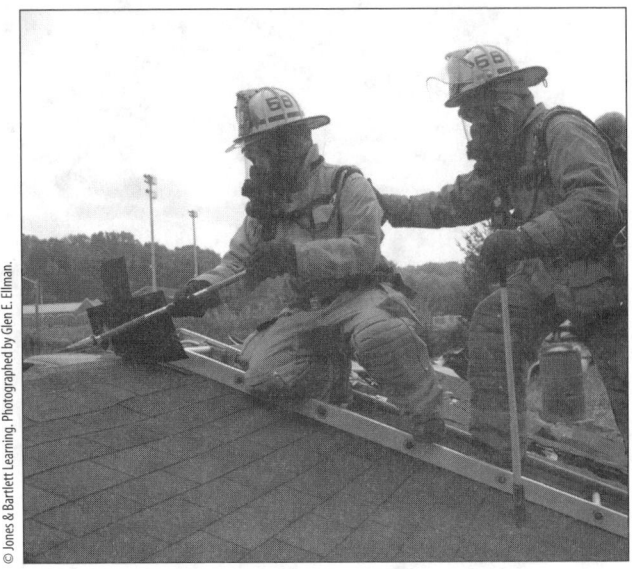

_____ Locate the roof supports.

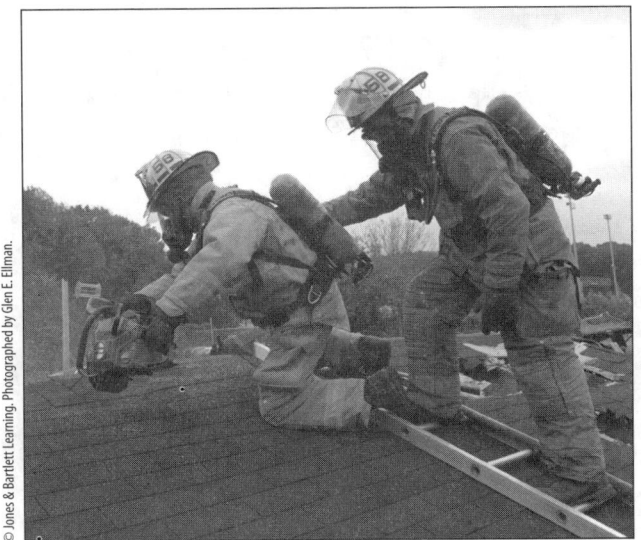

_____ Make the first cut vertically, at the farthest point away. Start at the roof peak in the area between the support members, and cut down to the bottom of the first plywood panel.

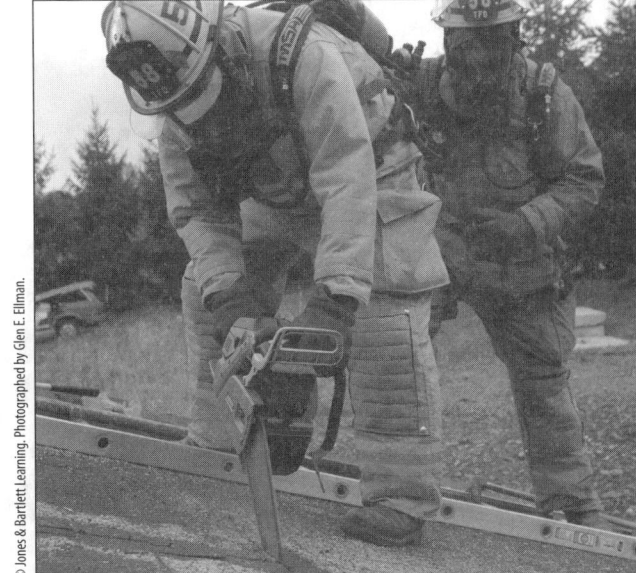

_____ Open the interior ceiling area below the opening by using the butt end of a pike pole. This hole should be the same size as the vent opening made in the roof decking.

166 Fundamentals of Fire Fighter Skills

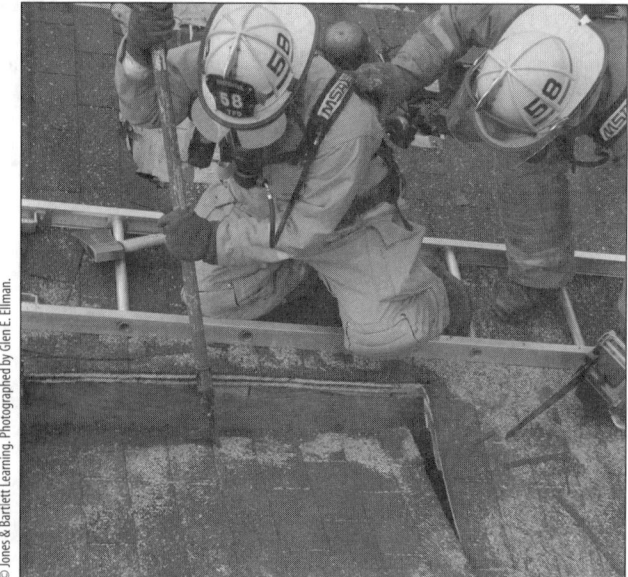

_____ Make parallel downward cuts between supports, moving horizontally along the roofline to make additional ventilation openings.

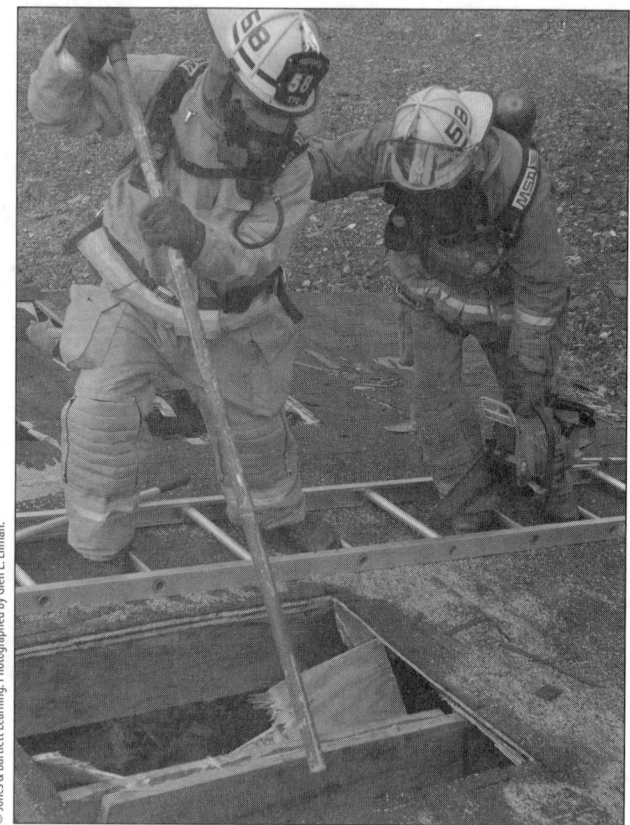

_____ Strike the nearest side of the roofing material with an axe or maul, pushing it in, using the support located at the center as a fulcrum. This causes one end of the roofing material to go downward into the opening and the other to rise up. If necessary, repeat this process on both sides of the peak, horizontally across the peak, or vertically toward the roof edge.

Skill Drill 13-13: Performing a Readiness Check on a Power Saw Fire Fighter I, NFPA 1001: 4.5.1
Test your knowledge of this skill drill by placing the photos below in the correct order. Number the first step with a "1," the second step with a "2," and so on.

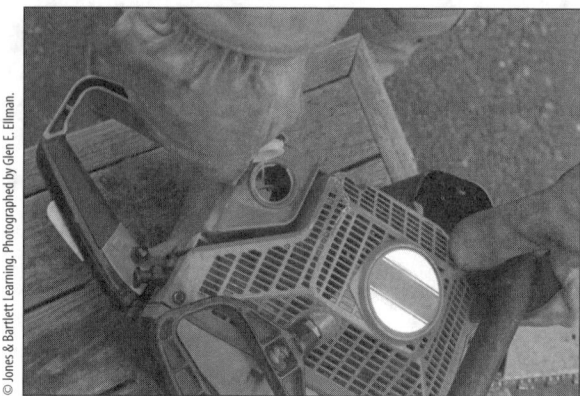

_____ Make certain that the stop switch functions. Record the results of the inspection.

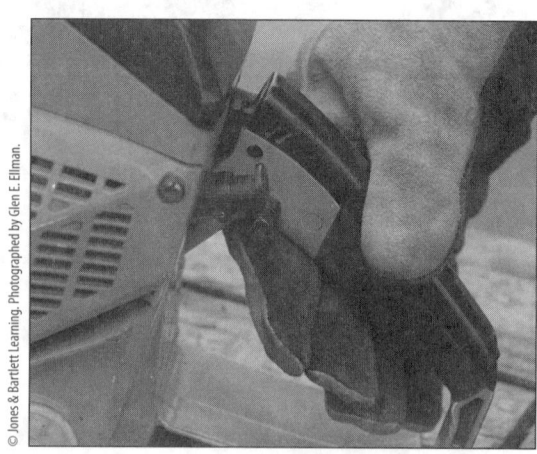

_____ Check the throttle trigger for smooth operation.

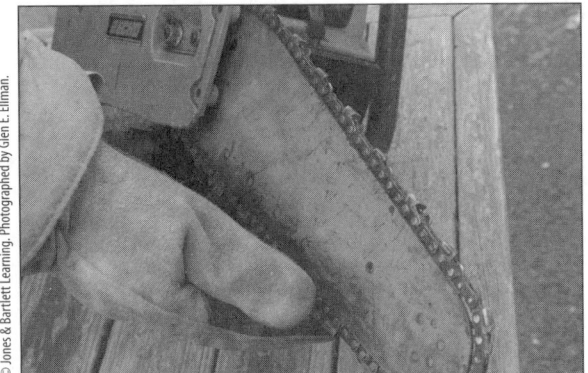

_____ Ensure that the saw, blade, air filter, and chain brake are clean and working. Inspect the blade for even wear, and lubricate the sprocket tip if needed.

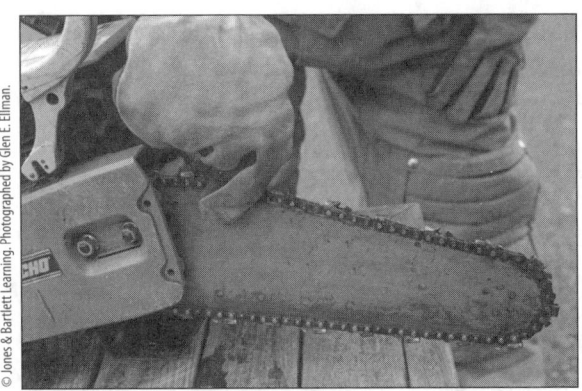

_____ Inspect the spark plugs.

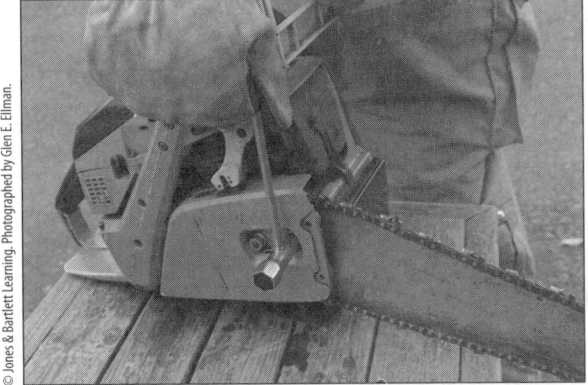

_____ Check for loose nuts and screws, and tighten them if needed. Check the starter and starter cord for wear.

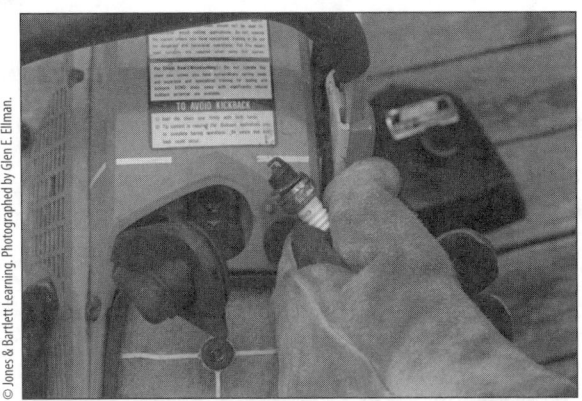

_____ Make certain that the fuel tank is full. Make certain that the bar and chain oil reservoirs are full.

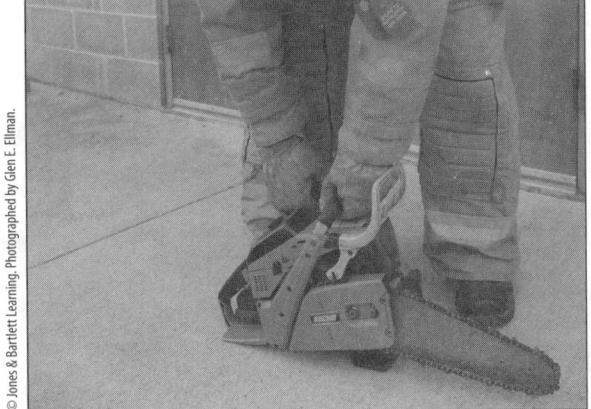

_____ Start the saw. Make certain that both the bar and the chain are being lubricated while the saw is running. Check the chain brake.

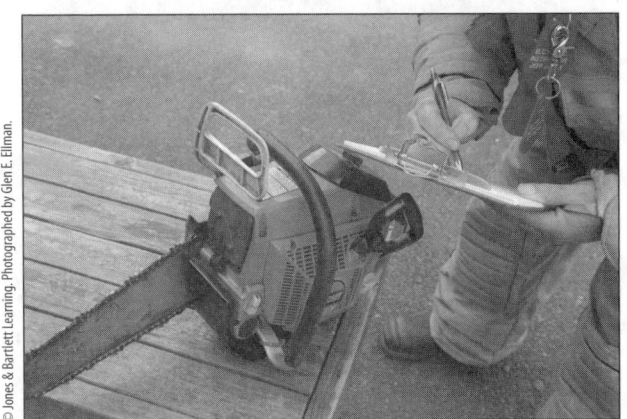

_____ Check the chain for wear, missing teeth, or other damage. Check the chain end for proper tension. Check the chain catcher.

Skill Drill 13-14: Maintaining a Power Saw Fire Fighter I, NFPA 1001: 4.5.1
Test your knowledge of this skill drill by placing the photos below in the correct order. Number the first step with a "1," the second step with a "2," and so on.

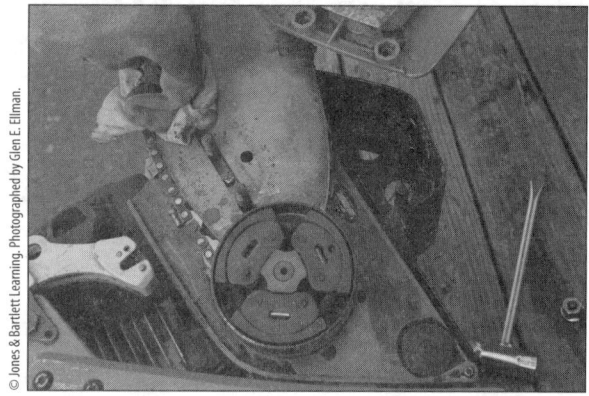

_____ Adjust the chain tension (make sure the bar and chain cool before adjusting).

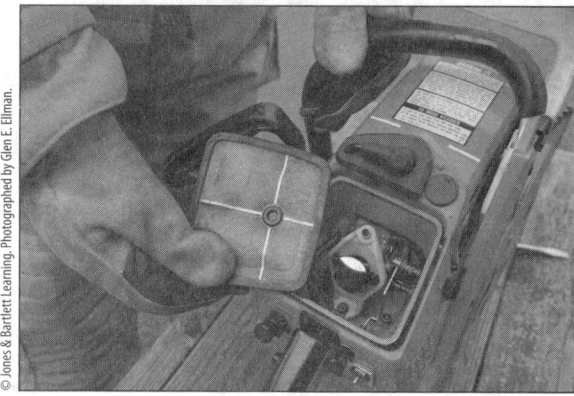

_____ Inspect the air filter and clean/replace as needed.

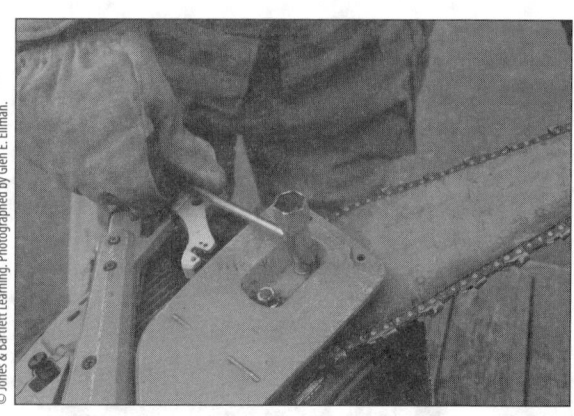

_____ Lubricate components as recommended by the manufacturer. Reinstall the bar and chain, flipping the bar over each time to help wear the bar evenly. Replace the clutch cover.

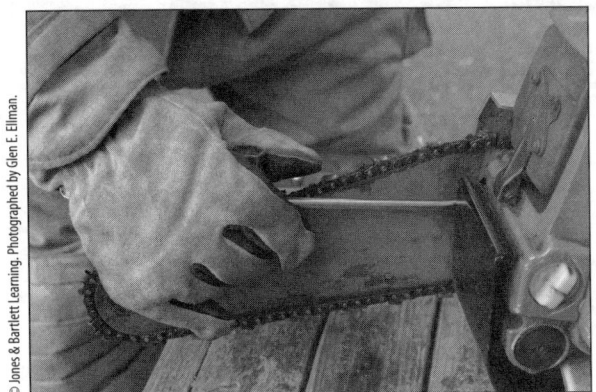

_____ Remove, clean, and inspect the clutch cover, bar, and chain for damage and wear. Replace if necessary.

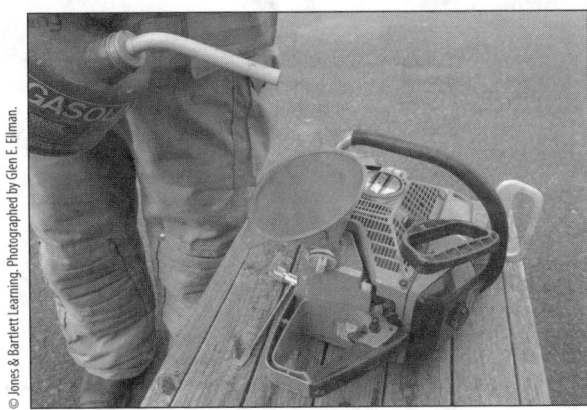

_____ Fill the power saw with fuel. Fill the bar and chain oil reservoirs.

Water Supply Systems

Workbook Activities

The following activities have been designed to help you. Your instructor may require you to complete some or all of these activities as a regular part of your fire fighter training program. You are encouraged to complete any activity your instructor does not assign to you, as a way to enhance your learning in the classroom.

Chapter Review

The following exercises provide an opportunity to refresh your knowledge of this chapter.

Matching

Match each of the terms in the left column to the appropriate definition in the right column.

_____ 1. Primary feeder
_____ 2. Static pressure
_____ 3. Reservoir
_____ 4. Distributor
_____ 5. Normal pressure
_____ 6. Water main
_____ 7. Shut-off valve
_____ 8. Dump valve
_____ 9. Residual pressure
_____ 10. Pitot gauge

A. Any valve that can be used to shut down water flow
B. Any underground water pipe
C. Amount of water available during normal consumption
D. A small-diameter underground water pipe, carries water to the user
E. The largest-diameter pipe in a water distribution system
F. Enables tankers to offload as much as 3000 gallons of water per minute
G. The pressure remaining in the system while water is flowing
H. A gauge used to determine the flow of water from a hydrant
I. A water storage facility
J. The pressure in a water pipe when there is no water flowing

Multiple Choice

Read each item carefully, and then select the best response.

_____ 1. What is the recommended minimum water pressure from a fire hydrant?
   A. 10 psi (69 kPa)
   B. 20 psi (138 kPa)
   C. 40 psi (276 kPa)
   D. 60 psi (414 kPa)

_____ 2. Fire department hoses can be connected to a hydrant by the
   A. valves.
   B. outlets.
   C. ports.
   D. taps.

CHAPTER 14

_____ 3. The flow or quantity of water moving through a pipe, hose, or nozzle is measured by
   A. volume.
   B. area.
   C. weight.
   D. mass.

_____ 4. Which type of hydrant includes a pipe with a strainer on one end and a connection for a hard suction hose on the other end that can be used to access static water sources?
   A. Dry hydrant
   B. Wet hydrant
   C. Static hydrant
   D. Straining hydrant

_____ 5. Which type of system may not require pumps because the water source, the treatment plant, and storage facilities are located on ground higher than the end users?
   A. Gravity-feed system
   B. Wet hydrant system
   C. Tanker shuttle system
   D. Static system

_____ 6. Hydrants should be positioned so that the connections, and especially the large steamer connection,
   A. are parallel to the water system.
   B. will not be damaged by passing traffic.
   C. are near waste storage areas.
   D. face the street.

_____ 7. What is the best indication of how much more water is available in the system while water is flowing?
   A. The elevation pressure
   B. The static pressure
   C. The residual pressure
   D. The potential pressure

_____ 8. If a large volume of water is needed for an extended period, tankers can be used to deliver water from a fill site to the scene, thereby creating
   A. a mobile water system.
   B. portable tanks.
   C. a mobile water supply apparatus.
   D. a tanker shuttle.

_____ 9. The water source, treatment plant, and distribution system are parts of a
   A. municipal water system.
   B. private water system.
   C. static water source.
   D. reservoir.

_____ 10. The pipes that deliver large quantities of water to a section of a town or city are the
   A. primary feeders.
   B. secondary feeders.
   C. direct mains.
   D. distributors.

_____ 11. To ensure that water flows to a fire hydrant from two or more directions, well-designed systems follow a
   A. mixed pattern.
   B. multiple-port pattern.
   C. grid pattern.
   D. center pattern.

_____ 12. Portable tanks typically hold between 600 and _____ gallons of water.
   A. 3000
   B. 5000
   C. 8000
   D. 10,000

_____ 13. A large opening on a fire hydrant that is used to allow as much water as possible to flow directly into the pump is a(n)
   A. outlet.
   B. steamer port.
   C. valve.
   D. drain.

_____ 14. The distribution system of underground pipes is known as
   A. reservoirs.
   B. piping.
   C. water mains.
   D. water traffic.

_____ 15. What are the first factors to check when inspecting hydrants?
   A. Stability and structural integrity
   B. Visibility and structural integrity
   C. Visibility and accessibility
   D. Stability and component location

_____ 16. A surge in pressure caused by suddenly stopping the flow of water is known as
   A. water surge
   B. friction loss
   C. pressure surge
   D. water hammer

_____ 17. The size of water mains depends on the amount of water needed for both normal consumption and
   A. heavy consumption.
   B. extended delays.
   C. fire protection.
   D. business operations.

_____ 18. Which unit is used to measure water pressure?
   A. Gallons
   B. Gallons per square inch
   C. Pounds per square inch
   D. Pounds

_____ 19. Most dry-barrel hydrants have _____ large valve(s) controlling the flow of water.
   A. one
   B. two
   C. three
   D. four

_____ 20. Water that is not moving has
   A. elevation pressure.
   B. static pressure.
   C. residual pressure.
   D. potential pressure.

Vocabulary

Define the following terms using the space provided.

1. Static water sources:

   _____
   _____
   _____

2. Tanker shuttle:

   _____
   _____
   _____

3. Dry-barrel hydrant:

   _____
   _____
   _____

4. Normal operating pressure:

   _____
   _____
   _____

5. Gravity-feed system:

   _____
   _____
   _____

Fill-In

Read each item carefully, and then complete the statement by filling in the missing word(s).

1. Most hydrants have an upright steel casing or _____ that is attached to the underground water distribution system.

2. The flow or quantity of water moving through a pipe is measured by its _____, usually in gallons per minute.

3. Elevation pressure can be created by _____.

4. The decrease in pressure that occurs when water moves through a pipe or hose is _____.

5. Water can be transported through long hose lines, pumper relays, or _____ water supply tankers.

6. Water that is not moving has _____ energy.

7. The importance of a dependable and adequate _____ _____ for fire-suppression operations is self-evident.

8. In many communities, hydrants are painted in bright reflective colors for increased _____.

9. Municipal water systems can draw water from human-made storage facilities called _____.

10. Hydrants are equipped with one or more _____ to control the flow of water through the hydrant.

11. Dry-barrel hydrants need to be either _____ opened or _____ closed.

12. _____ valves allow different water main sections to be turned off or isolated.

True/False

If you believe the statement to be more true than false, write the letter "T" in the space provided. If you believe the statement to be more false than true, write the letter "F."

1. _____ Volume and water pressure are synonymous.
2. _____ Generally, water pressure ranges from 40 psi to 60 psi (276 kPa to 414 kPa) at the delivery point.
3. _____ The Pitot gauge is used to measure flow pressure through an opening during a hydrant test.
4. _____ The basic plan for fighting most fires depends on having an adequate supply of water.
5. _____ Residual pressure is the amount of pressure that remains in the system when water is flowing.
6. _____ Elevated water storage towers are used to increase the efficiency of treatment facilities.
7. _____ Fire fighters must understand how to inspect and maintain a fire hydrant.
8. _____ The backup water supply for some municipal systems can be large enough to store enough water for several months or years of municipal use.
9. _____ The water department can often increase the flow of water within the system or to specific areas.
10. _____ When the hydrant valve is opened, the drain closes in a dry-barrel hydrant.

Short Answer

Complete this section with short written answers using the space provided.

1. List the duties that need to be included in a hydrant inspection.

   _____
   _____
   _____
   _____

2. Identify the two water sources fire fighters rely on.

   _____
   _____
   _____
   _____

3. Describe the differences between dry-barrel and wet-barrel hydrants.

   _____
   _____
   _____
   _____

Fire Alarms

The following real case scenarios will give you an opportunity to explore the concerns associated with water supply. Read each scenario, and then answer each question in detail.

1. You have just finished lunch. Your Lieutenant has scheduled you to inspect and maintain hydrants in a residential subdivision. Your engine arrives at the first hydrant. How should you proceed?

   _____
   _____
   _____
   _____
   _____
   _____

2. It is 3:00 on an August afternoon when your tanker (tender) is dispatched to a barn fire. The first engine on the scene reports a large barn that is 75 percent involved with multiple exposures. When you arrive on the scene, you are instructed to set up a portable tank at the top of the driveway for a tanker shuttle. The next-in engine will draft from the tank and hook into the supply line. Your department has metal frame portable tanks. How should you proceed?

   _____
   _____
   _____
   _____
   _____
   _____

Skill Drills

Skill Drill 14-1: Operating a Dry-Barrel Fire Hydrant Fire Fighter I, NFPA 1001: 4.3.15

Test your knowledge of this skill drill by placing the photos below in the correct order. Number the first step with a "1," the second step with a "2," and so on.

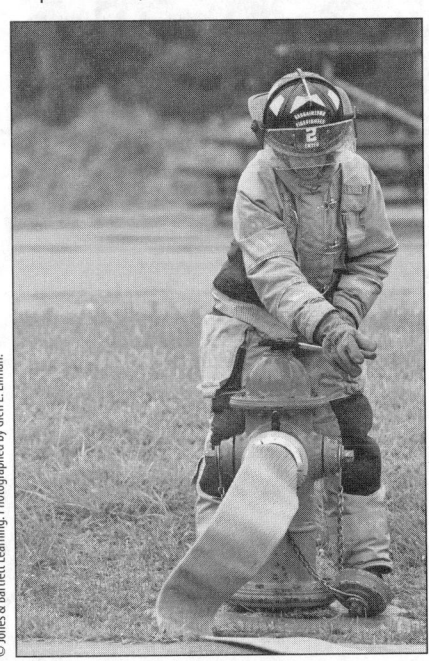

_____ When instructed to do so by your officer or the pump driver/operator, start the flow of water by turning the hydrant wrench to fully open the valve. This may take 12 or more turns depending on the type of hydrant.

176   Fundamentals of Fire Fighter Skills

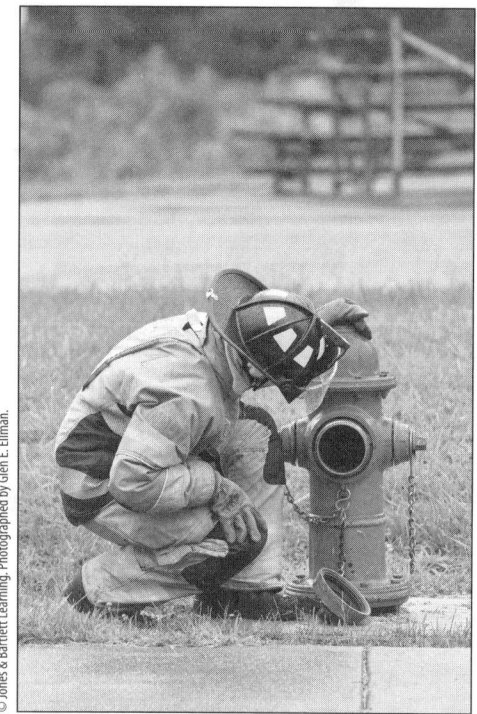

_____ Look inside the hydrant opening for debris.

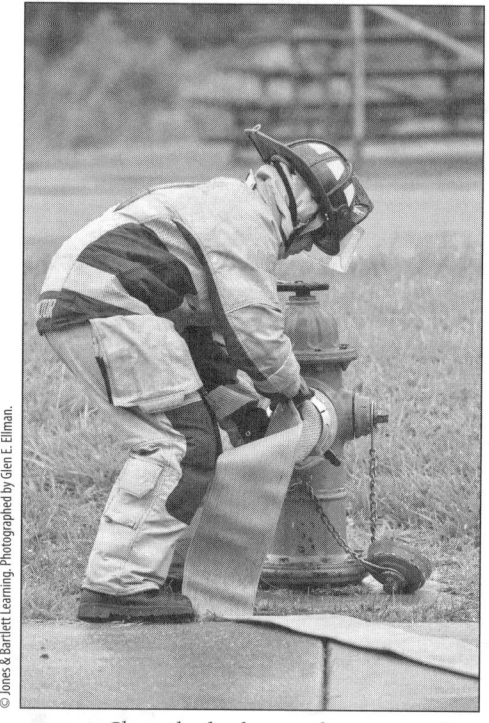

_____ Close the hydrant valve to stop the flow of water. Attach the hose or valve to the hydrant outlet.

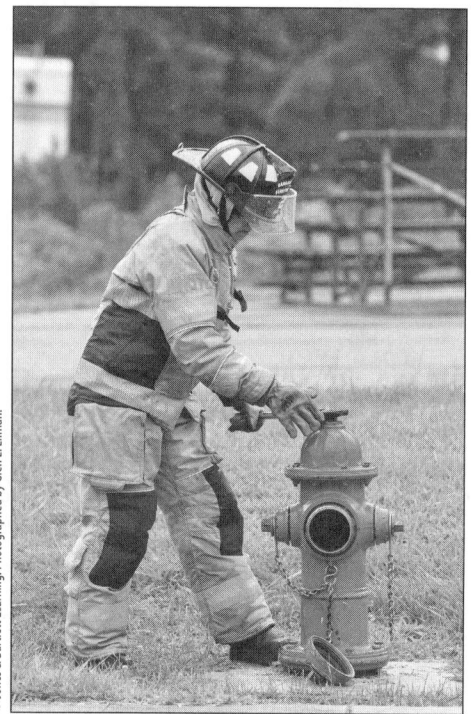

_____ Attach the hydrant wrench to the stem nut located on top of the hydrant. Check the top of the hydrant for an arrow indicating the direction to turn to open.

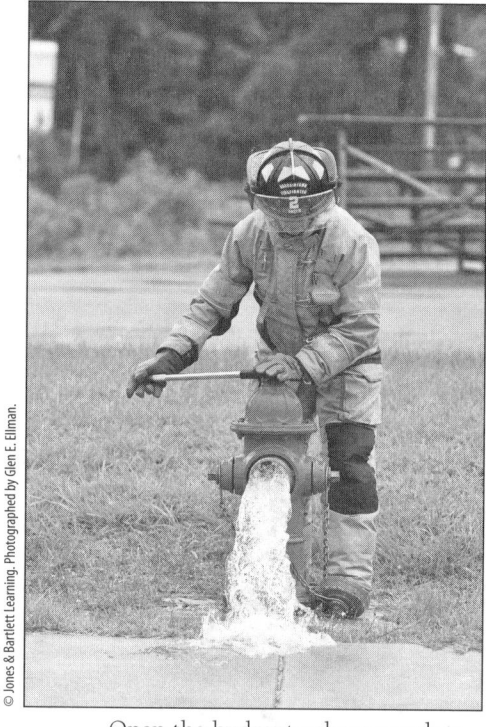

_____ Open the hydrant valve enough to verify flow of water and to flush out any debris that may be in the hydrant.

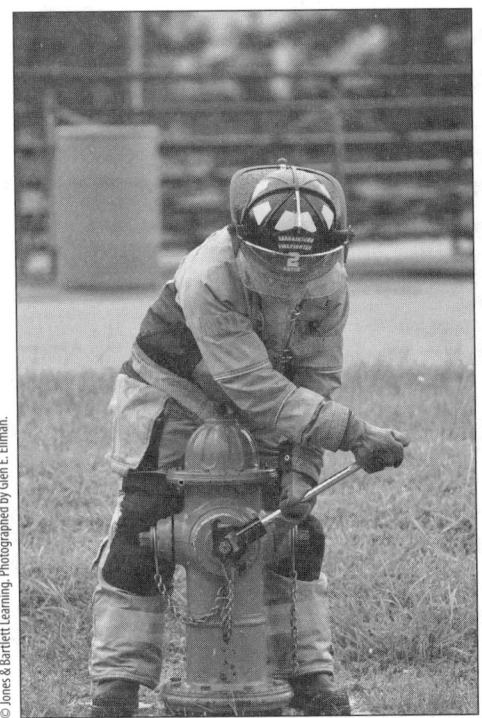

_____ Remove the cap from the outlet you will be using.

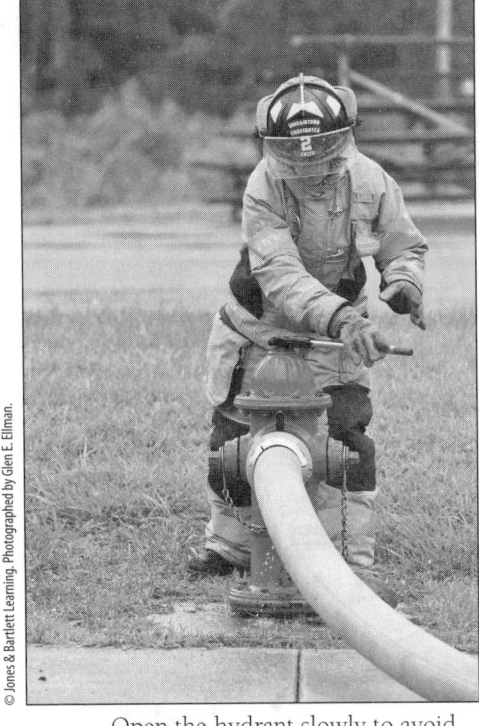

_____ Open the hydrant slowly to avoid a pressure surge. Once the flow of water has begun, you can open the hydrant valve more quickly. Make sure that you open the hydrant valve completely. If the valve is not fully opened, the drain hole will remain open.

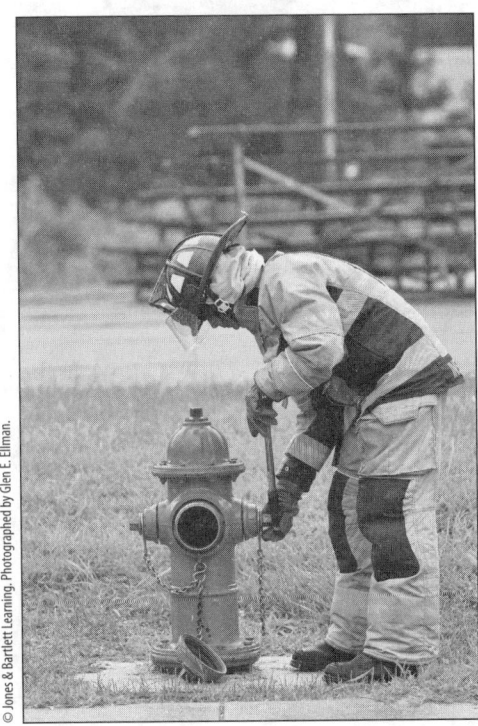

_____ Check that the remaining caps are snugly attached.

Skill Drill 14-2: Shutting Down a Dry-Barrel Fire Hydrant Fire Fighter I, NFPA 1001: 4.3.15

Test your knowledge of this skill drill by filling in the correct words in the photo captions.

1. Turn the hydrant wrench until the _____ _____ is closed.

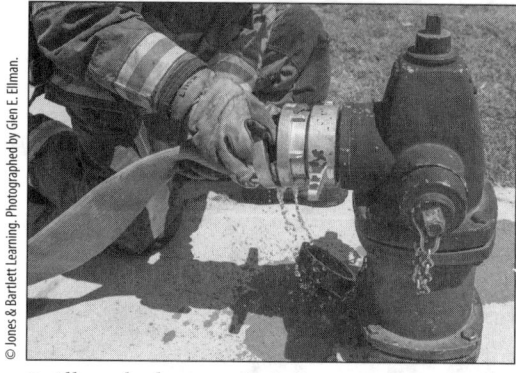

2. Allow the hose to drain by opening a drain valve or disconnecting a hose connection _____. Slowly disconnect the hose from the hydrant outlet, allowing any remaining pressure to escape.

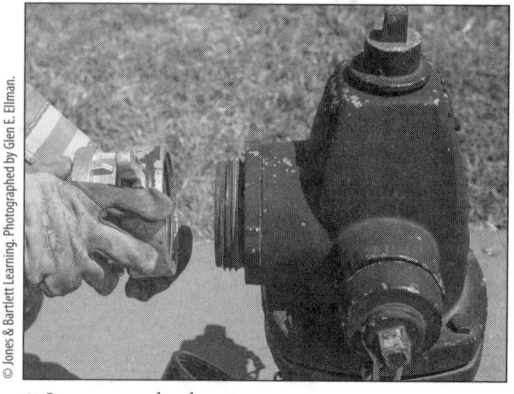

3. Leave one hydrant _____ open until the hydrant is fully drained.

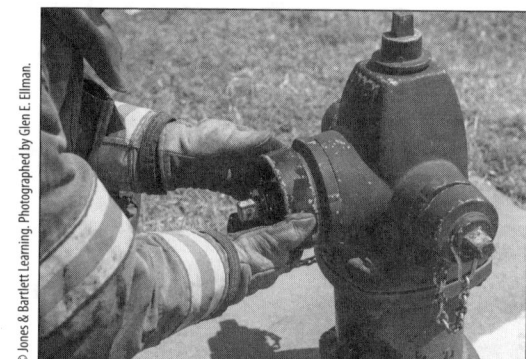

4. Replace the hydrant _____. Do not leave or replace the caps on a dry-barrel hydrant until you are sure the water has completely drained from the barrel. If you feel suction on your hand when you place it over the opening, the hydrant is still draining. In very cold weather, you may have to use a hydrant _____ to remove all of the water and prevent freezing.

Skill Drill 14-3: Operating a Wet-Barrel Fire Hydrant Fire Fighter I, NFPA 1001:4.3.15
Test your knowledge of this skill drill by filling in the correct words in the photo captions.

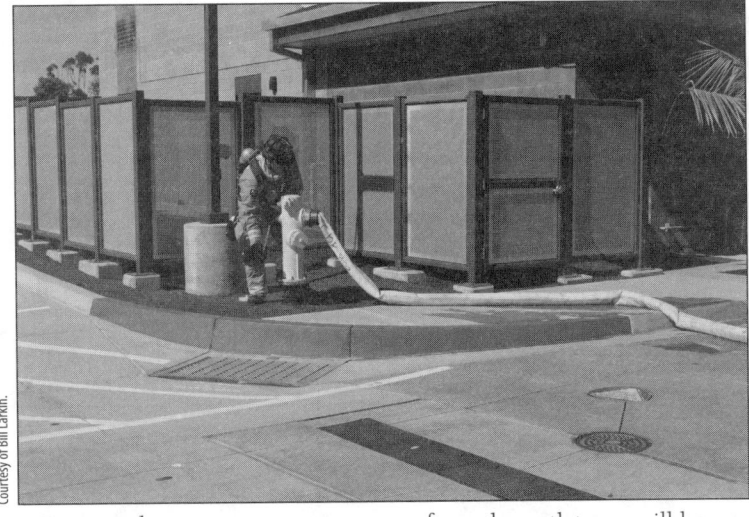

1. Remove the _____ from the outlet you will be using.

2. Look inside the hydrant opening for _____.

3. Check that the remaining caps are _____ attached.

4. Attach the hydrant wrench to the _____ _____ located behind the outlet you will be using. Check the hydrant for an _____ indicating the direction to turn to open.

5. Open the hydrant valve enough to verify _____ _____ _____ and to flush out any debris in the hydrant.

6. Close the hydrant valve to _____ the flow of water.

7. Attach the hose or valve to the hydrant _____.

8. When instructed to do so by your officer or the pump driver/operator, start the flow of water by turning the hydrant wrench to fully open the valve. This may take _____ or more turns, depending on the type of hydrant.

9. Open the hydrant slowly to avoid a _____ _____. Once the flow of water has begun, you can open the hydrant valve more quickly. Make sure you open the hydrant valve completely.

Skill Drill 14-4: Shutting Down a Wet-Barrel Fire Hydrant Fire Fighter I, NFPA 1001: 4.3.15
Test your knowledge of this skill drill by filling in the correct words in the photo captions.

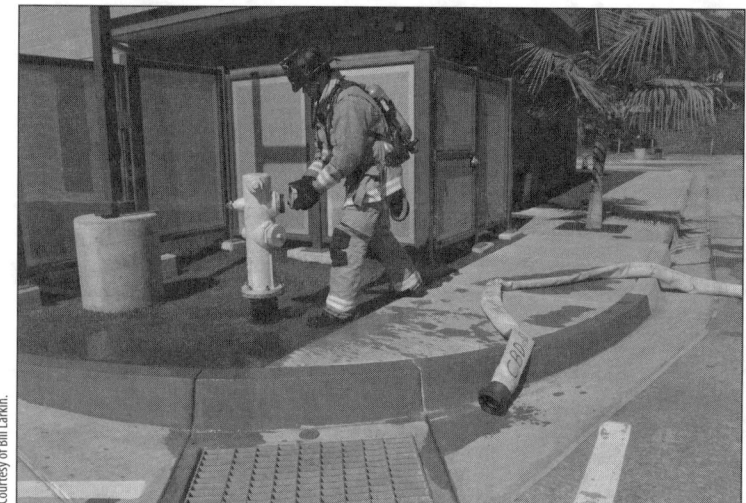

1. Turn the hydrant wrench until the valve _____ the outlet you are using is closed.

2. Allow the hose to drain by opening a drain valve or disconnecting a hose connection downstream. Slowly disconnect the hose from the _____ _____, allowing any remaining pressure to escape.

3. Replace the _____ cap.

Skill Drill 14-5: Conducting a Fire Hydrant Flow Test Fire Fighter I
Test your knowledge of this skill drill by placing the photos below in the correct order. Number the first step with a "1," the second step with a "2," and so on.

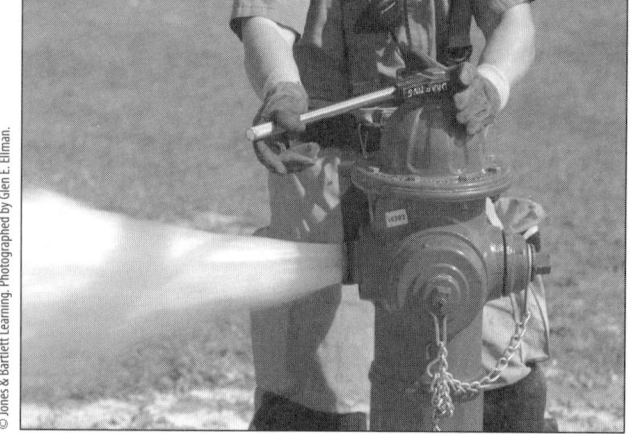

_____ Move to the second hydrant, remove one of the discharge caps, and open the second hydrant.

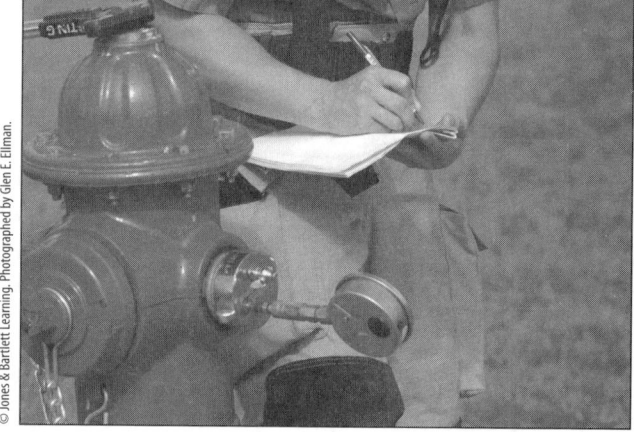

_____ Open the hydrant valve to fill the hydrant barrel. No water should be flowing. Record the initial pressure reading on the gauge. This is the static pressure.

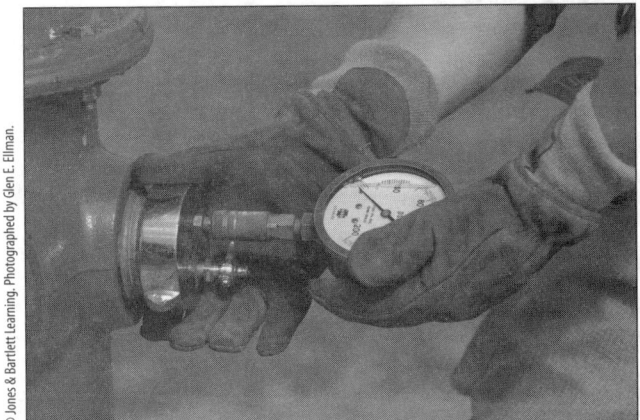

_____ Remove the cap from the hydrant port, open the hydrant, and allow water to flow until it runs clear. Close the hydrant valve. Place a cap gauge on one of the outlets of the first hydrant.

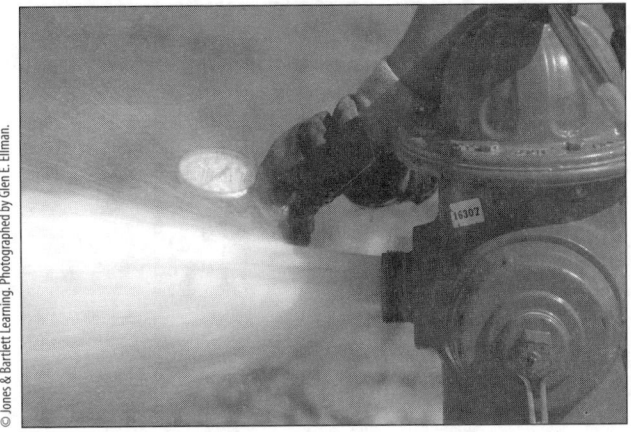

_____ Place the Pitot gauge one-half the diameter of the orifice away from the opening, and record this pressure as the Pitot pressure. At the same time, fire fighters at the first hydrant should record a second pressure reading. This is the residual pressure. Use the recorded pressure readings to calculate or look up the flow rates at 20 psi (138 kPa) residual pressure. Document your findings.

Skill Drill 14-6: Assisting the Pump Driver/Operator with Drafting Fire Fighter I, NFPA 1001: 4.3.15

Test your knowledge of this skill drill by placing the photos below in the correct order. Number the first step with a "1," the second step with a "2," and so on.

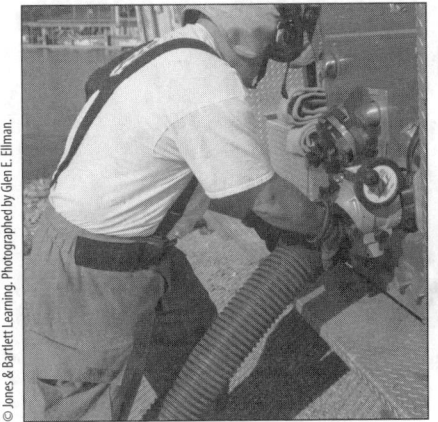

_____ Connect the other end of the suction hose to the fire pump.

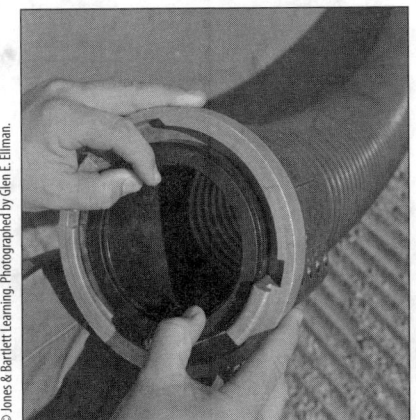

_____ After the pump driver/operator has positioned the engine at the draft site, inspect the swivel gaskets on the female coupling for damage or debris.

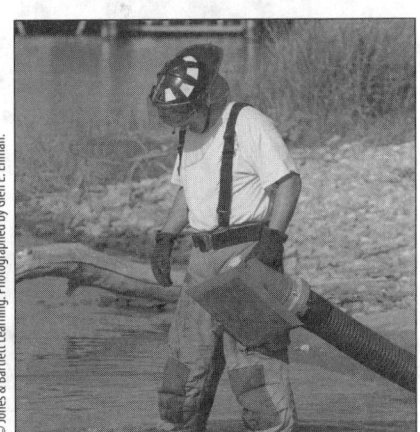

_____ Advance the suction hose assembly into position with the strainer in the water.

182 FUNDAMENTALS OF FIRE FIGHTER SKILLS

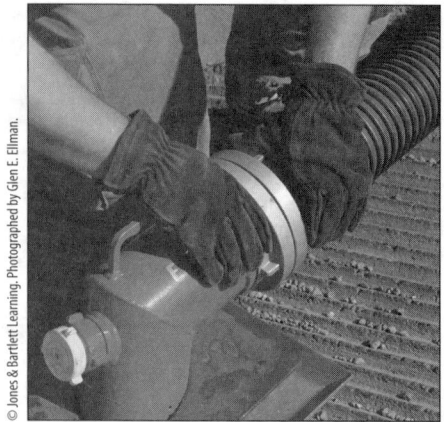

_____ Connect each section of suction hose together, and connect the strainer to the end of the hose that will be placed in the water.

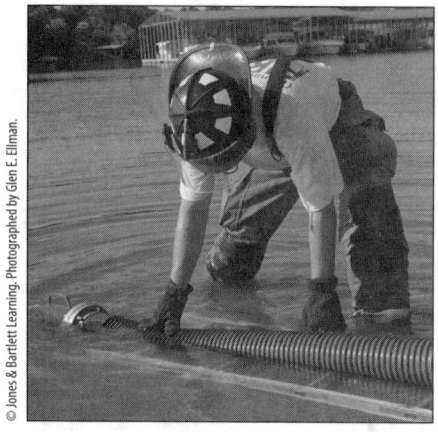

_____ Ensure that the strainer assembly has at least 24 in. (0.5 m) of water in all directions around the strainer.

Skill Drill 14-7: Setting Up a Portable Tank Fire Fighter I, NFPA 1001: 4.3.15
Test your knowledge of this skill drill by placing the photos below in the correct order. Number the first step with a "1," the second step with a "2," and so on.

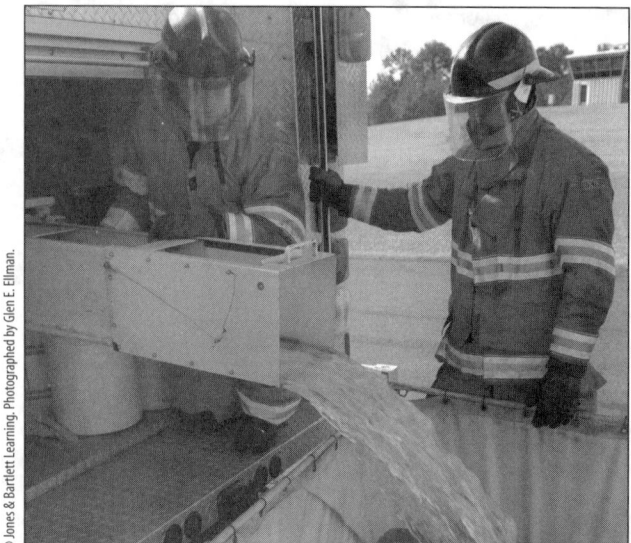

_____ The second fire fighter helps the tanker driver discharge water into the portable tank. If the tank is self-expanding, the fire fighters may need to hold the collar until the water level is high enough for the tank to support itself.

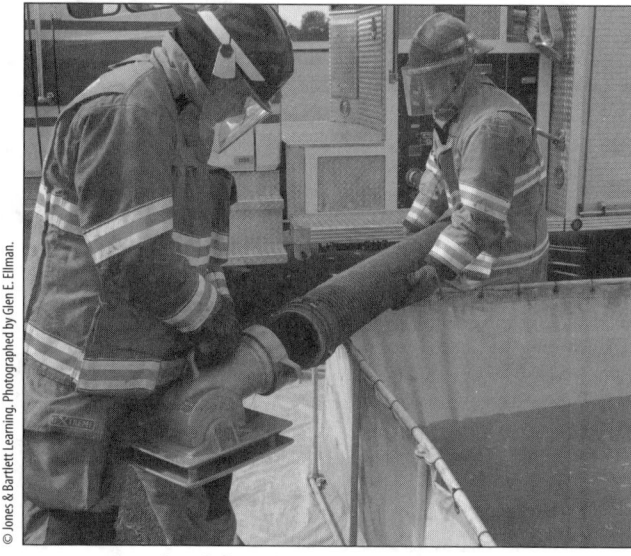

_____ One fire fighter helps the pump driver/operator place the strainer on the end of the suction hose, put the suction hose into the tank, and connect it to the engine.

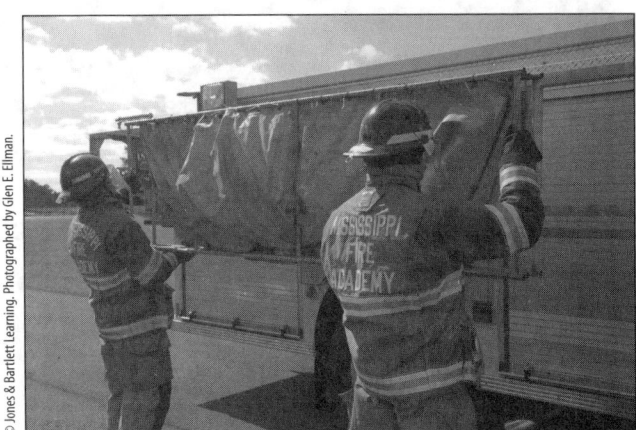 _____ Two fire fighters lift the portable tank off the apparatus. This tank may be mounted on a side rack or on a hydraulic rack that lowers it to the ground. Place the portable tank on as level ground as possible beside the engine. The pump driver/operator will indicate the best location.

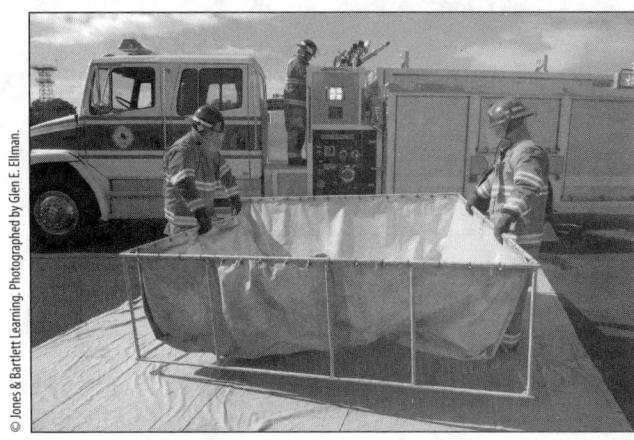 _____ Expand the tank (metal-frame type), or lay it flat (self-expanding type).

Fire Hose, Appliances, and Nozzles

Workbook Activities

The following activities have been designed to help you. Your instructor may require you to complete some or all of these activities as a regular part of your fire fighter training program. You are encouraged to complete any activity your instructor does not assign to you, as a way to enhance your learning in the classroom.

Chapter Review

The following exercises provide an opportunity to refresh your knowledge of this chapter.

Matching

Match each of the terms in the left column to the appropriate definition in the right column.

_____ 1. Adjustable-gallonage fog nozzle   **A.** Produces fine droplets of water

_____ 2. Attack engine   **B.** Used to deliver a flat screen of water that then forms a protective sheet of water on the surface of an exposed building

_____ 3. Cellar nozzle   **C.** A device used to temporarily stop the flow of water in a hose line

_____ 4. Hose clamp   **D.** Has a limited flow, in the range of 40 to 50 gpm

_____ 5. Booster hose   **E.** A nozzle that allows the operator to select a desired flow from several settings

_____ 6. Water curtain nozzle   **F.** Attachments to the discharge end of attack hoses

_____ 7. Fixed-gallonage fog nozzle   **G.** A nozzle used to fight fires in cellars and other inaccessible places

_____ 8. Breakaway type nozzle   **H.** Delivers a preset flow at the rated discharge pressure

_____ 9. Wye   **I.** Used to make a hole in automobile sheet metal, aircraft, or building walls so as to extinguish fires behind these surfaces

_____ 10. Smooth-bore nozzle   **J.** Can be separated between the shut-off and the tip

_____ 11. Fog-stream nozzle   **K.** The engine from which the attack lines have been pulled

_____ 12. Nozzles   **L.** Extinguishes a fire with less air movement and less disturbance of the thermal layering than does a fog stream

_____ 13. Piercing nozzle   **M.** A device used to split a single hose into two separate lines

CHAPTER 15

Multiple Choice

Read each item carefully, and then select the best response.

_____ 1. The part or layer of a fire hose that prevents water from leaking out of the hose is the
   A. inner jacket.
   B. hose liner.
   C. outer jacket.
   D. reinforcement liner.

_____ 2. Threaded hose couplings are used on most hoses up to_____ in diameter.
   A. 3 in
   B. 2 ½ in
   C. 4 in
   D. 5 in

_____ 3. Which nozzles separate the water into fine droplets?
   A. Smooth-bore nozzles
   B. Fog-stream nozzles
   C. Breakaway nozzles
   D. Aeration nozzles

_____ 4. A 1¾-in handline hose is generally considered to flow
   A. 60–90 gallons of water per minute.
   B. 120–180 gallons of water per minute.
   C. 250–300 gallons of water per minute.
   D. over 300 gallons of water per minute.

_____ 5. The notch or cut on the outside of one of the lugs on a hose coupling that indicates the position of the first thread of the coupling is known as a
   A. Thread indicator.
   B. Storz indicator.
   C. Higbee indicator.
   D. National standard thread indicator.

_____ 6. Attack lines can be either multiple-jacket or _____ construction.
   A. rubber-covered
   B. linen
   C. vinyl
   D. quadruple jacket

_____ 7. The NFPA recommends that a fire pumper carry at least _____ feet of 2½-in or larger supply hose.
   A. 500
   B. 800
   C. 1000
   D. 1500

_____ 8. Attack hose must be tested annually at a pressure of at least _____ psi.
   A. 150
   B. 200
   C. 300
   D. 400

_____ 9. The three groups of nozzles are low-volume, master-stream, and
   A. high-volume nozzles.
   B. secondary-stream nozzles.
   C. apparatus nozzles.
   D. handline nozzles.

_____ 10. A booster hose is generally considered to flow
   A. 40–50 gallons of water per minute.
   B. 60–90 gallons of water per minute.
   C. 125–150 gallons of water per minute.
   D. over 200 gallons of water per minute.

_____ 11. Which type of hose roll is used for general transportation of hose and rack storage?
   A. Single-doughnut roll
   B. Straight roll
   C. Forward roll
   D. Double-doughnut roll

_____ 12. Bresnan distributor nozzles are used to fight fires in
   A. warehouses.
   B. open spaces.
   C. inaccessible places.
   D. defensive attacks.

_____ 13. Which nozzle allows the operator to select a desired flow from several settings?
   A. Fixed-gallonage fog
   B. Adjustable-gallonage fog
   C. Automatic-adjusting fog
   D. Distributor

_____ 14. Which nozzle is used to make a hole in automobile sheet metal?
   A. Cellar
   B. Bresnan
   C. Piercing
   D. Smooth bore

_____ 15. Which nozzle is used on deck guns, portable monitors, and ladder pipes?
   A. Low volume
   B. Handline
   C. Master stream
   D. Straight bore

_____ 16. A 2½-in handline hose is generally considered to flow
   A. 100 gallons of water per minute.
   B. 150 gallons of water per minute.
   C. 200 gallons of water per minute.
   D. 250 gallons of water per minute.

_____ 17. A device that is placed over a leaking section of hose to stop a leak is known as a
   A. hose clamp.
   B. hose reducer.
   C. hose jacket.
   D. hose sleeve.

_____ 18. Which type of hose roll forms its own carrying loop?
   A. Single doughnut roll
   B. Straight roll
   C. Self-locking twin-doughnut roll
   D. Twin-doughnut roll

Vocabulary
Define the following terms using the space provided.

1. Handline nozzle:

   _____
   _____
   _____

2. Smooth-bore nozzle:

   _____
   _____
   _____

3. Fixed-gallonage fog nozzle:

   _____
   _____
   _____

4. Siamese connection:

   _____
   _____
   _____

Fill-In
Read each item carefully, and then complete the statement by filling in the missing word(s).

1. Examples of _____ damage to fire hose includes damage from battery acid, gasoline, and motor oil.

2. A(n) _____ fire hose is often used for fighting wildland and ground fires.

3. A(n) _____ hose is usually carried on a hose reel that holds 150 or 200 ft (46 to 61 m) of rubber hose.

4. Large-diameter hose (LDH) has a limited role as a(n) _____ _____ tool.

5. A _____. _____ hose is a short section of rigid hose that is used to draft water from a static source.

6. A visual hose inspection should be performed at least _____.

7. Each length of fire hose should be tested at least _____ according to the procedures listed in NFPA 1962.

8. A double-female adapter is used to join two _____ hose couplings.

9. The hoses used to discharge water from an attack engine onto the fire are called _____ _____.

10. Fire fighters can add hose to the discharge end of the hose if the nozzle is a(n) _____ _____ nozzle.

True/False

If you believe the statement to be more true than false, write the letter "T" in the space provided. If you believe the statement to be more false than true, write the letter "F."

1. _____ The straight stream from a fog-stream nozzle breaks up faster and does not have the reach of a solid stream.
2. _____ The advantage of booster hose is its large flow.
3. _____ A disadvantage of forestry hose is that it is limited to a maximum of 200 ft in length.
4. _____ A single-jacket hose is constructed with only one layer of woven fiber.
5. _____ Female hose couplings are manufactured in two pieces.
6. _____ The most common type of lugs on a hose coupling are pin lugs.
7. _____ Supply hose is tested annually to a pressure of at least 200 psi.
8. _____ Most fire hose is dried before being placed back on the fire apparatus.
9. _____ A wye is an appliance that combines two or more hose lines into one.
10. _____ A deck gun is permanently mounted on a vehicle.

Short Answer

Complete this section with short written answers using the space provided.

1. List the items that should be included on a hose record.

   _____

   _____

   _____

   _____

2. Describe the difference between a wye and a siamese connection.

   _____

   _____

   _____

   _____

3. List the six types of valves.

   _____

   _____

   _____

   _____

4. Describe the difference between soft sleeve hose and hard suction hose.

   _____

   _____

   _____

   _____

Fire Alarms

The following real case scenarios will give you an opportunity to explore the concerns associated with fire hoses, nozzles, streams, and foam. Read each scenario, and then answer each question in detail.

1. Your station has been assigned two new recruit fire fighters. Your officer asks you to review with them the basic steps for cleaning fire hoses. Which items should you cover?

   _____
   _____
   _____
   _____
   _____
   _____

2. Your engine company has just completed testing six new lengths of fire hose. Your Captain asks you to complete the hose record for each length. Which items should you make sure are included in the record?

   _____
   _____
   _____
   _____
   _____
   _____

Skill Drills

Skill Drill 15-1: Replacing the Swivel Gasket Fire Fighter I, NFPA 1001: 4.5.2
Test your knowledge of this skill drill by filling in the correct words in the photo captions.

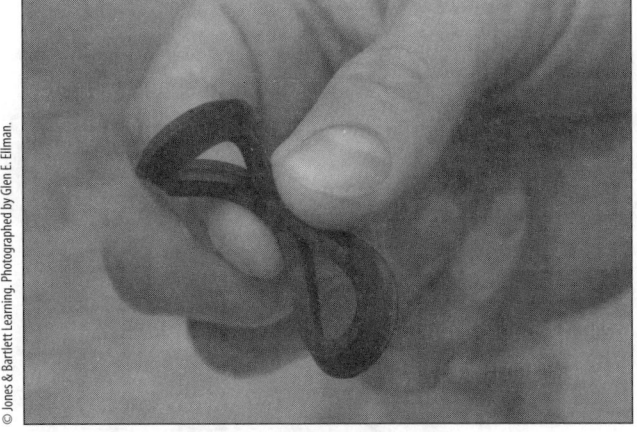

1. Fold the new swivel gasket in half by bringing the _____ and the _____ together to create two loops.

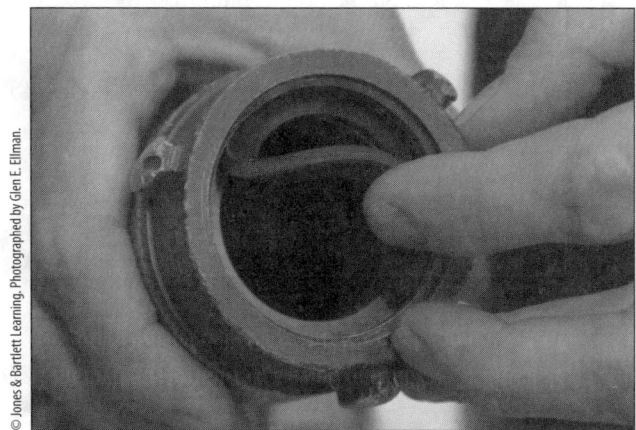

2. Place either of the two loops inside the hose _____, and position it against the gasket seat.

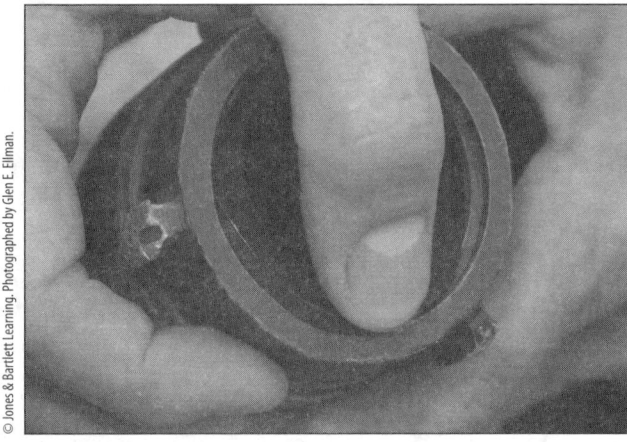

3. Using the thumb, push the remaining unseated portions of the _____ _____ into the hose coupling until the entire swivel gasket is properly positioned against the gasket seat inside the coupling.

Skill Drill 15-2: Performing the One-Fire Fighter Foot-Tilt Method of Coupling a Fire Hose Fire Fighter I, NFPA 1001: 4.3.10
Test your knowledge of this skill drill by filling in the correct words in the photo captions.

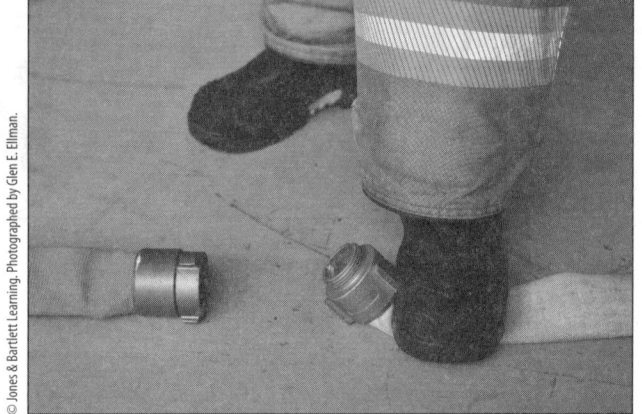

1. Place one foot on the hose behind the _____ coupling. Push down with your foot to tilt the _____ coupling upward.

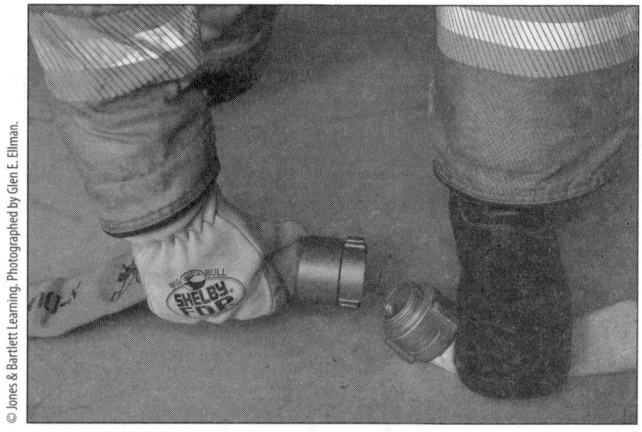

2. Place one hand behind the _____ coupling, and grasp the hose.

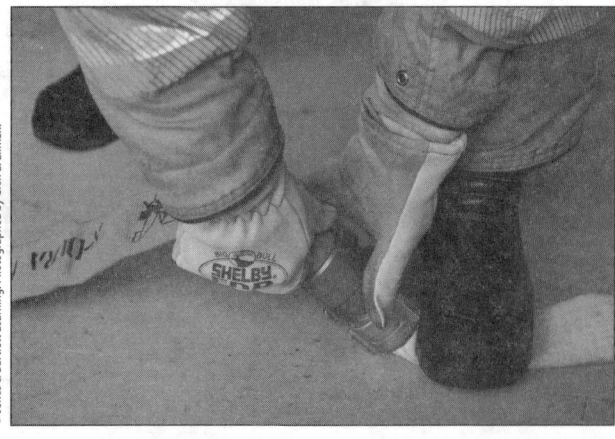

3. Place the other hand on the _____ of the female coupling. Bring the two couplings together and align the _____ indicators. Turn the female coupling counterclockwise until it clicks, which indicates that the threads are aligned. Rotate the swivel in a clockwise direction to connect the hose.

Skill Drill 15-3: Performing the Two-Fire Fighter Method of Coupling a Fire Hose Fire Fighter I, NFPA 1001: 4.3.10

Test your knowledge of this skill drill by placing the photos below in the correct order. Number the first step with a "1," the second step with a "2," and so on.

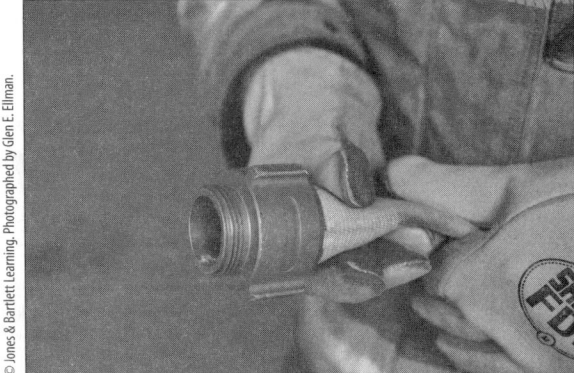

_____ Pick up the male coupling. Grasp it directly behind the coupling, and hold it tightly against the body.

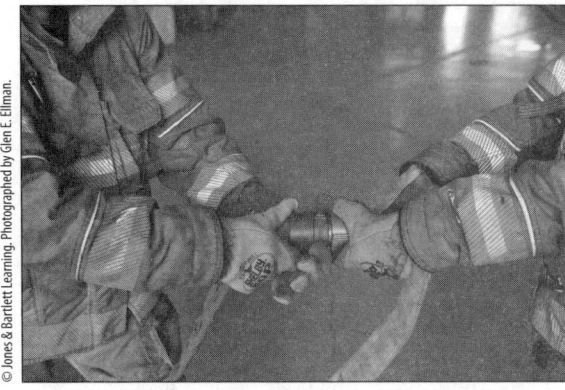

_____ The second fire fighter turns the female coupling counterclockwise until it clicks, which indicates that the threads are aligned, and then turns the female coupling swivel clockwise to couple the hose.

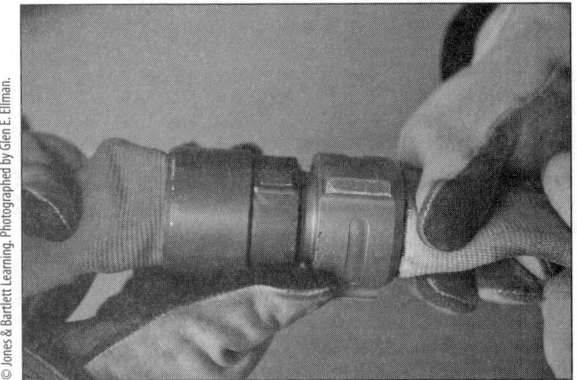

_____ The second fire fighter brings the female coupling to the male coupling and aligns the female coupling with the male coupling, using the Higbee indicators for easy alignment.

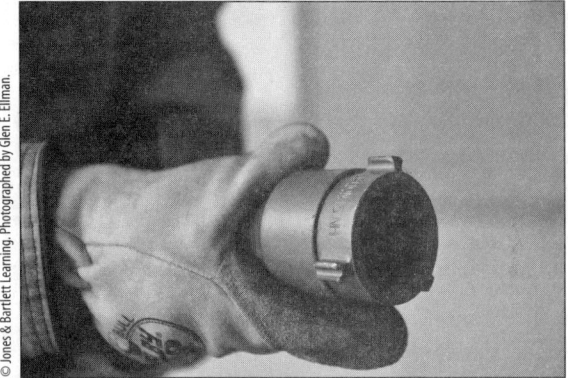

_____ The second fire fighter holds the female coupling firmly with both hands.

Skill Drill 15-6: Uncoupling a Hose with Spanner Wrenches Fire Fighter I, NFPA 1001: 4.3.10
Test your knowledge of this skill drill by placing the photos below in the correct order. Number the first step with a "1," the second step with a "2," and so on.

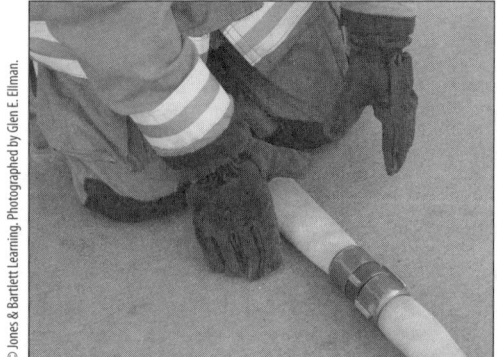

_____ With the connection on the ground, straddle the connection above the female coupling.

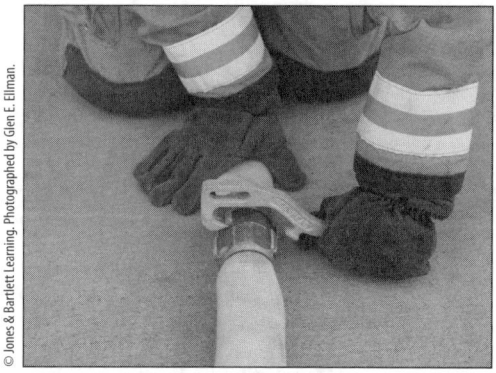

_____ Place one spanner wrench on the swivel of the female coupling, with the handle of the wrench to the left.

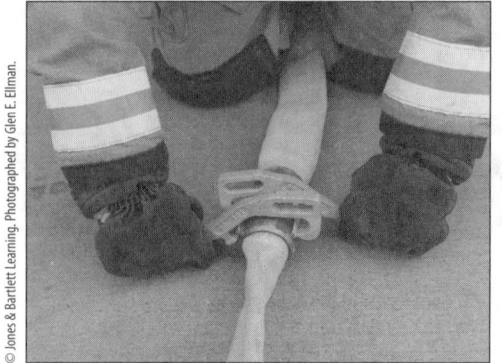

_____ Push both spanner wrench handles down toward the ground, loosening the connection.

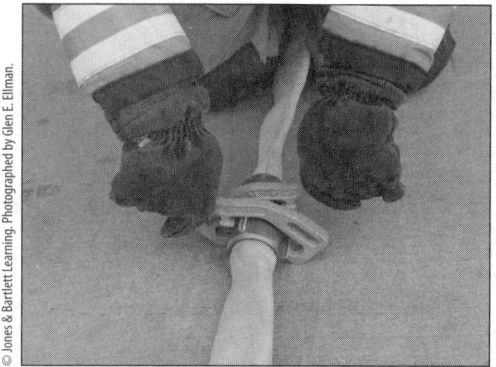

_____ Place the second spanner wrench on the male coupling, with the handle of the wrench to the right.

Skill Drill 15-9: Performing a Straight or Storage Hose Roll Fire Fighter I, NFPA 1001: 4.5.2
Test your knowledge of this skill drill by filling in the correct words in the photo captions.

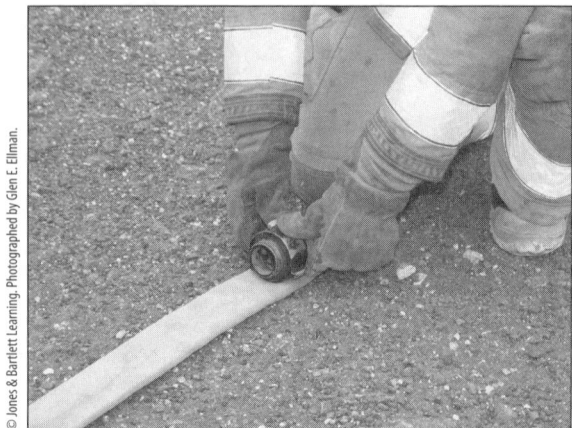

1. Lay the hose flat and in a _____ line.

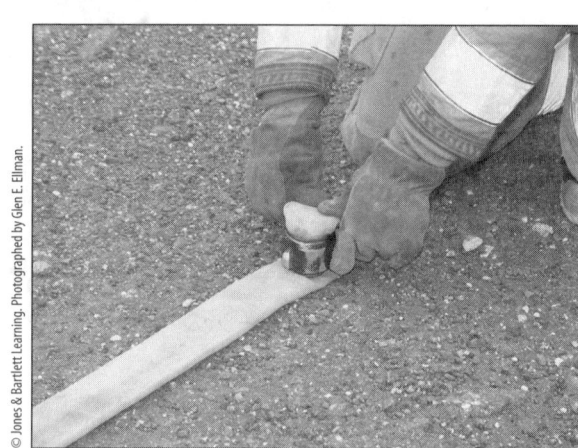

2. Fold the _____ coupling over on top of the hose.

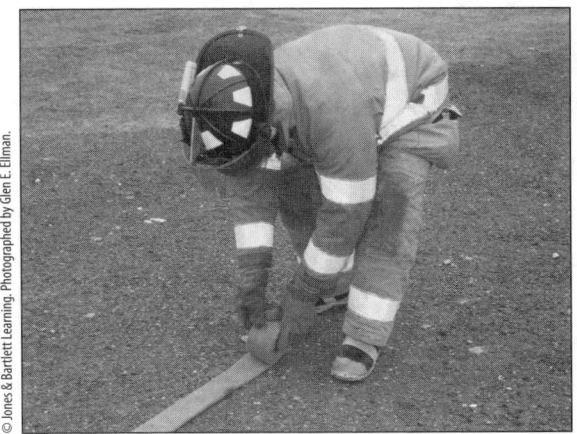

3. Roll the hose to the _____ coupling.

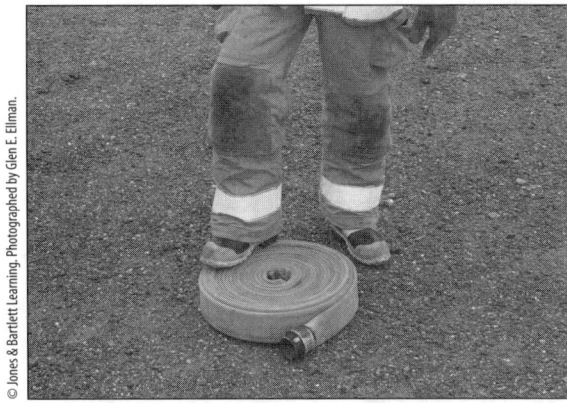

4. Set the hose roll on its side, and tap any protruding hose flat with a foot. With this arrangement, the _____ coupling is at the center of the roll, and the _____ coupling is on the outside of the roll.

Skill Drill 15-11: Performing a Twin-Doughnut Hose Roll Fire Fighter I, NFPA 1001: 4.5.2

Test your knowledge of this skill drill by placing the photos below in the correct order. Number the first step with a "1," the second step with a "2," and so on.

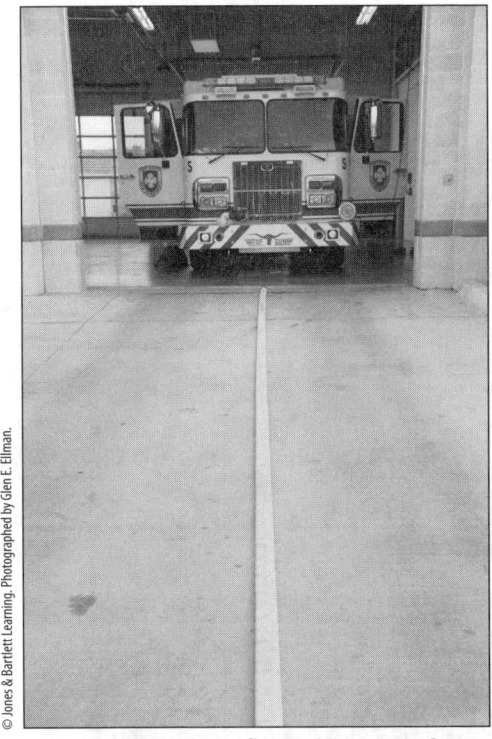

_____ Lay the hose flat and in a straight line.

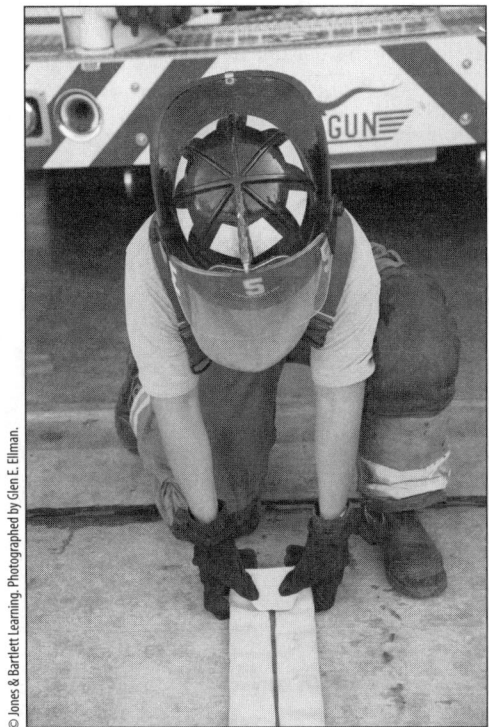

_____ Fold the far end over, and roll both sections of hose toward the couplings, creating a double roll.

194 Fundamentals of Fire Fighter Skills

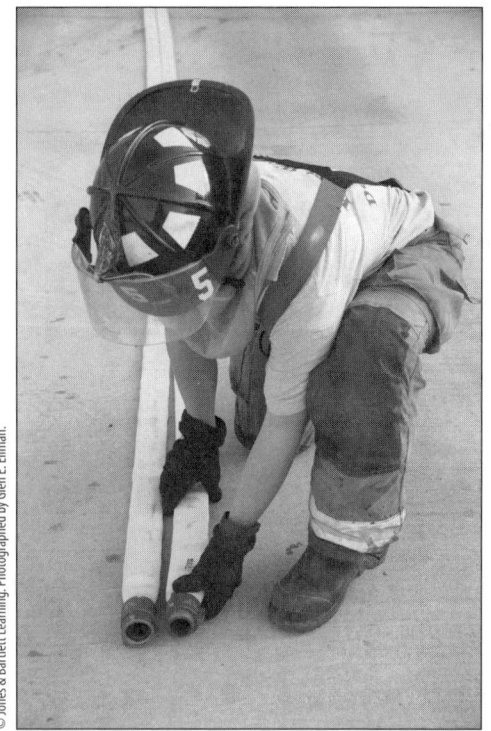

_____ Bring the male coupling alongside the female coupling.

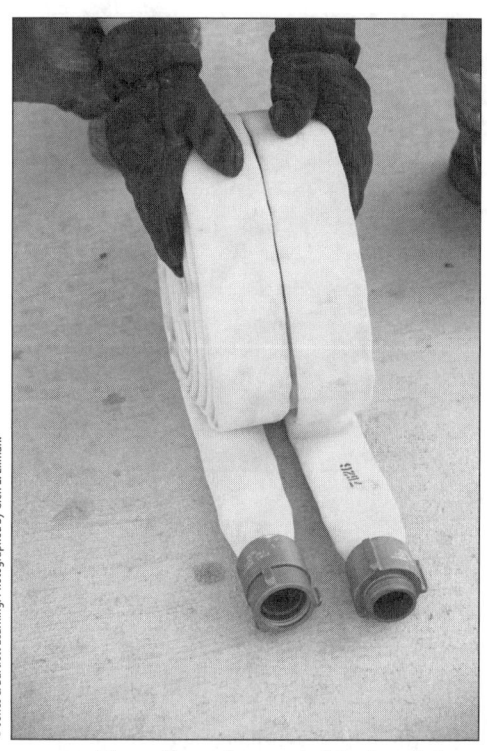

_____ The roll can be carried by hand, by a rope, or by a hose strap.

Skill Drill 15-12: Performing a Self-Locking Twin-Doughnut Hose Roll Fire Fighter I, NFPA 1001: 4.5.2
Test your knowledge of this skill drill by placing the photos below in the correct order. Number the first step with a "1," the second step with a "2," and so on.

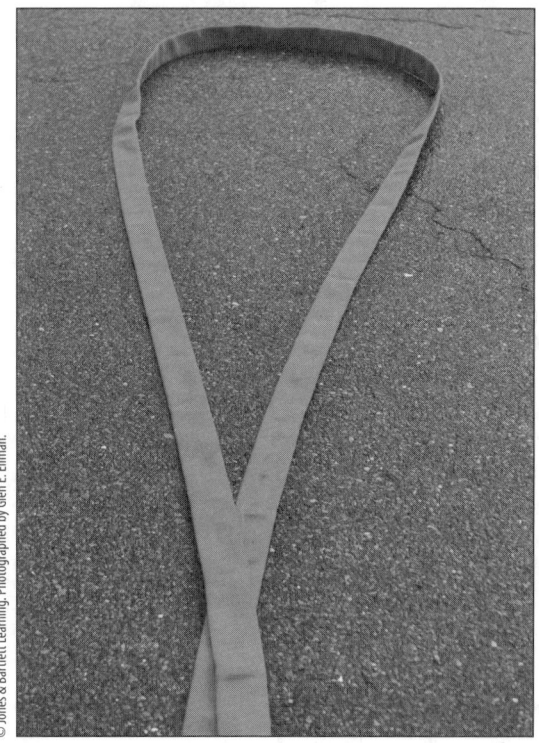

_____ Move one side of the hose over the other, creating a loop. This creates the carrying shoulder loop.

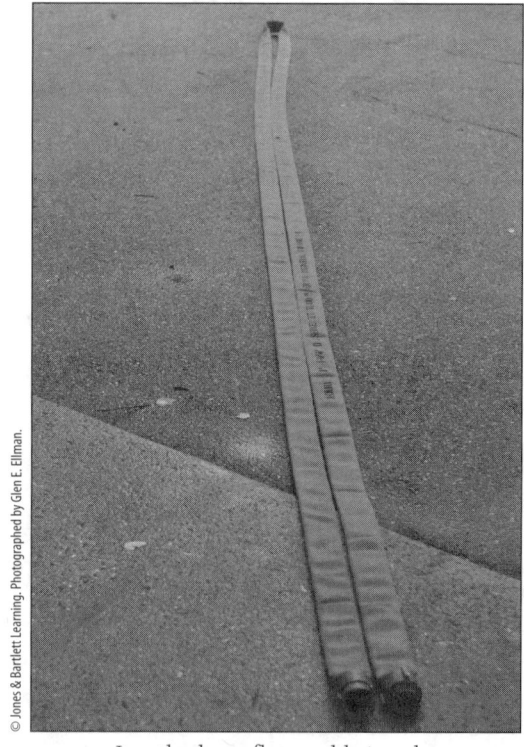

_____ Lay the hose flat, and bring the couplings alongside each other.

Chapter 15 Fire Hose, Appliances, and Nozzles

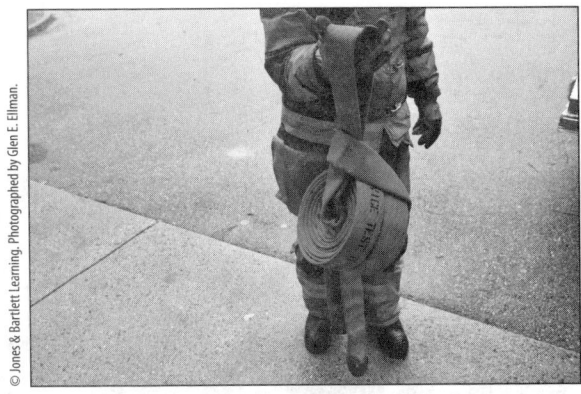

_____ The finished result is the self-locking twindoughnut roll.

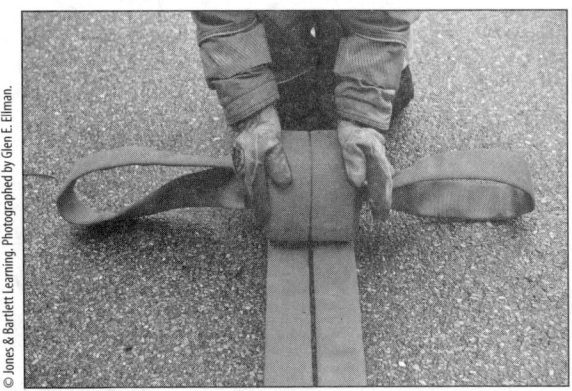

_____ From the point where the hose crosses, begin to roll the hose toward the couplings.

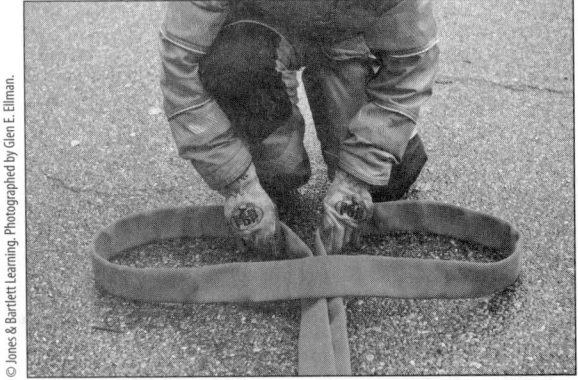

_____ Bring the loop back toward the couplings to the point where the hose crosses.

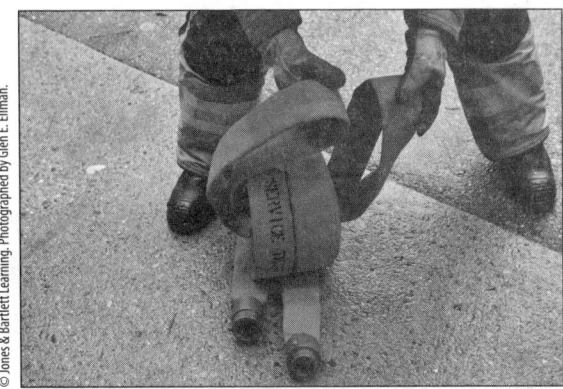

_____ Position the loops so that one is larger than the other. Pass the larger loop over the couplings and through the smaller loop, which secures the rolls together and forms the shoulder loop.

Skill Drill 15-14: Operating a Smooth-Bore Nozzle Fire Fighter I, NFPA 1001: 4.3.10
Test your knowledge of this skill drill by filling in the correct words in the photo captions.

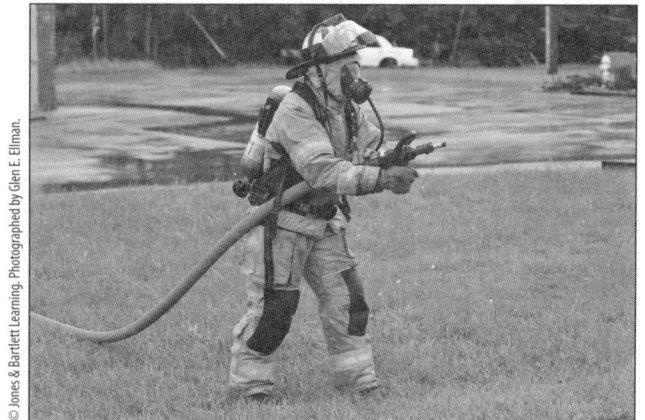

1. Select the desired tip size, and attach it to the _____ _____-_____ _____. Attain a stable stance (if standing).

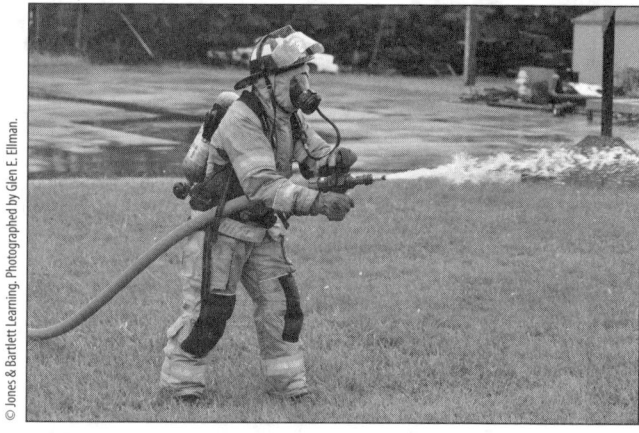

2. Slowly open the _____, allowing water to flow.

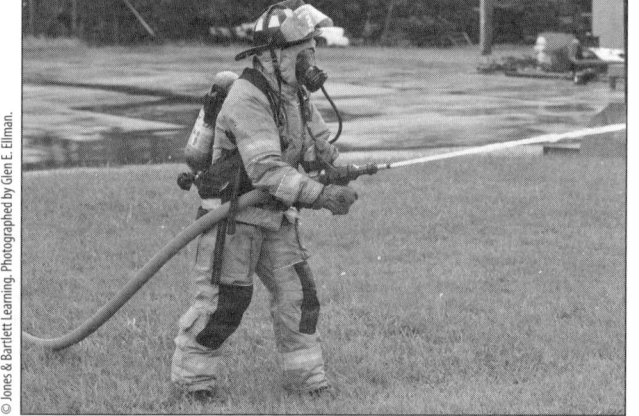

3. Open the valve completely to achieve maximum _____.

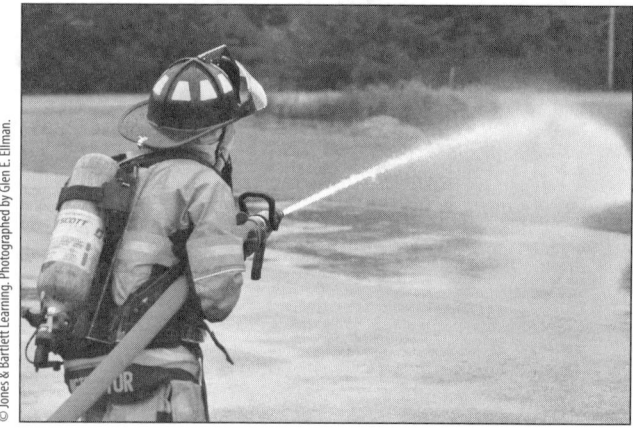

4. Direct the _____ to the desired location.

Skill Drill 15-15: Operating a Fog-Stream Nozzle Fire Fighter I, NFPA 1001: 4.3.10

Test your knowledge of this skill drill by filling in the correct words in the photo captions.

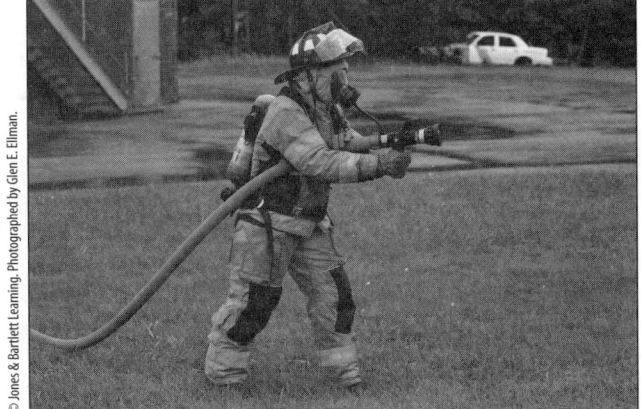

1. Select the desired nozzle. Attain a _____ _____ (if standing).

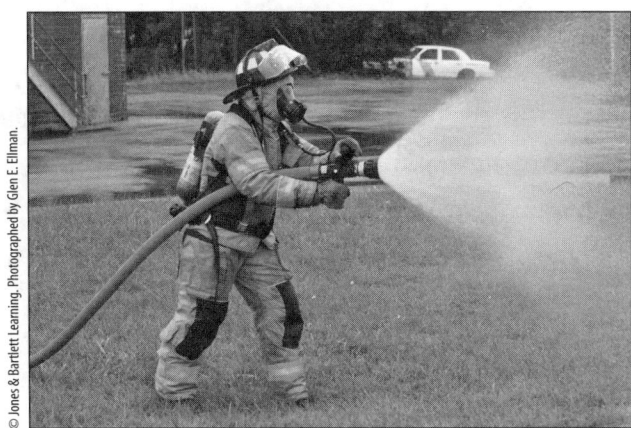

2. Slowly open the valve, and allow water to _____.

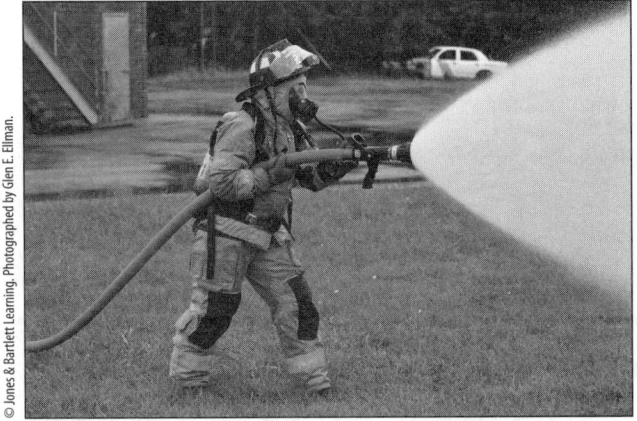

3. Open the _____ completely.

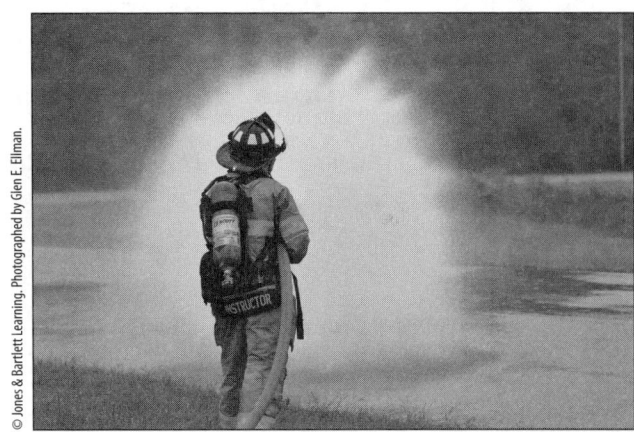

4. Select the desired water _____ by rotating the _____ of the nozzle. Apply water where needed.

Supply Line and Attack Line Evolutions

Workbook Activities

The following activities have been designed to help you. Your instructor may require you to complete some or all of these activities as a regular part of your fire fighter training program. You are encouraged to complete any activity your instructor does not assign you, as a way to enhance your learning in the classroom.

Chapter Review

The following exercises provide an opportunity to refresh your knowledge of this chapter.

Matching

Match each of the terms in the left column to the appropriate definition in the right column.

_____ 1. Attack line operations
_____ 2. Breakaway nozzle
_____ 3. Combination hose load
_____ 4. Dutchman
_____ 5. Forward hose lay
_____ 6. Handline
_____ 7. Preconnected flat load
_____ 8. Reverse hose lay
_____ 9. Split hose bed
_____ 10. Supply line operations

A. Hose load where the female end of the hose line is preconnected
B. Delivery of water from a water supply source to an attack engine
C. Laying a supply line from the water source to the attack engine
D. Delivery of water from an attack engine to a handline
E. A hose and nozzle that can be held and directed by hand
F. A nozzle and tip that can be separated from the shut-off valve
G. Laying a supply line from the attack engine to the water source
H. Hose load used when one long hose is needed
I. Hose load which can lay out one or two supply lines
J. Short fold placed in a hose when loading it into the hose bed

Multiple Choice

Read each item carefully, and then select the best response.

_____ 1. How should attack lines be loaded in the hose bed?
   A. Nozzle toward the cab
   B. Shut off toward the cab
   C. In a manner that ensures they can be quickly stretched from the attack engine to the fire
   D. Dutchman fold toward the cab

_____ 2. When is a preconnected flat load ready for use?
   A. When the load is finished and the nozzle is attached
   B. When the loop is added
   C. When the female end is attached to the discharge
   D. When the adapter is added

CHAPTER 16

_____ 3. To perform an interior attach, an attack line is usually advanced in how many stages?
   A. One stage
   B. Two stages
   C. Three stages
   D. Four stages

_____ 4. The end of the hose bed closest to the tailboard is known as the
   A. traverse.
   B. front.
   C. rear.
   D. bumper.

_____ 5. The forward hose lay is most often used by the
   A. second arriving engine company.
   B. first arriving tanker (tender).
   C. first arriving hose wagon.
   D. first arriving engine company.

_____ 6. A hose lay that is used where hose must be laid in two different directions is known as the
   A. split hose lay.
   B. hydrant hose lay.
   C. forward hose lay.
   D. combination hose lay.

_____ 7. The three basic hose loads for supply hose are the
   A. reverse, forward, combination.
   B. preconnect, horseshoe, triple-layer.
   C. flat, horseshoe, accordion.
   D. minuteman, accordion, flat.

_____ 8. The _____ hose load is accomplished by placing the hose around the perimeter of the hose bed in a U-shape.
   A. triple-layer
   B. horseshoe
   C. basic
   D. forward

_____ 9. Soft sleeve hose is most often used for
   A. drafting water from a static water source.
   B. connecting the discharge of one fire pump to the suction side of another fire pump.
   C. rural water supply evolutions.
   D. transporting water from a fire hydrant to the suction side of the fire pump.

_____ 10. A type of fire nozzle that can be used to add extra hose to the discharge end of the attack line is known as a
   A. combination nozzle.
   B. breakaway nozzle.
   C. leader line nozzle.
   D. smooth bore nozzle.

_____ 11. Places along a hose line where the hose is changing direction, turning a corner, or going through a doorway are known as
   A. kinks.
   B. catch points.
   C. friction points.
   D. corner bends.

_____ 12. A type of fire attack that is a combination of offensive, exterior, and interior operations is known as a
   A. transitional attack.
   B. combination attack.
   C. preconnect attack.
   D. flow path attack.

_____ 13. A type of hose carry that is used to transport full lengths of hose over a longer distance than is practical to drag the hose is known as a
   A. flat carry.
   B. shoulder carry.
   C. triple-layer carry.
   D. rapid carry.

_____ 14. A fire department connection (FDC) is provided so that
   A. the fire department can bypass the standpipe system.
   B. the capacity of the building's fire pump can be tested.
   C. attack hose lines can be attached at each floor in a high-rise building.
   D. the fire department can pump water into the standpipe and sprinkler system.

_____ 15. The _____ hose load is performed with the hose placed on its edge and laid side to side in the hose bed.
   A. accordion
   B. flat
   C. horseshoe
   D. reverse

_____ 16. A _____ hose load is used when one long hose line is needed.
   A. single
   B. flat
   C. combination
   D. split

_____ 17. The most commonly used attack lines are the
   A. 1½" (38 mm).
   B. 1¾" (45 mm).
   C. 2½" (65 mm).
   D. 3" (76 mm).

_____ 18. A type of hose load that is suited for departments that generally respond to fires in one- or two-story single-family dwellings is the
   A. forward load.
   B. horseshoe load.
   C. flat load.
   D. triple-layer load.

_____ 19. When loading fire hose, a short fold in the hose close to the coupling is known as a(n)
   A. Dutchman.
   B. Short fold.
   C. Reverse fold.
   D. Hose turn.

_____ 20. Preconnected hose lines are used for
   A. supply lines.
   B. standpipe operations.
   C. attack lines.
   D. small trash fires.

Labeling

Label the following diagram with the correct terms.

1. Two engines perform a split hose lay.

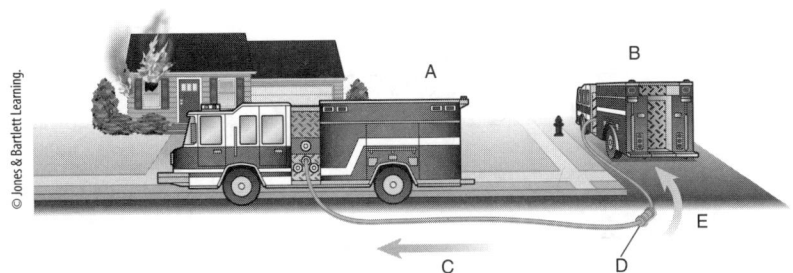

A. _____

B. _____

C. _____

D. _____

E. _____

2. Three basic hose loads are used to load supply hose onto the apparatus.

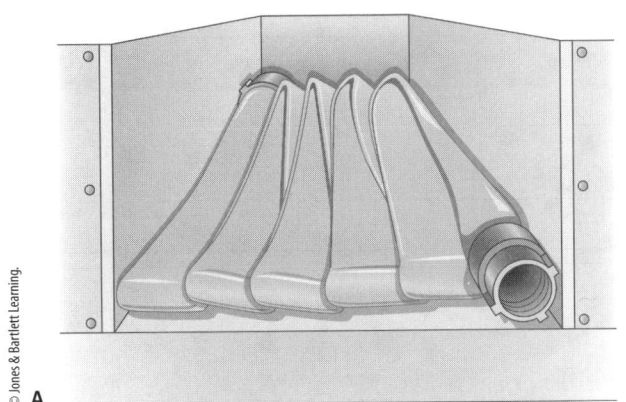

A _____

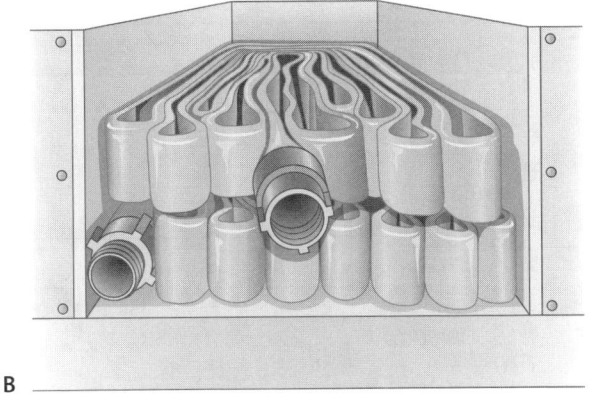

B _____

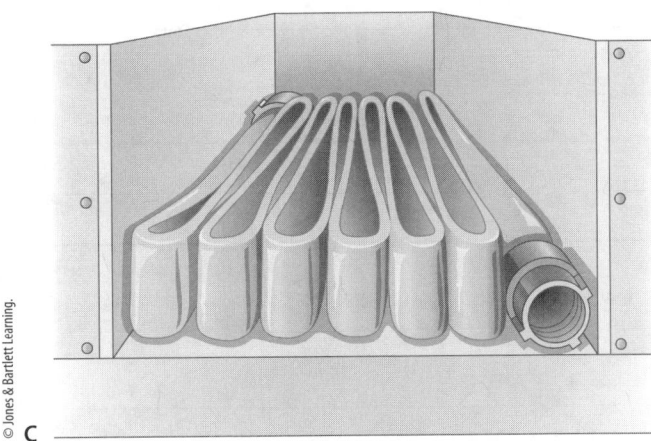

C _____

A. _____

B. _____

C. _____

Vocabulary

Define the following terms using the space provided.

1. Accordion hose load:
   _____
   _____
   _____

2. Forward hose lay:
   _____
   _____
   _____

3. Reverse hose lay:
   _____
   _____
   _____

4. Combination hose load:
   _____
   _____
   _____

5. Dutchman:
   _____
   _____
   _____

6. Split hose bed:
   _____
   _____
   _____

7. Split hose lay:
   _____
   _____
   _____

8. Horseshoe hose load:
   _____
   _____
   _____

9. Flat hose load:
_____
_____
_____

10. Triple-layer load:
_____
_____
_____

Fill-In
Read each item carefully, and then complete the statement by filling in the missing word(s).

1. The objective of laying supply hose is to deliver water from a water supply source to a(n) _____.

2. The _____ hose lay is most often used by the first arriving engine company at the scene of a fire.

3. A _____ hydrant valve ensures that the supply hose can be charged with water immediately using pressure from the hydrant, yet still allows for a second engine to connect to the hose line later to provide pump pressure.

4. The _____ hose load is the easiest loading technique to implement and can be used for any size of attack or supply hose.

5. A fire department connection on a building is provided so that the fire department can pump water into the _____ and _____ systems.

6. Booster hose should not be used for _____ or _____ fires.

7. Attack lines are used for three different types of hose evolutions: offensive, defensive, and _____.

8. When advancing attack lines from the attack engine to the door, when the attack line has been laid out to the entry point, the hose should be flaked out in a _____ pattern.

9. To perform the _____ hose lay, the supply engine stops close to the attack engine, and the supply hose is pulled from the bed of the supply engine and connected to the suction side of the pump on the attack engine.

10. The accordion hose load is not recommended for _____ hose because this kind of hose tends to collapse when placed on its side.

True/False
If you believe the statement to be more true than false, write the letter "T" in the space provided. If you believe the statement to be more false than true, write the letter "F."

1. _____ If a hose line has to be advanced up a ladder, it should be done before the line is charged.

2. _____ The forward hose lay is most often used by the second arriving engine company at the scene of a fire.

3. _____ The reverse hose lay is laid out from the fire to the water source.

4. _____ The split hose bed is used when one long hose line is needed.

5. _____ Soft sleeve hose is used to draft water from a static water source.

6. _____ A Siamese appliance can be used to split one larger hose line into two smaller ones.

7. _____ A defensive attack is conducted from the exterior of the building.

8. _____ Ideally, a hose line crew consists of at least three members at the nozzle and a fourth at the door.

9. _____ Booster hose is especially suited for attacking vehicle fires.

10. _____ The objective of moving hose is to move as much hose as possible.

Short Answer

Complete this section with short written answers using the space provided.

1. List the four purposes of a split hose bed.

   _____
   _____
   _____
   _____

2. Identify the criteria used in determining which techniques to use when advancing attack lines from the attack engine to the door.

   _____
   _____
   _____
   _____

3. Describe the difference between a forward hose lay and a reverse hose lay.

   _____
   _____
   _____
   _____

4. Describe the procedure for replacing a defective section of hose.

   _____
   _____
   _____
   _____

Fire Alarms

The following real case scenarios will give you an opportunity to explore the concerns associated with water supply. Read each scenario, and then answer each question in detail.

1. Your engine company is dispatched to a reported structure fire. Upon arrival, you find a one-story single-family house with heavy dark smoke coming out of the house in Division A. Your officer tells you to get a 1¾" (45-mm) hose line to the front door while she completes the size up. How should you proceed?

   _____
   _____
   _____
   _____

2. Today is your first day as the assigned Driver/Operator for your engine company. In the early evening, you are dispatched to a reported structure fire in a commercial occupancy. As you are getting close to the scene, your officer advises that your company will be the second arriving engine and you need to do a reverse hose lay to provide water supply for the attack engine. How should you proceed?

___

Skill Drills

Skill Drill 16-1: Performing a Forward Hose Lay Fire Fighter I, NFPA 1001: 4.3.15

Test your knowledge of this skill drill by placing the photos below in the correct order. Number the first step with a "1," the second step with a "2," and so on.

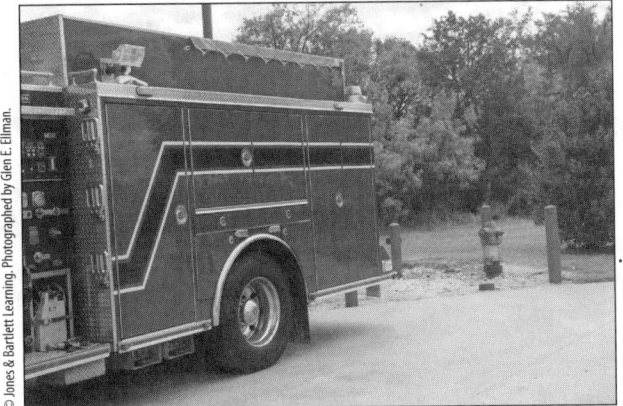

_____ The pump driver/operator stops the fire apparatus 10 ft (3 m) from the fire hydrant.

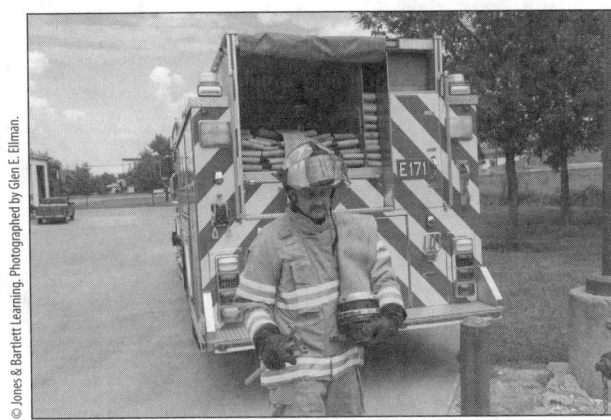

_____ Step off of the apparatus carrying the hydrant wrench and all necessary tools. Grasp enough hose to reach to and loop around the fire hydrant. Loop the end of the hose around the fire hydrant, or secure the hose as specified in the local standard operating procedure (SOP). Do not stand between the hose and the fire hydrant. Never stand on the hose.

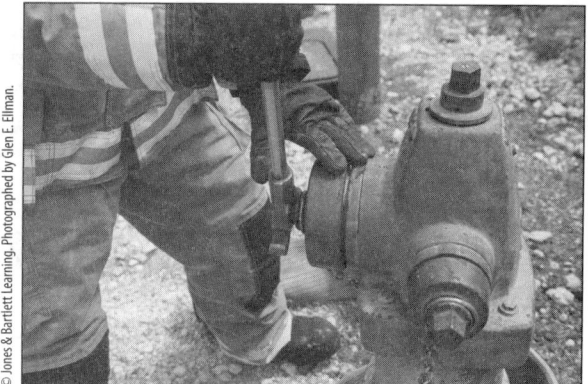

_____ Once the apparatus has moved off and a length of supply hose has been removed from the apparatus and is lying on the ground, remove the appropriate-size fire hydrant cap from the outlet nearest to the fire. Follow the local SOP for checking the operating condition of the fire hydrant.

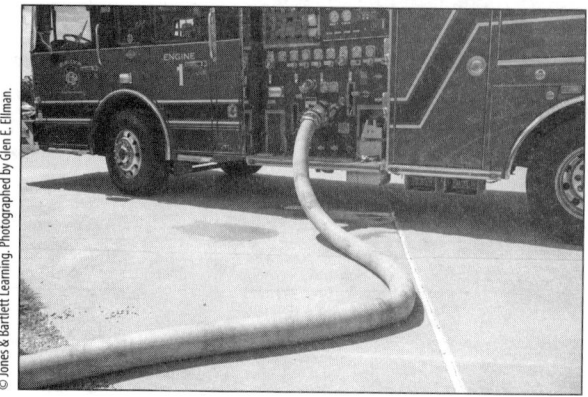

_____ Follow the hose back to the engine, and remove any kinks from the supply hose.

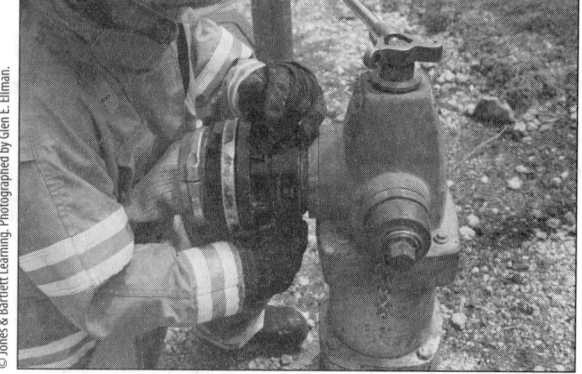

_____ Attach the supply hose to the outlet on the fire hydrant. An adaptor may be needed if a large-diameter hose with Storz-type couplings is used.

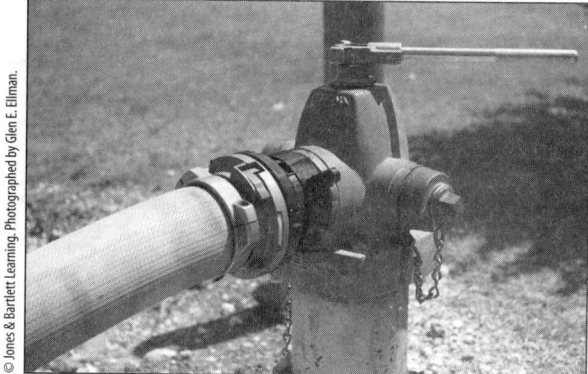

_____ When the pump driver/operator signals to charge the hose by prearranged hand signal, radio, or air horn, open the hydrant valve slowly and completely.

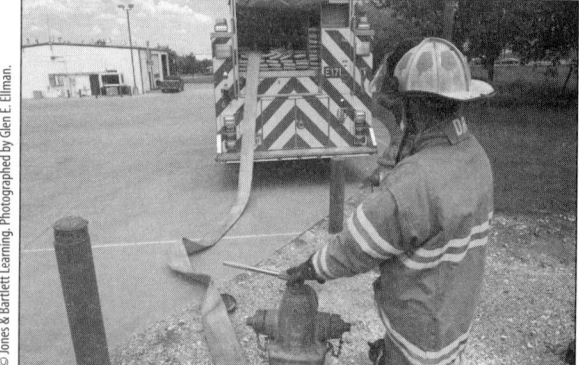

_____ Signal the pump driver/operator to proceed to the fire once the hose is secured.

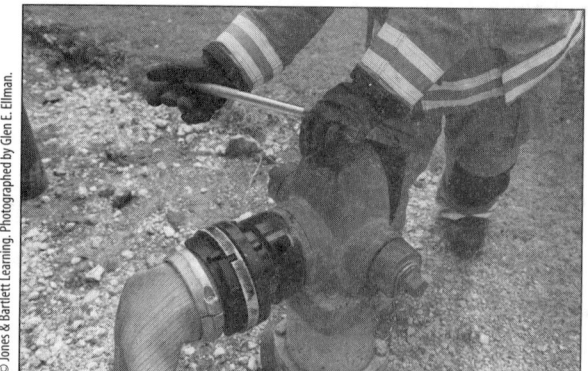

_____ Attach the hydrant wrench to the stem nut on the fire hydrant. Check the top of the hydrant for an arrow indicating the direction to turn to open. The pump driver/operator uncouples the hose and attaches the end of the supply hose to the suction side of the pump on the attack engine or clamps the hose closed to the fire pump, depending on the local SOP.

Skill Drill 16-2: Attaching a Fire Hose to a Four-Way Hydrant Valve Fire Fighter I, NFPA 1001: 4.3.15
Test your knowledge of this skill drill by placing the photos below in the correct order. Number the first step with a "1," the second step with a "2," and so on.

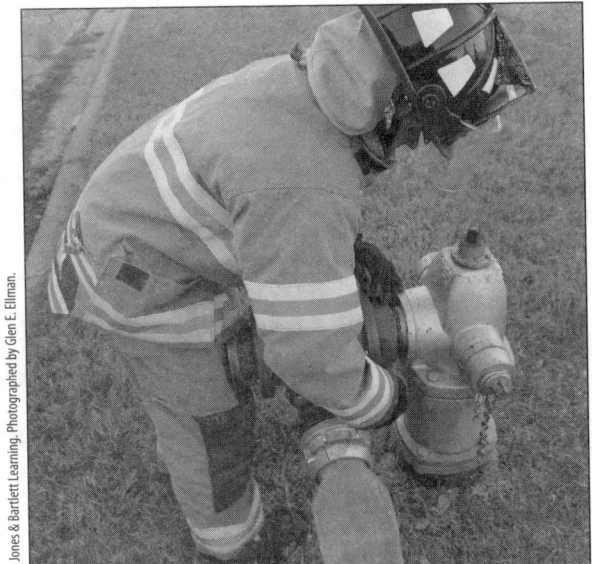

_____ Once enough hose has been removed from the apparatus and is lying on the ground, remove the steamer port (large-diameter port) from the fire hydrant. Follow the local SOP for checking the operating condition of the fire hydrant. Attach the four-way hydrant valve to the fire hydrant outlet (an adaptor may be needed). Attach the hydrant wrench to the fire hydrant. The attack engine driver/operator uncouples the hose and attaches the end of the supply line to the suction side of the pump on the attack engine. The attack engine driver/operator signals by prearranged hand signal, radio, or air horn to charge the supply line. Open the hydrant valve slowly and completely.

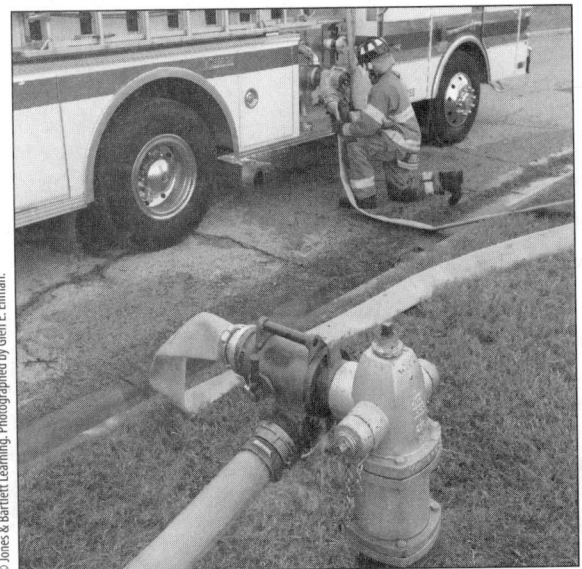

_____ The supply engine driver/operator attaches a hose from the four-way hydrant valve outlet to the suction side of the pump on the supply engine.

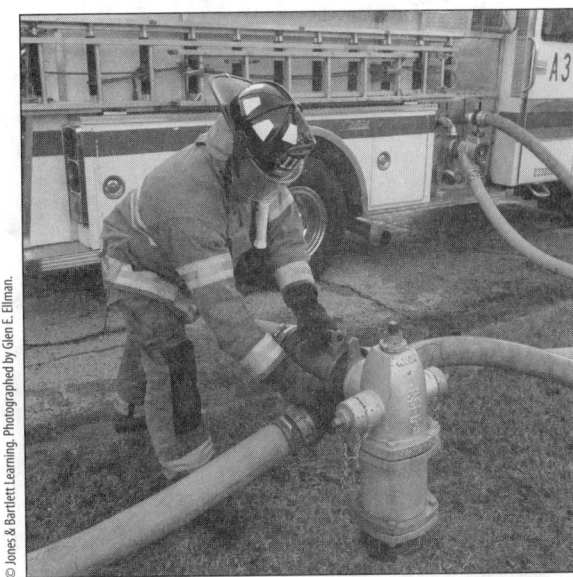

_____ Change the position of the four-way hydrant valve to direct the flow of water from the fire hydrant through the supply engine and into the supply line.

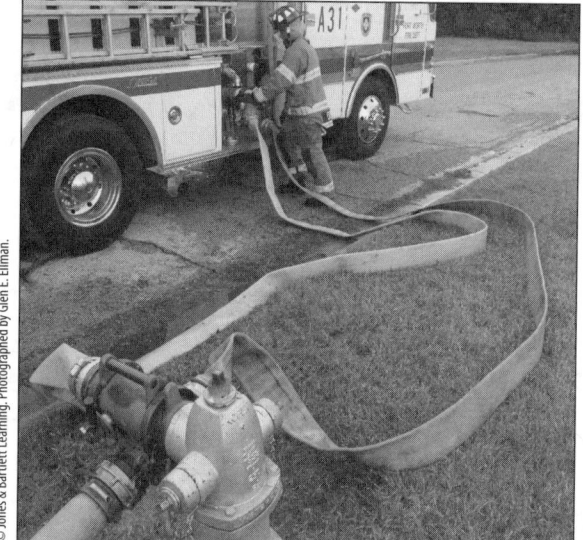

_____ The supply engine driver/operator attaches a second hose to the inlet side of the four-way hydrant valve and connects the other end to the discharge side of the pump on the supply engine.

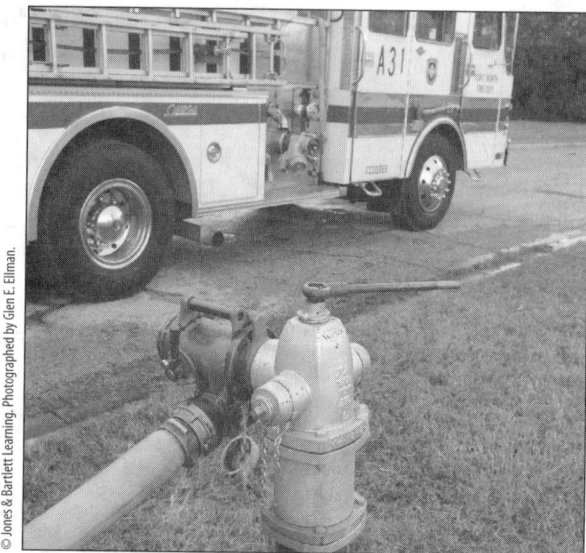

_____ Initially, the attack engine is supplied with water from the fire hydrant. When the supply engine arrives at the fire scene, the supply engine driver/operator stops at the fire hydrant that has the four-way valve.

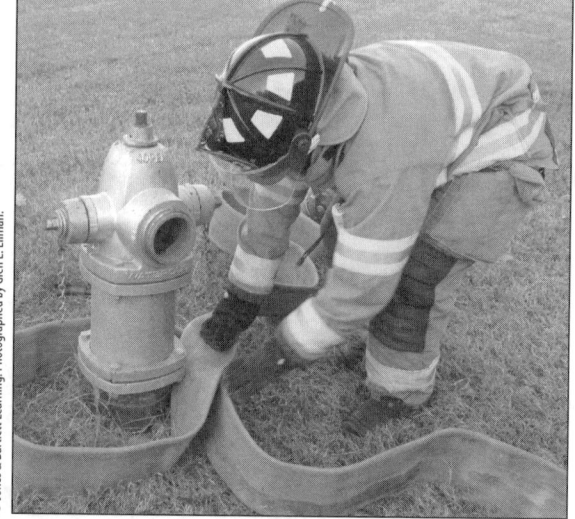

_____ Stop the attack engine 10 ft (3 m) past the fire hydrant to be used. Grasp the four-way hydrant valve, the attached hose, and enough hose to reach to and loop around the fire hydrant. Carry the four-way hydrant valve from the apparatus, along with the hydrant wrench and any other needed tools. Loop the end of the hose around the fire hydrant or secure the hose with a rope as specified in the local SOP. Do not stand between the fire hydrant and hose. Signal the attack engine driver/operator to proceed to the fire.

Skill Drill 16-5: Performing a Flat Hose Load Fire Fighter I, NFPA 1001: 4.5.2
Test your knowledge of the skill drill by filling in the correct words in the photo captions.

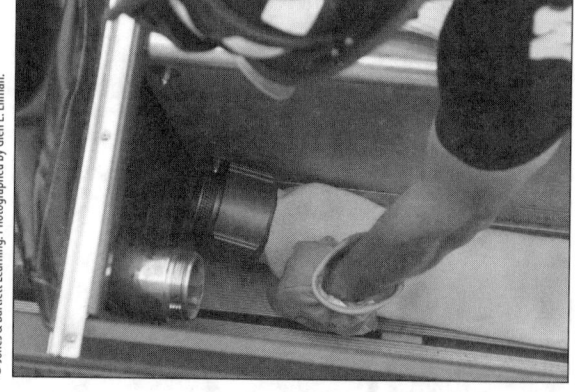

If you are loading supply hose with threaded couplings, determine whether the hose will be used for a forward hose lay or a reverse hose lay. To set up the hose for a forward hose lay, place the _____ hose coupling in the hose bed first. To set up the hose for a reverse hose lay, place the _____ hose coupling in the hose bed first. Start the hose load with the coupling at the front end of the hose bed.

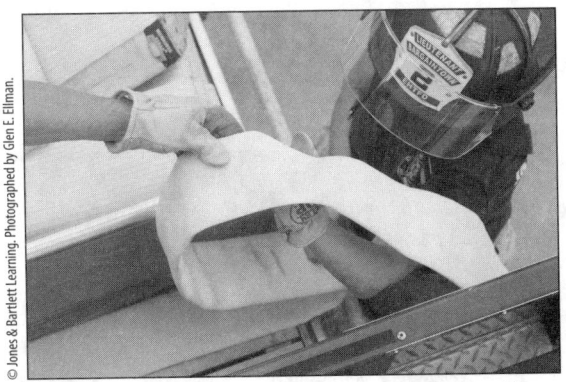

_____ the hose back on itself at the rear of the hose bed.

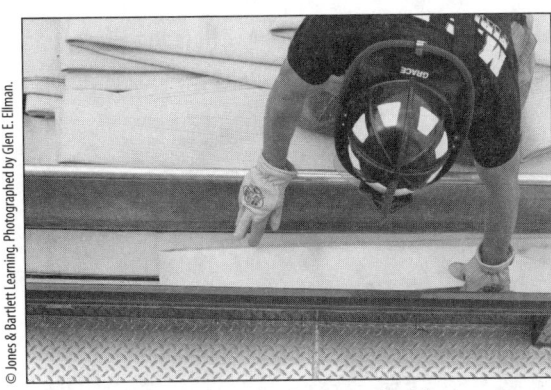

Run the hose back to the front end of the hose bed on top of the previous length of hose. Fold the hose back on itself so that the _____ of the hose is on the previous length.

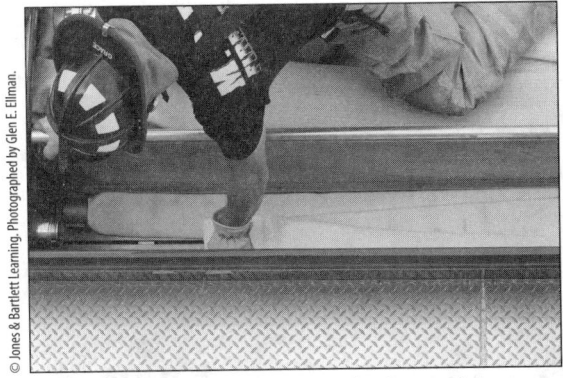

While laying the hose back to the front of the hose bed, _____ the hose to the _____ of the previous fold.

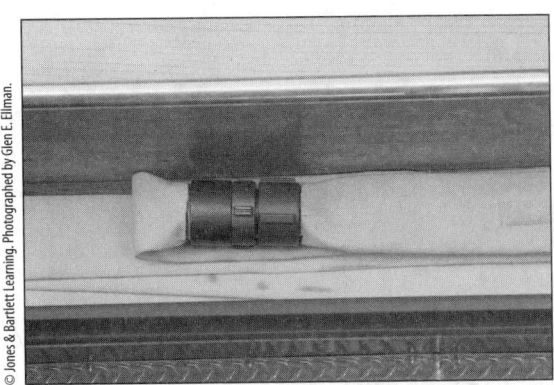

Continue to lay the hose in neat folds until the whole hose bed is covered with a layer of hose. To make this hose load neat, make every other layer of hose slightly _____, or alternate the folds. This keeps the ends from getting too high at the folds. Continue to load the layers of hose until the required amount of hose is loaded.

Skill Drill 16-8: Attaching a Soft Sleeve Hose to a Fire Hydrant Fire Fighter I, NFPA 1001: 4.3.15
Test your knowledge of this skill drill by filling in the correct words in the photo captions.

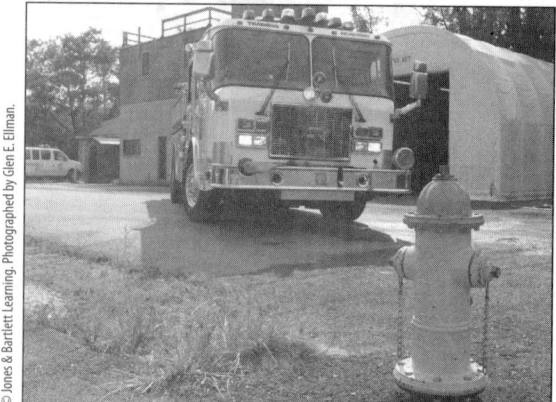

The pump driver/operator positions the apparatus so that the **suction** side of the pump on the attack engine is the correct distance from the fire hydrant. Remove the hose from the hose bed along with any needed adaptors and the hydrant wrench.

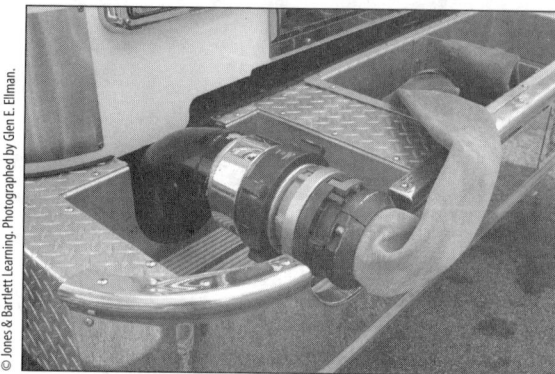

Attach the soft sleeve hose to the suction side of the pump on the attack engine if it is not already attached. In some departments, this end of the hose is preconnected. It may be necessary to use an _____.

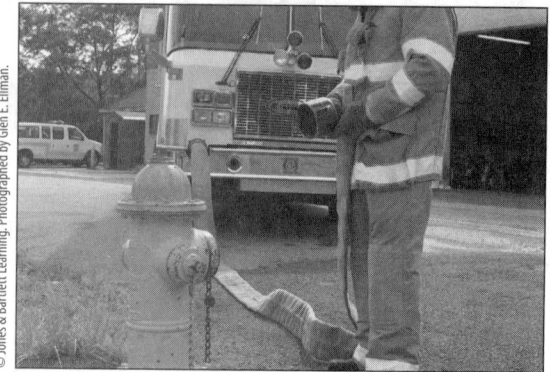

_____ the hose.

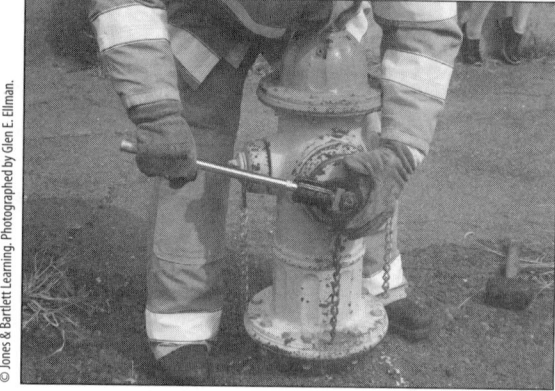

Remove the large fire hydrant _____. Check the fire hydrant for proper operation.

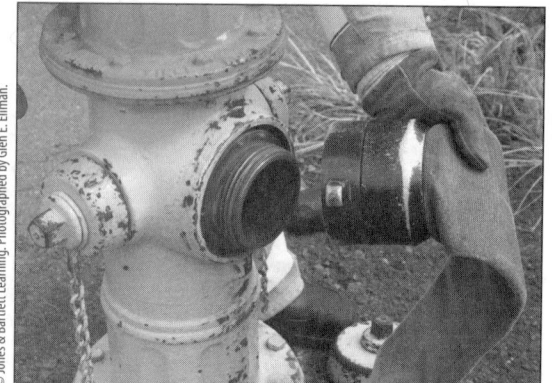

Attach the soft sleeve hose to the fire _____.

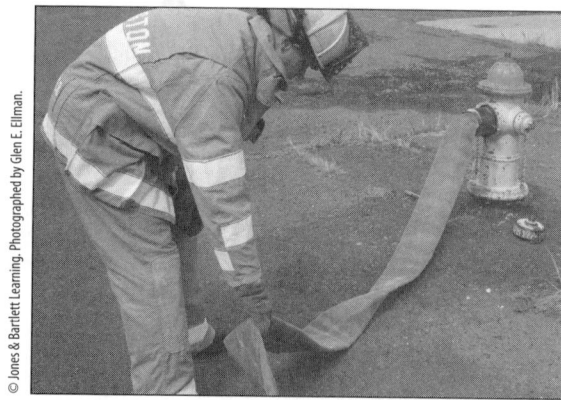

Ensure that there are no kinks or sharp bends in the hose that might _____ the flow of water.

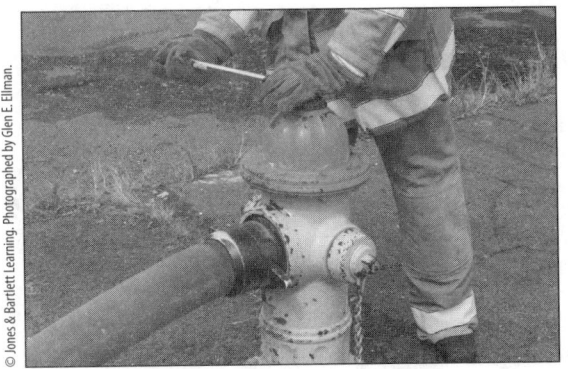

Open the fire hydrant valve slowly when indicated by the driver/operator. Check all connections for _____. Tighten the couplings if necessary.

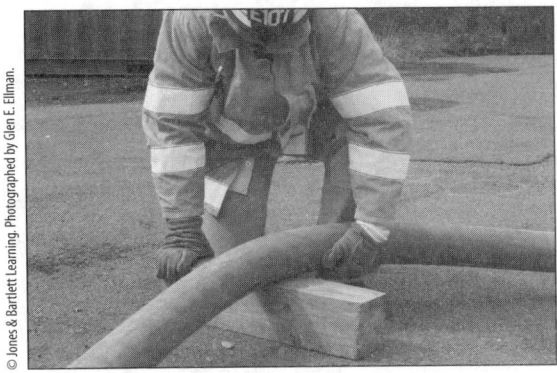

Where required, place _____ _____ under the hose where it contacts the ground to prevent mechanical abrasion.

Skill Drill 16-12: Connecting a Hose Line to Supply a Fire Department Connection Fire Fighter I, NFPA 1001: 4.3.15
Test your knowledge of this skill drill by filling in the correct words in the photo captions.

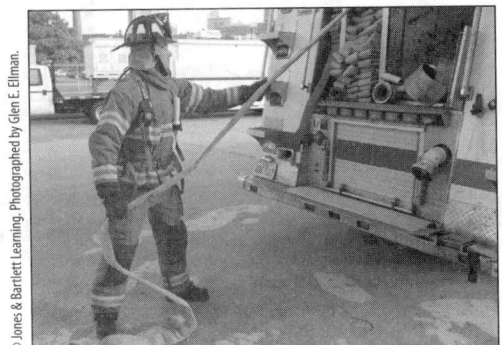

Locate the fire department connection (FDC) to the standpipe or sprinkler system. Extend a hose line from the _____ side of the pump on the engine to the FDC using the size of hose required by the fire department's SOPs. Some fire departments use a single hose line, whereas others call for two or more lines to be connected.

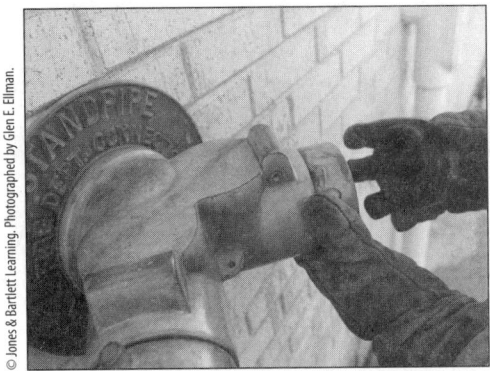

Remove the caps on the standpipe inlet. Some caps are _____ into the connections and must be _____. Other caps are designed to break away when struck with a tool such as a hydrant wrench or spanner wrench.

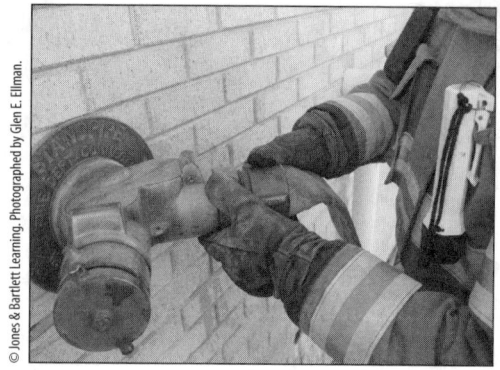

Visually inspect the _____ of the connection on the FDC to ensure it does not contain any debris that might obstruct the water flow. Never stick your hand or fingers inside the connections; fire fighters have been injured from sharp debris left inside these connections. Attach the hose line to the _____. Notify the pump driver/operator when the connection has been completed.

Skill Drill 16-17: Performing a Triple-Layer Hose Load Fire Fighter I, NFPA 1001: 4.5.2
Test your knowledge of this skill drill by filling in the correct words in the photo captions.

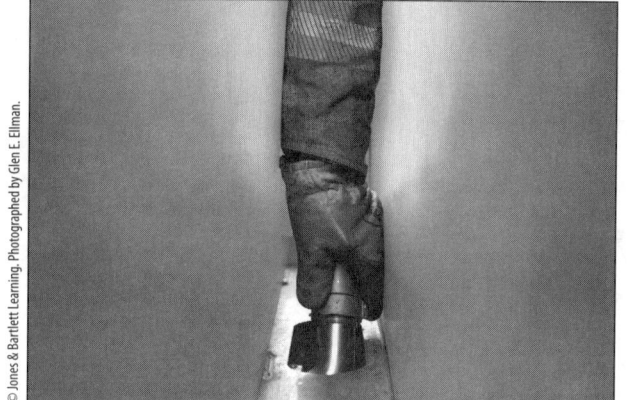

Attach the female end of the hose to the _____ discharge outlet.

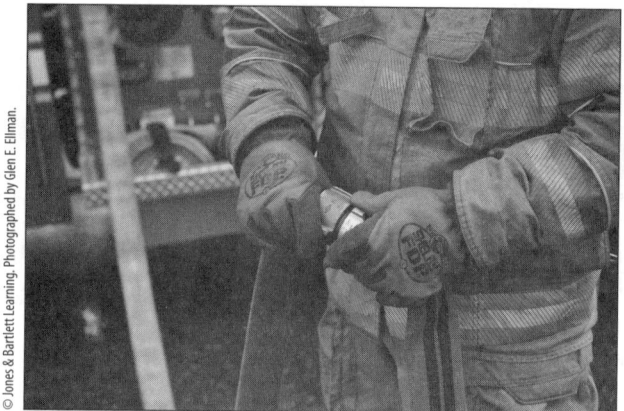

Connect the sections of hose _____.

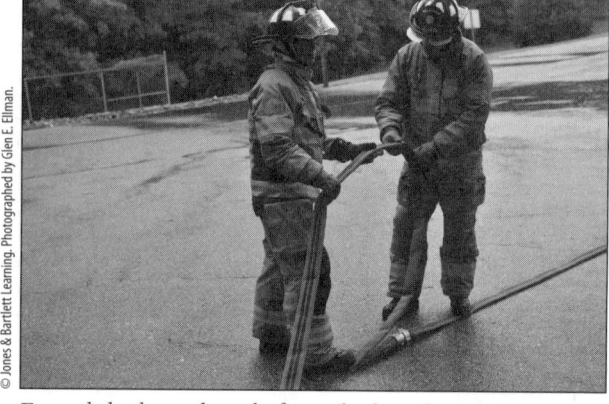

Extend the hose directly from the hose bed. Pick up the hose _____-_____ of the distance from the preconnect discharge outlet to the hose nozzle.

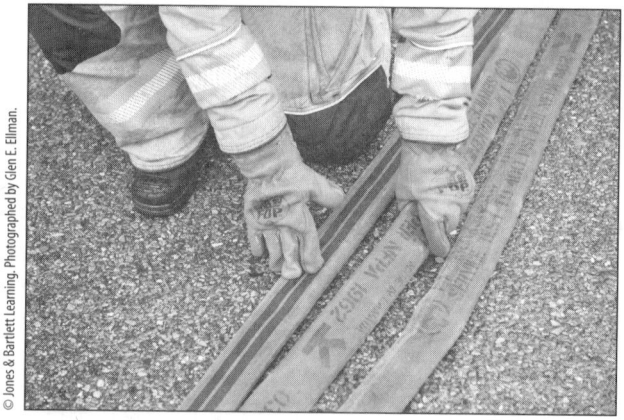

Carry the hose back to the apparatus, forming a _____-layer loop.

Pick up the entire length of _____ _____. (This will take at least two fire fighters).

Lay the triple-folded hose in the hose bed in an _____-_____ with the nozzle on top.

Skill Drill 16-19: Unloading and Advancing Wyed Lines Fire Fighter I, NFPA 1001: 4.3.10
Test your knowledge of this skill drill by placing the photos below in the correct order. Number the first step with a "1," the second step with a "2," and so on.

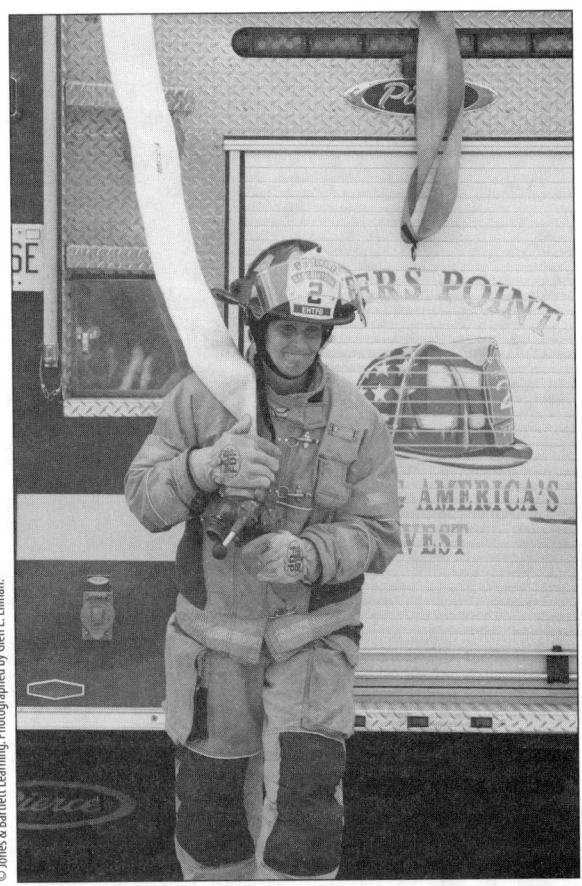

_____ Grasp the wye that is attached to the end of a 2½-in. (65-mm) attack line, and pull it from the bed.

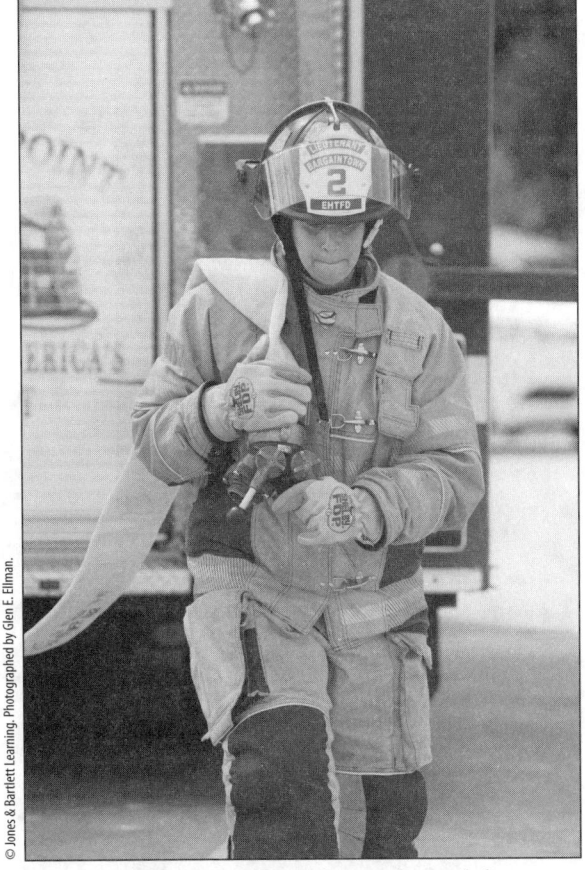

_____ Advance the 2½-in. (65-mm) attack line toward the fire.

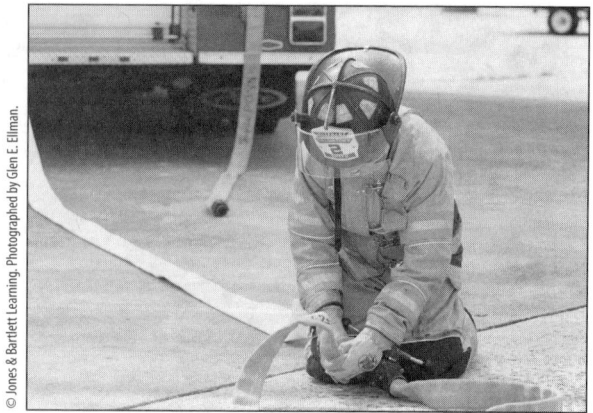

_____ Attach the female end of a second 1¾-in. (45-mm) attack line to the second outlet of the gated wye. The individual ¾-in. (45-mm) attack lines can now be extended to the desired positions.

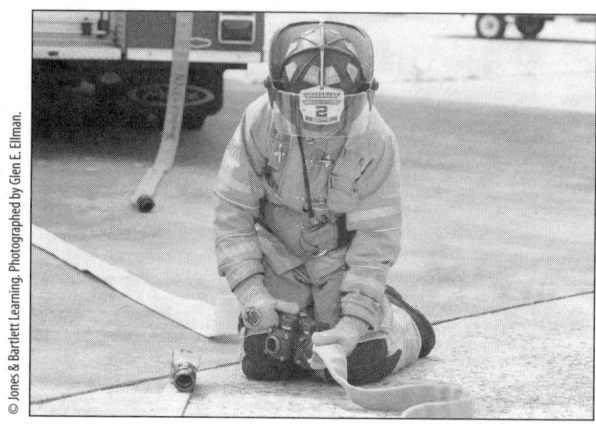

_____ Attach the female end of a 1¾-in. (45-mm) attack line to one outlet on the gated wye.

Skill Drill 16-22: Advancing an Uncharged Attack Line up a Ladder Fire Fighter I, NFPA 1001: 4.3.10
Test your knowledge of this skill drill by filling in the correct words in the photo captions.

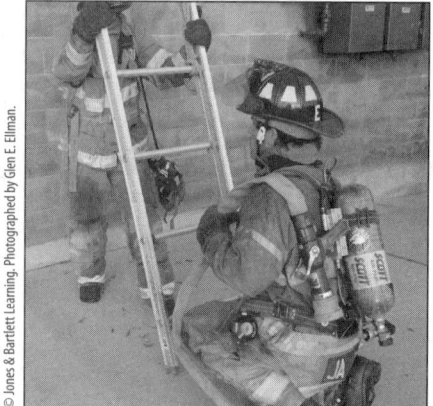

If a hose line needs to be advanced up a ladder, it should be advanced before it is _____. Advance the hose line to the ladder. Pick up the nozzle; place the hose over the chest, with the nozzle draped over the shoulder. Climb up the ladder with the uncharged hose line.

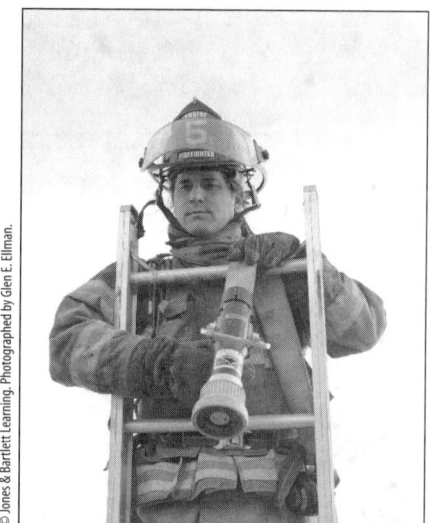

Once the first fire fighter reaches the first _____ section of the ladder, a second fire fighter shoulders the hose to assist advancing the hose line up the ladder. To avoid overloading of the ladder, enforce a limit of one fire fighter per fly section. The nozzle is placed over the top rung of the ladder and advanced into the fire area.

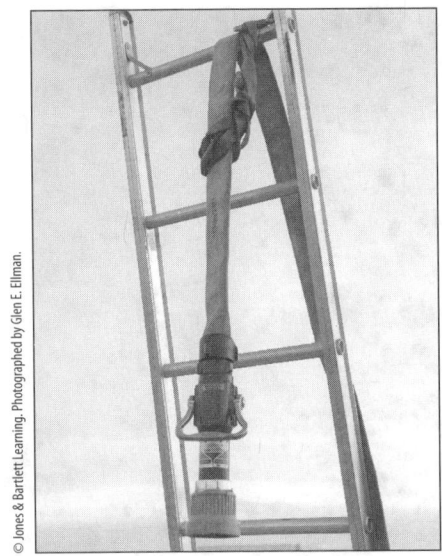

Additional hose can be fed up the ladder until sufficient hose is in position. The hose can be secured to the ladder with a _____ _____ to support its weight and keep it from becoming dislodged.

Skill Drill 16-24: Connecting and Advancing an Attack Line from a Standpipe Outlet Fire Fighter I, NFPA 1001: 4.3.10
Test your knowledge of this skill drill by placing the photos below in the correct order. Number the first step with a "1," the second step with a "2," and so on.

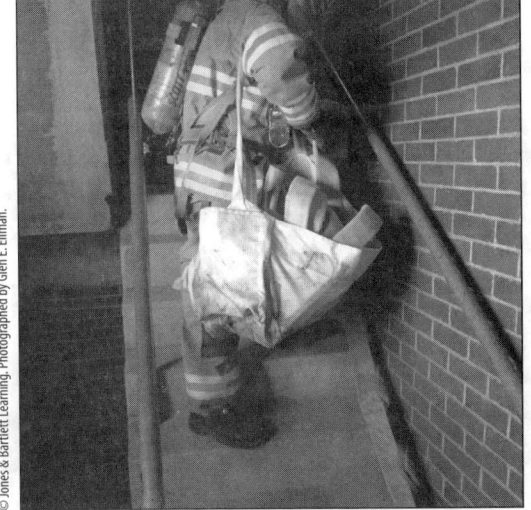

_____ Flake the hose up the stairs to the floor above the fire floor or along a hallway outside the fire compartment. It is better to have too much hose than not enough hose.

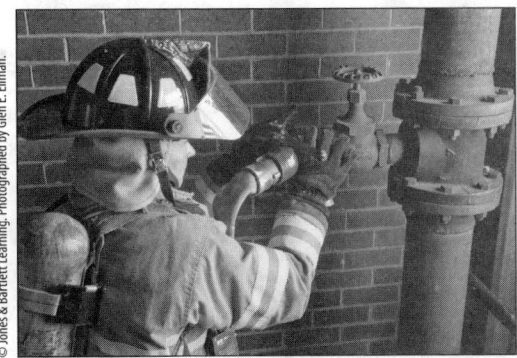

_____ Remove the cap from the standpipe outlet. Open the standpipe valve to flush the standpipe. Attach the proper adaptor or an appliance such as a gated wye to the standpipe outlet.

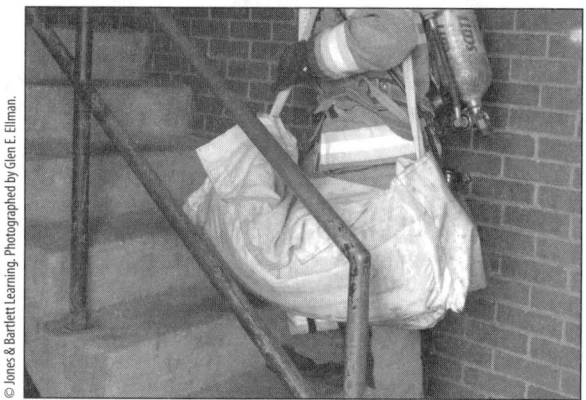

_____ Carry a standpipe hose bundle to the standpipe outlet that is one floor below the fire.

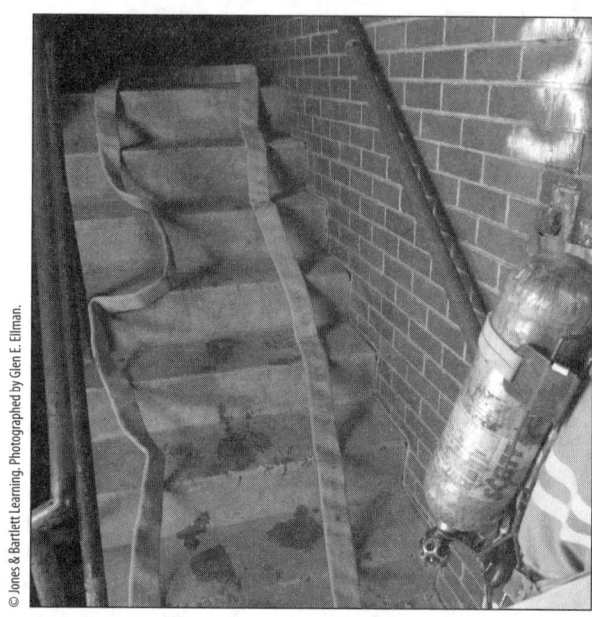

_____ Extend the hose back down to the fire floor and prepare for the fire attack.

Skill Drill 16-26: Draining a Hose Fire Fighter I, NFPA 1001: 4.5.2

Test your knowledge of this skill drill by placing the photos below in the correct order. Number the first step with a "1," the second step with a "2," and so on.

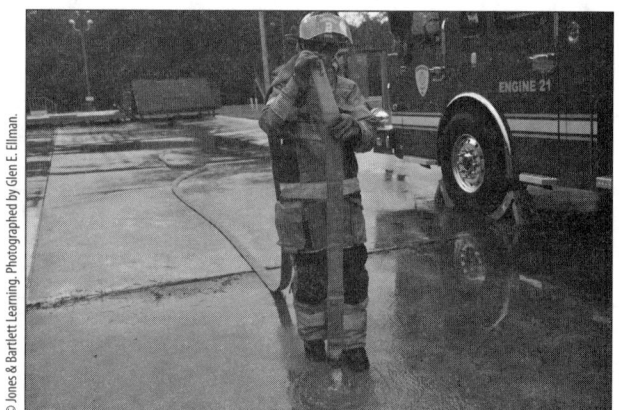

_____ Continue down the length until the entire hose is on the shoulder.

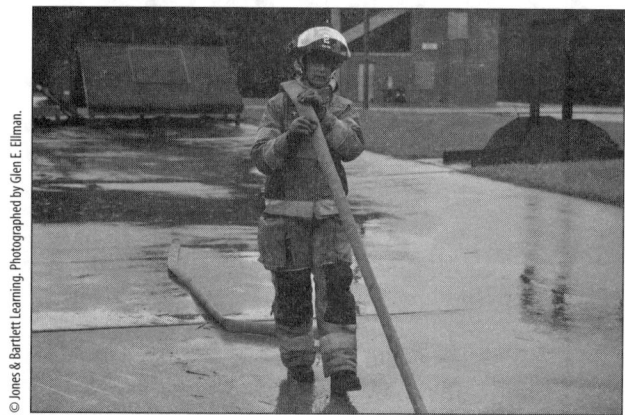

_____ Move down the length of hose, laying it on the ground or folding it back and forth over the shoulder.

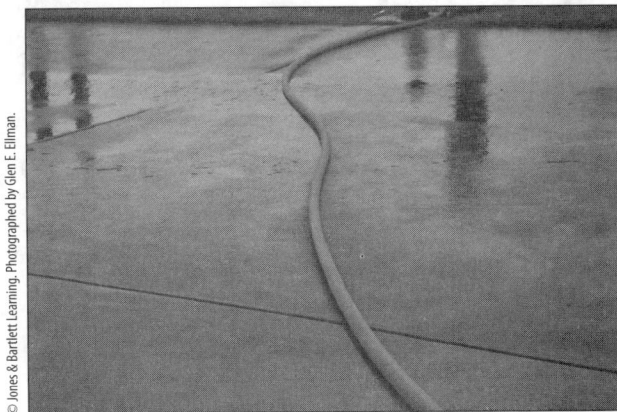
_____ Lay the section of hose straight on a flat surface.

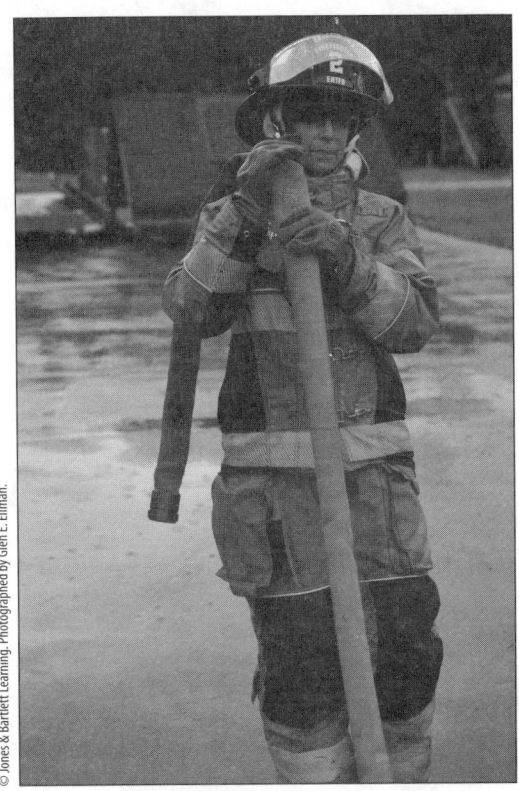
_____ Starting at one end of the hose, lift the hose to shoulder level.

Fire Suppression

Workbook Activities

The following activities have been designed to help you. Your instructor may require you to complete some or all of these activities as a regular part of your fire fighter training program. You are encouraged to complete any activity your instructor does not assign you, as a way to enhance your learning in the classroom.

Chapter Review

The following exercises provide an opportunity to refresh your knowledge of this chapter.

Matching

Match each of the terms in the left column to the appropriate definition in the right column.

_____ 1. Alternative fuel
_____ 2. Defensive operation
_____ 3. Direct attack
_____ 4. Hybrid electric vehicle
_____ 5. Offensive operation
_____ 6. Solar panels
_____ 7. Solid stream
_____ 8. Fog stream
_____ 9. Transitional attack
_____ 10. Combination attack

A. Attack that uses both indirect and direct attack methods
B. Type of steam with greater reach and penetrating power
C. Combines a brief exterior attack followed by an interior attack
D. Type of operation conducted from exterior of building
E. Term used to describe thermal collectors or photovoltaic (PV) modules
F. Used when fire fighters advance hose lines toward a building
G. Type of fire attack that delivers water directly to the base of the fire
H. Vehicle fuel other than gasoline or diesel
I. Vehicle that uses both a battery-powered motor and a liquid-fueled engine
J. A fire stream that divides water into droplets

Multiple Choice

Read each item carefully, and then select the best response.

_____ 1. The type of fire attack used in situations where the fire is heavily involved and the level of risk to fire fighters is high is known as a(n)
　　A. offensive attack.
　　B. defensive attack.
　　C. transitional attack.
　　D. combination attack.

_____ 2. When fighting fires in piled or stacked materials, the greatest danger to fire fighters is
　　A. the possibility that the materials will collapse.
　　B. a sudden flashover.
　　C. rapid fire spread.
　　D. the release of flammable vapors.

CHAPTER 17

_____ 3. A type of vehicle that uses anything other than petroleum-based motor fuel is known as a(n)
   A. dual-fuel vehicle.
   B. battery electric vehicle.
   C. hybrid vehicle.
   D. alternative-fuel vehicle.

_____ 4. When deploying a portable monitor, what determines the number of hose lines needed?
   A. The size of the smooth bore tip being used
   B. The distance between the monitor and the building
   C. The volume of water to be delivered
   D. The size of the fire pump

_____ 5. Which nozzle separates the water into fine droplets?
   A. Smooth-bore nozzles
   B. Fog-stream nozzles
   C. Breakaway nozzles
   D. Cellar nozzles

_____ 6. The most commonly used master stream devices flow between _____ and _____ gpm.
   A. 50 and 2500
   B. 250 and 2000
   C. 500 and 1000
   D. 350 and 1500

_____ 7. Only Class _____ extinguishing agents should be used for energized electrical equipment involved in a fire.
   A. A
   B. B
   C. C
   D. K

_____ 8. The objective of a(n) _____ attack is to apply water to the hot gases by sweeping the ceiling with water to cool the gases and droplets.
   A. defensive
   B. indirect
   C. blitz
   D. offensive

_____ 9. A type of vehicle fuel that is derived from agricultural products such as grains or grasses is known as
   A. biofuel.
   B. agrifuel.
   C. hybrid fuel.
   D. blended fuel.

_____ 10. _____ fires are one of the most common types of fires handled by fire departments.
   A. Structure
   B. Electrical
   C. Dumpster
   D. Vehicle

_____ 11. What is considered the lowest safe operating angle for portable monitors?
   A. 15 degrees
   B. 30 degrees
   C. 35 degrees
   D. 60 degrees

_____ 12. A type of fire attack that employs both the indirect and direct attack methods is known as a
   A. transitional attack.
   B. combination attack.
   C. preconnect attack.
   D. flow path attack.

_____ 13. A type of fire nozzle that has a greater reach and penetrating power is a
   A. booster stream nozzle.
   B. combination nozzle.
   C. fog nozzle.
   D. smooth-bore nozzle.

_____ 14. When two fire fighters are operating a large handline, the backup fire fighter should be positioned approximately _____ behind the nozzle operator.
   A. 2 ft (0.6 m)
   B. 3 ft (0.9 m)
   C. 5 ft (1.5 m)
   D. 8 ft (2.4 m)

_____ 15. A by-product of burning wood that coats the inside of a chimney and builds up over time is known as
   A. ash.
   B. soot.
   C. creosote.
   D. carbon.

Labeling

Label the following diagram with the correct terms.

1. Fog-stream nozzles produce straight streams or multiple fog streams.

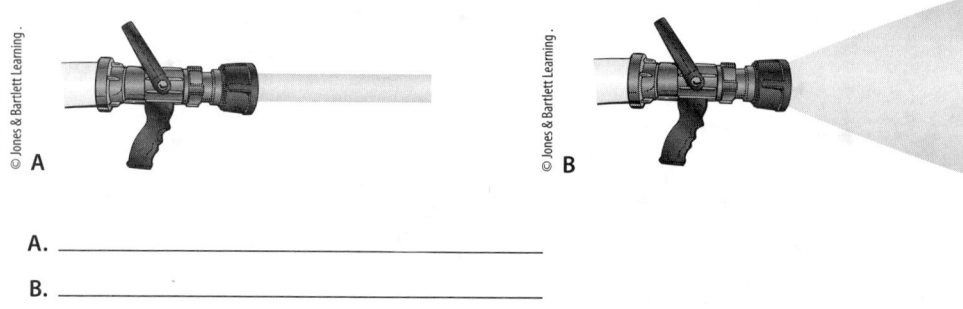

A. _____

B. _____

2. Roof vents will affect how fires grow and spread.

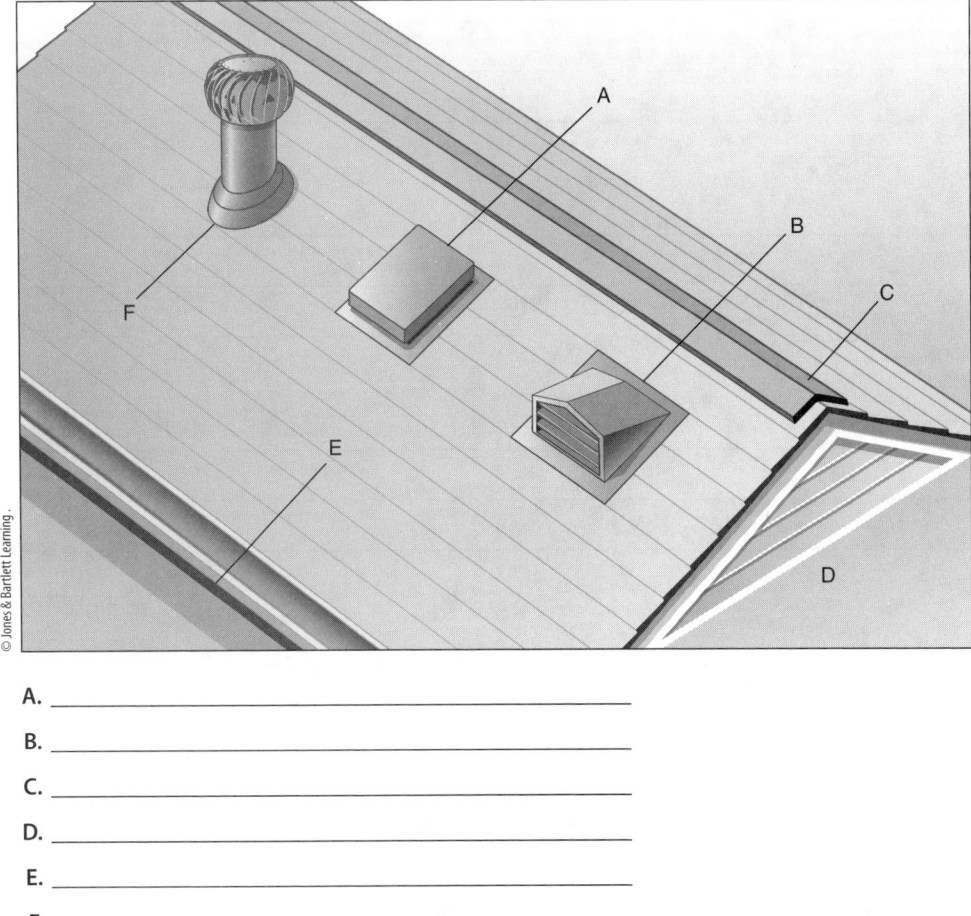

A. _____

B. _____

C. _____

D. _____

E. _____

F. _____

Vocabulary

Define the following terms using the space provided.

1. Solar photovoltaic (PV) systems:

_____
_____
_____

2. Hybrid electric vehicle:

_____
_____
_____

3. Fuel cells:

_____
_____
_____

Fundamentals of Fire Fighter Skills

4. Offensive operation:

_____
_____
_____

5. Defensive operation:

_____
_____
_____

6. Ladder pipe:

_____
_____
_____

7. Soffit:

_____
_____
_____

8. Alternative-fuel vehicle:

_____
_____
_____

9. Conventional vehicle:

_____
_____
_____

10. Combination attack:

_____
_____
_____

Fill-In

Read each item carefully, and then complete the statement by filling in the missing word(s).

1. The decision regarding the type of fire attack is made by the _____.

2. A combination attack begins with an indirect attack and continues with a(n) _____ attack.

3. A _____ is permanently mounted on a vehicle.

4. When attacking a vehicle fire, fire fighters should approach from a(n) _____ position, moving in at a _____ degree angle.

5. A fire in the trunk area of an automobile can be assessed by first using the pick of a _____ tool.

6. Liquified _____ gas is also known as propane.

7. One consideration when selecting and operating nozzles is the amount of _____ that is moved along with the water.

8. At least _____ team members are needed to advance and maneuver a 2½-in. (65-mm) handline inside a building.

9. Attic fires that start outside often start as a _____ fire.

10. _____ is often the primary objective at lumberyard fires.

True/False

If you believe the statement to be more true than false, write the letter "T" in the space provided. If you believe the statement to be more false than true, write the letter "F."

1. _____ A master stream device can be either manually operated or directed by remote control.
2. _____ There is usually a single switch that will disable a photovoltaic (PV) system.
3. _____ Most of the vehicles on the road today are conventional vehicles that use internal combustion engines.
4. _____ One of the biggest hazards faced by fire fighters when fighting vehicle fires is the dangers posed by traffic.
5. _____ A straight stream has a shorter reach than a fog stream, given similar water flow rates and nozzle pressure.
6. _____ Master stream devices are used when large quantities of water are needed to control a large fire.
7. _____ A defensive attack is conducted from the exterior of the building.
8. _____ Battery electric vehicles also have a liquid-fueled engine.
9. _____ Lumberyard fires are often prime candidates for defensive firefighting operations.
10. _____ Master streams are used mainly during offensive operations.

Short Answer

Complete this section with short written answers using the space provided.

1. List three locations where an attic fire can start.

_____
_____
_____
_____

2. Identify four of the challenges presented by basement fires.

_____
_____
_____
_____

3. Describe the challenges of fires in buildings during construction, renovation, or demolition.

___

4. Describe the difference between battery electric vehicles and hybrid electric vehicles.

___

Fire Alarms

The following real case scenarios will give you an opportunity to explore the concerns associated with water supply. Read each scenario, and then answer each question in detail.

1. Your engine company is dispatched to a reported chimney fire. Upon arrival, you find a two-story single-family house with smoke coming out of the chimney and light smoke on the first floor. Your size-up confirms that the fire is confined to the chimney. How should you proceed with the fire attack?

___

2. You are assigned as the fire fighter on an engine company that will be the third arriving engine at a large lumberyard fire. As you get closer to the scene, your officer advises that your company will be setting up the portable monitor in Division D of the building. Upon arrival, how should you proceed?

___

Skill Drills

Skill Drill 17-1: Performing the Transitional Attack Fire Fighter I, NFPA 1001: 4.3.10

Test your knowledge of this skill drill by placing the photos below in the correct order. Number the first step with a "1," the second step with a "2," and so on.

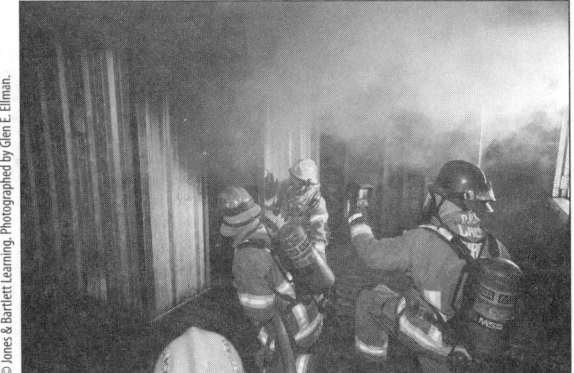

_____ Shut the nozzle off, and reassess the fire conditions. Confirm that ventilation has been completed.

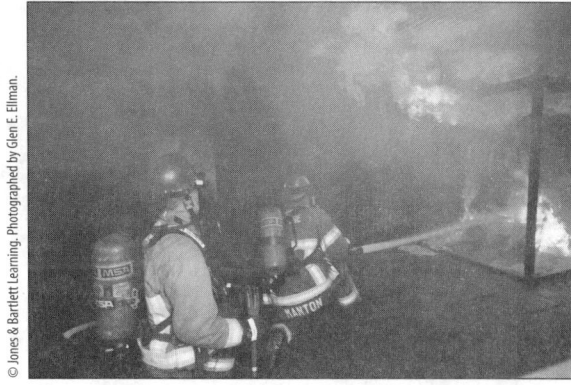

_____ If it is safe to do so, advance into the fire compartment and apply water to the base of the fire. If it is not safe to advance into the fire compartment, apply water from a safe location such as a hallway, adjoining room, or doorway, until the room begins to darken.

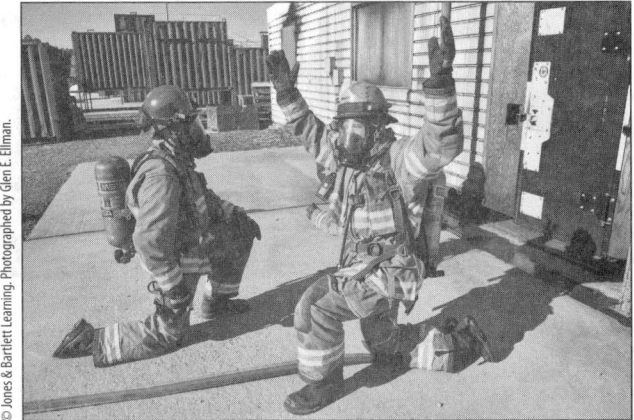

_____ Notify the pump driver/operator that you are ready for water. Open the nozzle to purge air from the system, and make sure water is flowing. If using an adjustable nozzle, ensure that it is set to the proper nozzle pattern for entry. Shut down the nozzle until you are in a position to apply water.

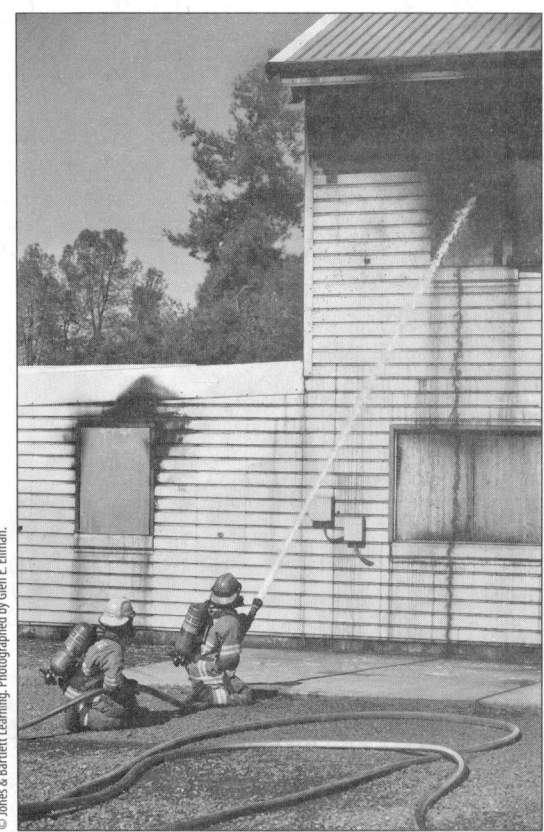

_____ If fire has vented from a door or window, apply a straight stream through the top of the opening from a safe, exterior location so it deflects off the ceiling. Evaluate the effectiveness of the hose stream before transitioning to an interior fire attack.

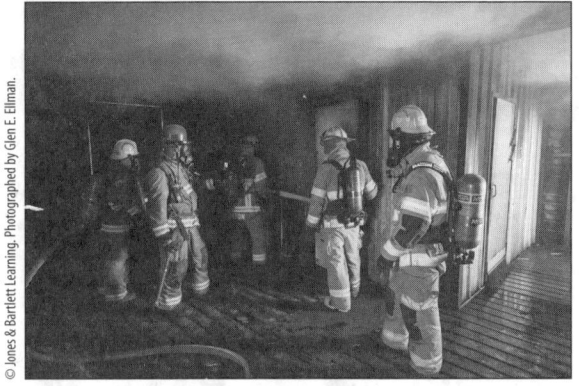 _____ Locate and extinguish hot spots until the fire is completely extinguished.

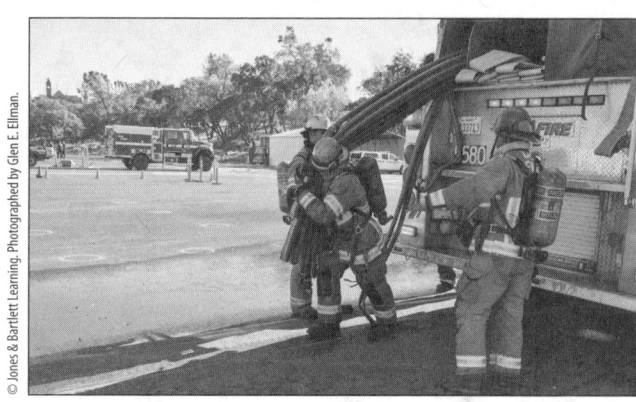 _____ Don full personal protective equipment (PPE) and self-contained breathing apparatus (SCBA). Select the proper handline to be used to attack the fire based on the fire's size, location, and type. Advance the hose line from the apparatus to the entry point of the structure. Flake out excess hose in front of the entry point.

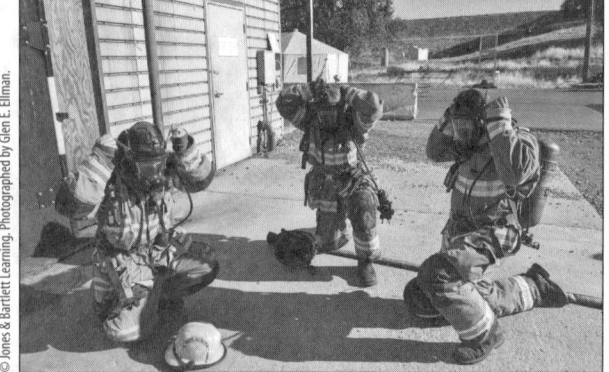 _____ Don the face piece, and activate the SCBA and personal alert safety system (PASS) device prior to entering the building.

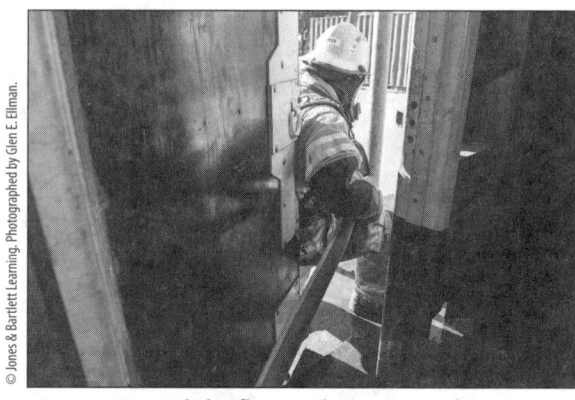 _____ Control the flow path as crews advance toward the fire.

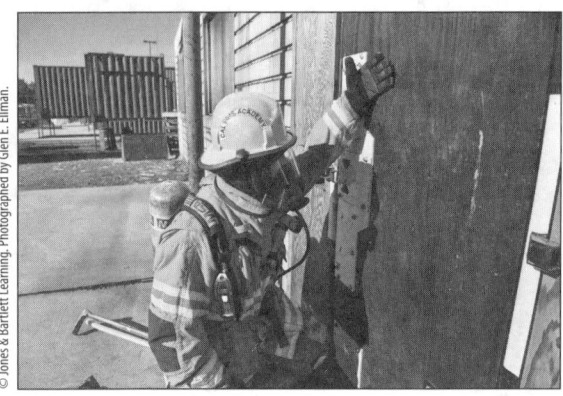 _____ Check the entry door for heat before making entry.

Skill Drill 17-2: Performing a Direct Attack Fire Fighter I, NFPA 1001: 4.3.10

Test your knowledge of this skill drill by placing the photos below in the correct order. Number the first step with a "1," the second step with a "2," and so on.

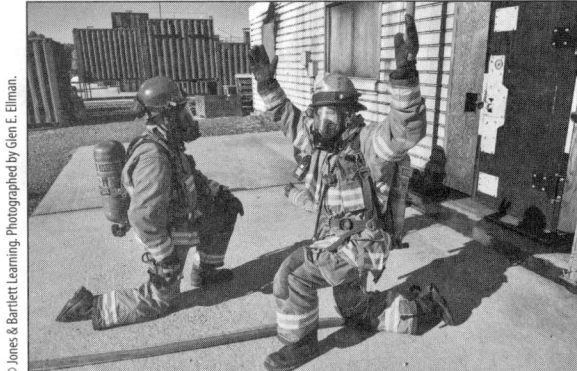

_____ Notify the pump driver/operator that you are ready for water.

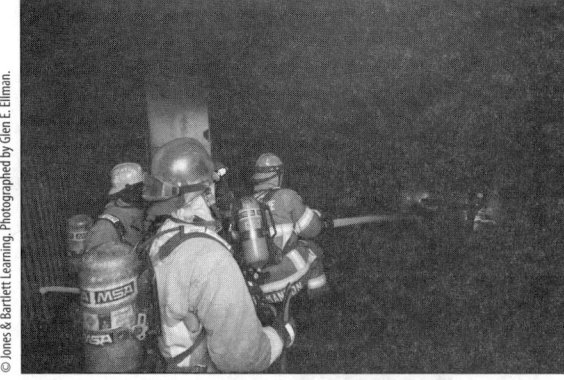

_____ Shut the nozzle off, and reassess the fire conditions. Confirm that ventilation has been completed. Locate and extinguish hot spots until the fire is completely extinguished.

_____ Open the nozzle to purge air from the system, and make sure water is flowing. If using an adjustable nozzle, ensure that it is set to the proper nozzle pattern for entry. Shut down the nozzle until you are in a position to apply water.

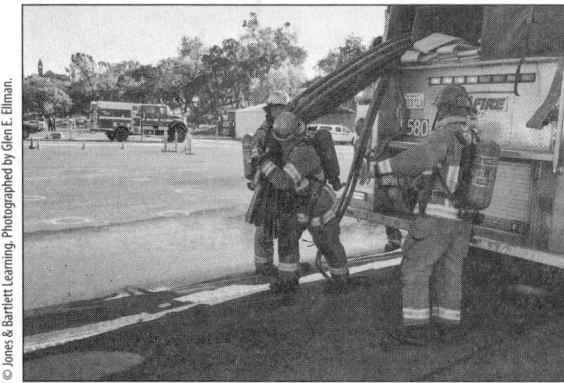

_____ Don full PPE and SCBA. Select the proper handline to be used to attack the fire based on the fire's size, location, and type. Advance the hose line from the apparatus to the entry point of the structure. Flake out excess hose in front of the entry point.

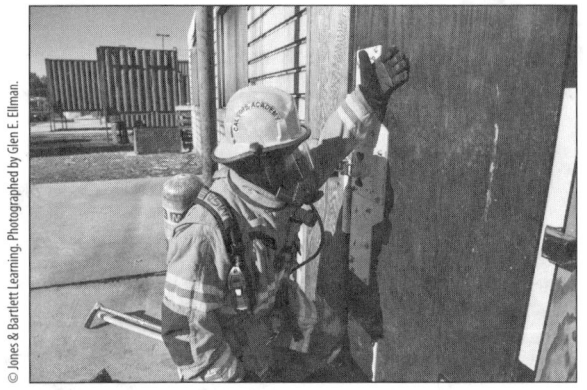

_____ Check the entry door for heat before making entry.

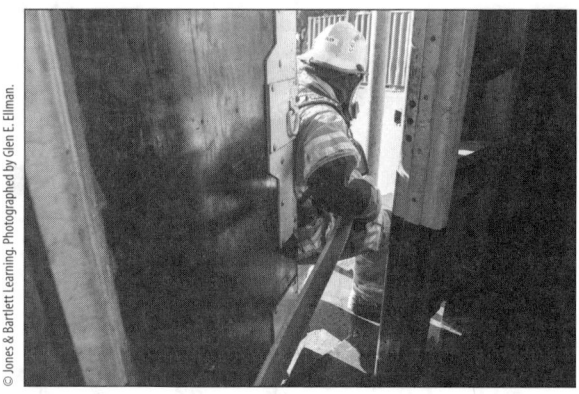

_____ Control the flow path as crews advance toward the fire.

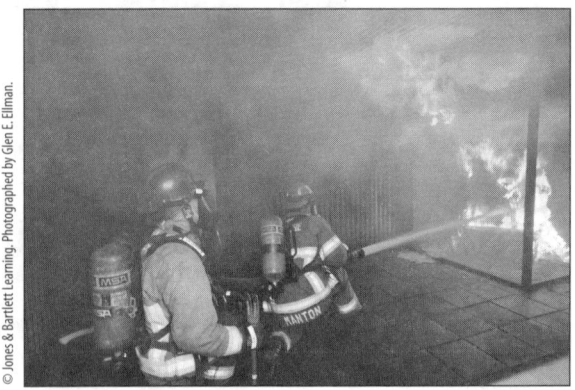

_____ If it is safe to do so, advance into the fire compartment, and apply water to the base of the fire.

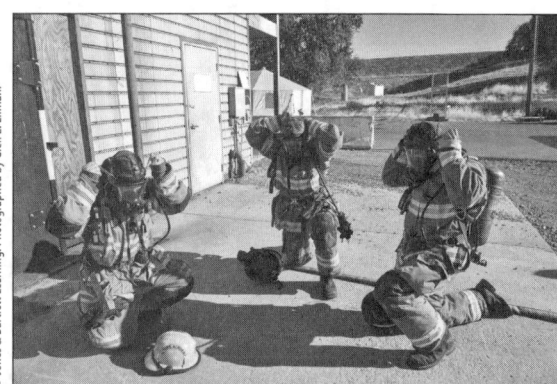

_____ Don the face piece, and activate the SCBA and PASS device prior to entering the building.

Skill Drill 17-3: Performing an Indirect Attack Fire Fighter I, NFPA 1001: 4.3.10

Test your knowledge of this skill drill by placing the photos below in the correct order. Number the first step with a "1," the second step with a "2," and so on.

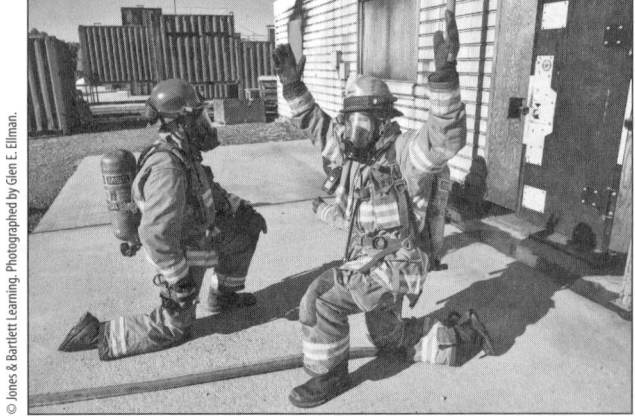

_____ Notify the pump driver/operator that you are ready for water.

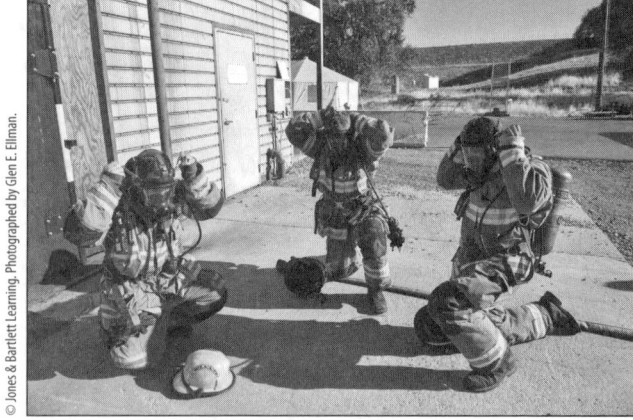

_____ Don the face piece, and activate the SCBA and PASS device prior to entering the building.

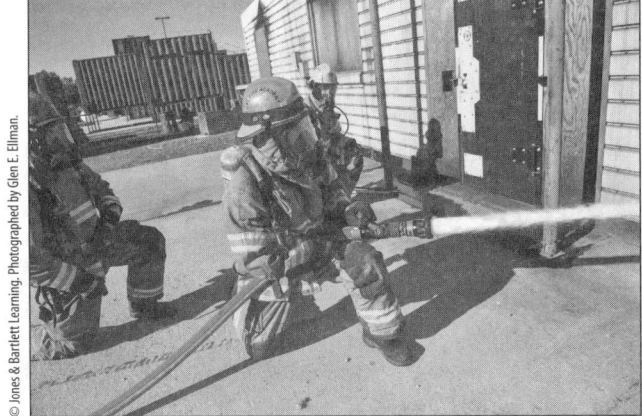

_____ Open the nozzle to purge air from the system, and make sure water is flowing. If using an adjustable nozzle, ensure that it is set to the proper nozzle pattern for entry. Shut down the nozzle until you are in a position to apply water.

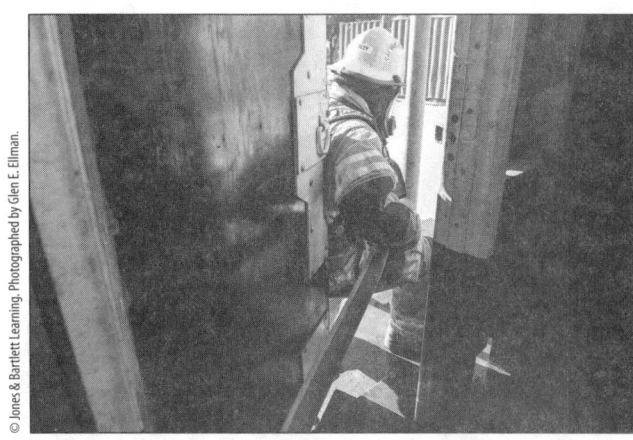

_____ Control the flow path as crews advance toward the fire.

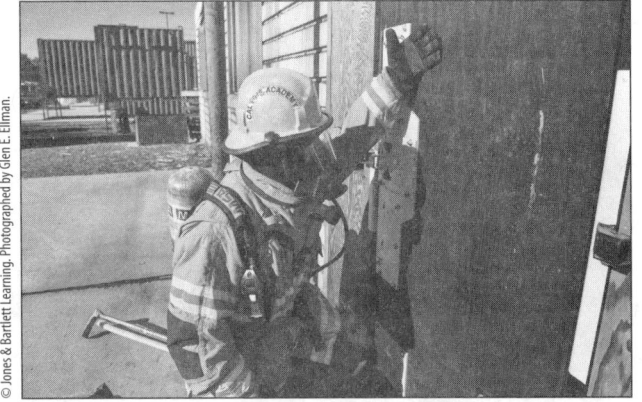

_____ Check the entry door for heat before making entry.

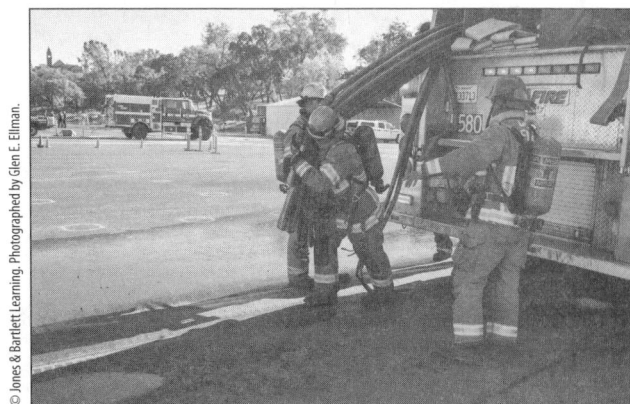

_____ Don full PPE and SCBA. Select the proper handline to be used to attack the fire based on the fire's size, location, and type. Advance the hose line from the apparatus to the entry point of the structure. Flake out excess hose in front of the entry point.

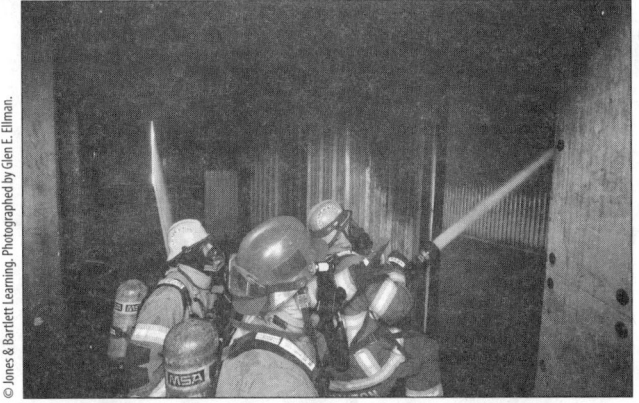

_____ From the safest location, such as a hallway, adjoining room, or doorway, apply water to the superheated gases at the ceiling, and move the stream back and forth. Flow water until the room begins to darken.

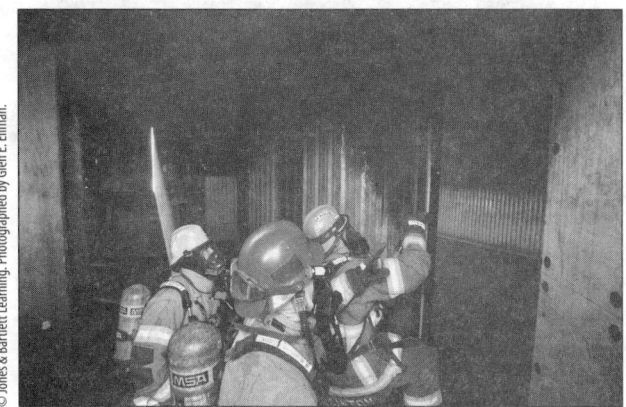

_____ Shut the nozzle off, and reassess the fire conditions. Confirm that ventilation has been completed. Locate and extinguish hot spots until the fire is completely extinguished.

Skill Drill 17-4: Performing a Combination Attack Fire Fighter I, NFPA 1001:4.3.10
Test your knowledge of this skill drill by filling in the correct words in the photo captions.

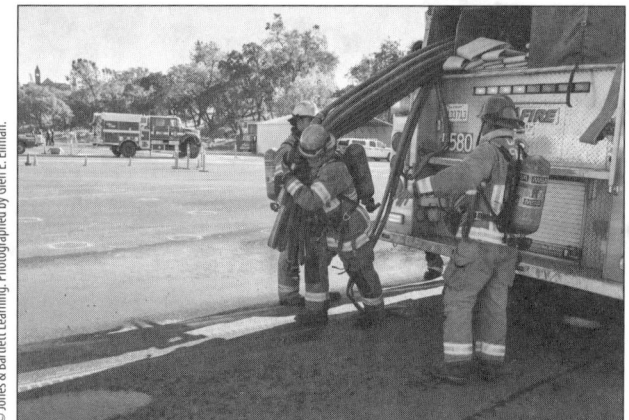

Don full _____ and _____. Select the proper handline to be used to attack the fire based on the fire's size, location, and type. Advance the hose line from the apparatus to the entry point of the structure. Flake out excess hose in front of the entry point.

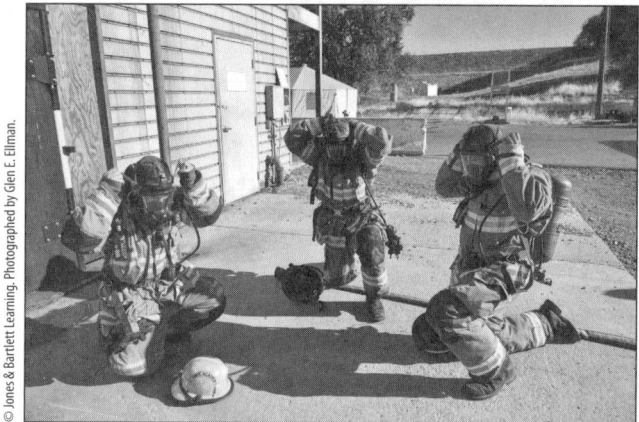

Don the face piece, and activate the SCBA and _____ device prior to entering the building.

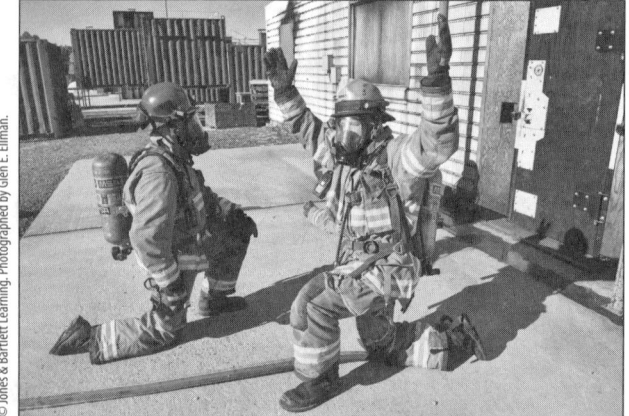

Notify the pump driver/operator that you are ready for _____.

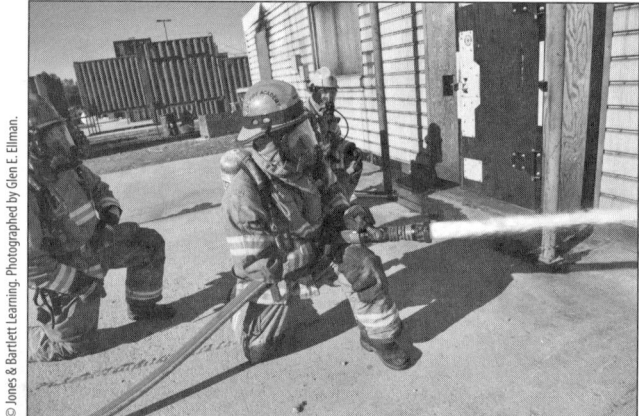

Open the nozzle to purge air from the system, and make sure water is flowing. If using an adjustable nozzle, ensure it is set to the proper nozzle _____ for entry. Shut down the nozzle until you are in a position to apply water.

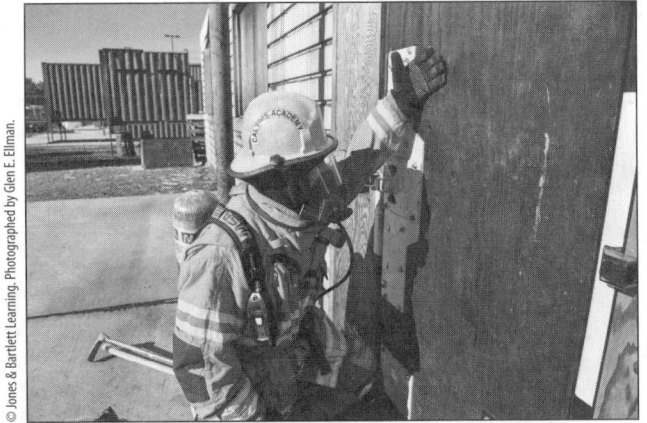
Check the entry door for _____ before making entry.

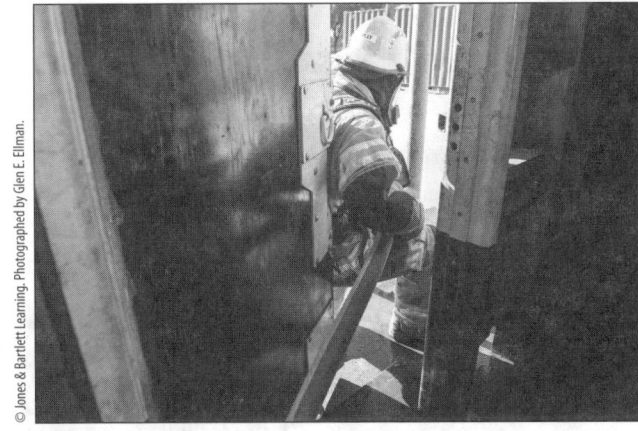
Control the _____ _____ as crews advance toward the fire.

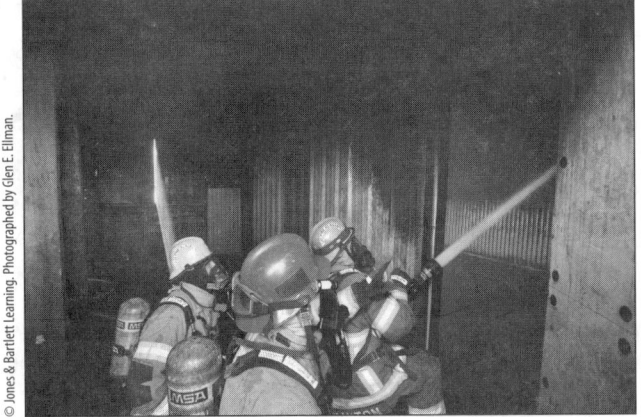
From the safest location, such as a hallway, adjoining room, or doorway, apply water to the superheated gases at the ceiling, and move the stream back and forth. Flow water until the room begins to _____.

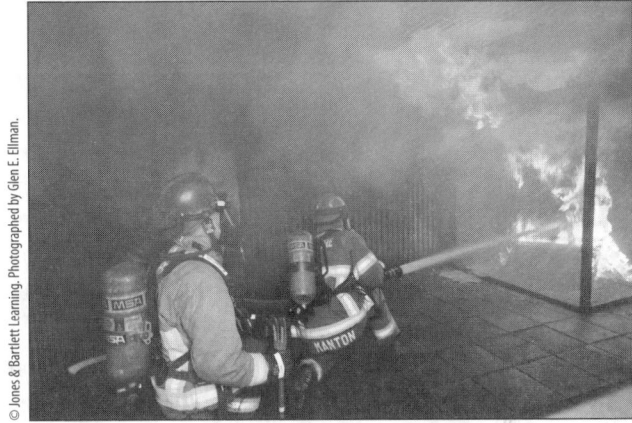
If it is safe to do so, advance into the fire compartment, and apply water to the _____ of the fire.

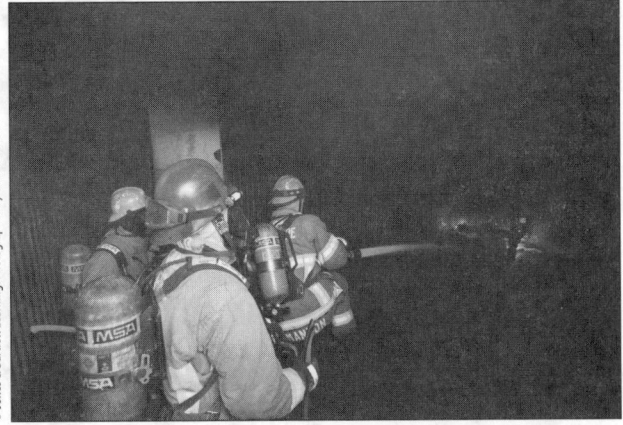
Shut the nozzle off, and reassess the fire conditions. Confirm that _____ has been completed. Locate and extinguish hot spots until the fire is completely extinguished.

Skill Drill 17-5: Performing the One-Fire Fighter Method for Operating a Large Handline Fire Fighter I, NFPA 1001: 4.3.8
Test your knowledge of this skill drill by filling in the correct words in the photo captions.

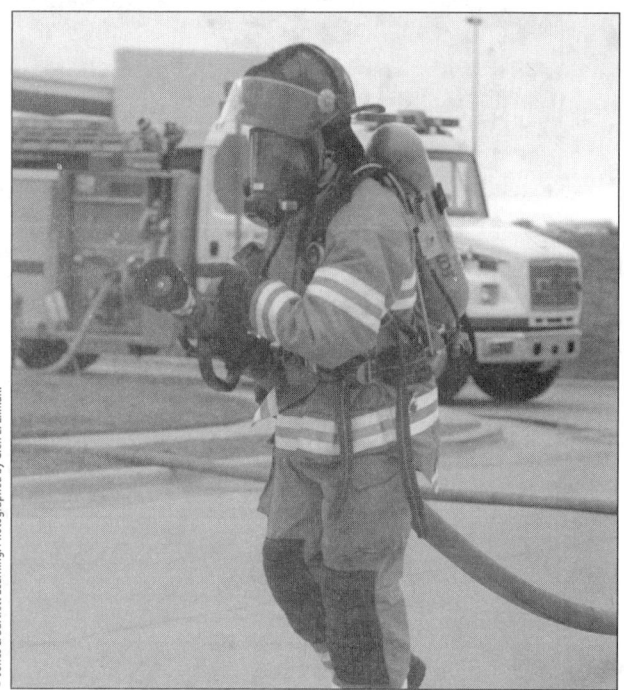

Select the correct size of fire hose for the task to be performed. While wearing full PPE and SCBA, advance the hose into the position from which you plan to attack the fire. Signal that you are ready for water. Open the nozzle to allow _____ to escape and to ensure that water is _____, and then close the nozzle.

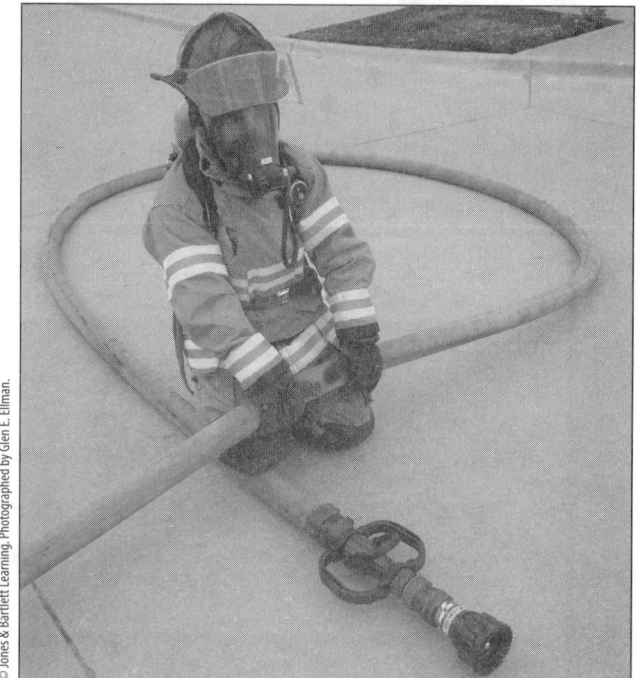

Make a _____ with the hose. Ensure that the nozzle is under the hose line that is coming from the fire apparatus. Using rope or a strap, secure the hose sections together where they cross, or use your body weight to kneel or sit on the hose line at the point where the hose crosses itself.

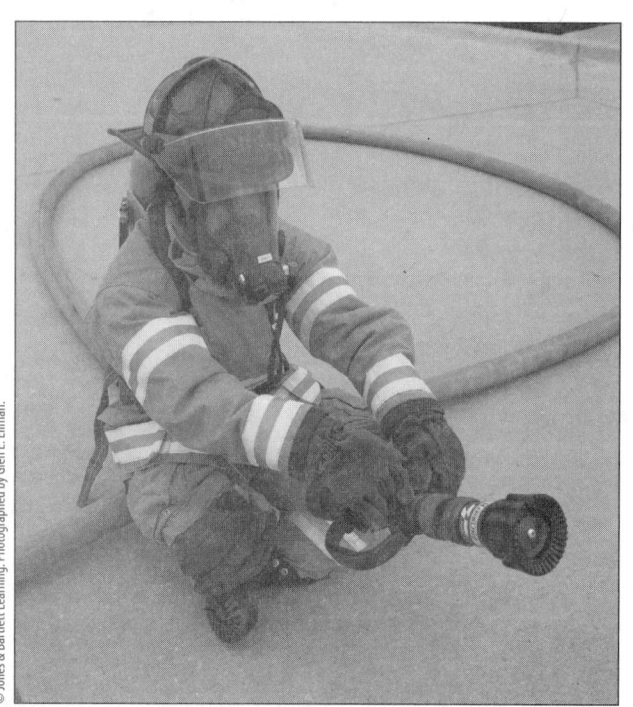

Allow enough hose to extend past the section where the line crosses itself for _____.

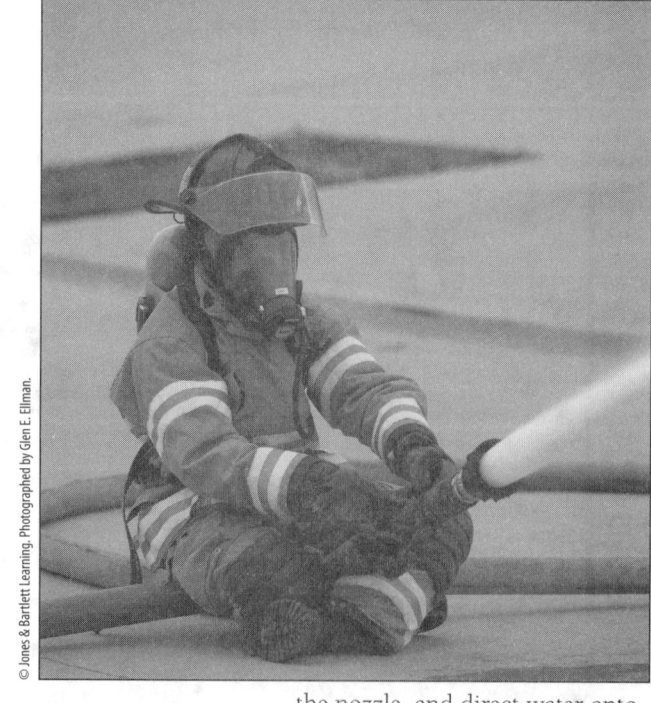

_____ the nozzle, and direct water onto the designated area.

Skill Drill 17-6: Performing the Two-Fire Fighter Method for Operating a Large Handline Fire Fighter I, NFPA 1001: 4.3.8
Test your knowledge of this skill drill by filling in the correct words in the photo captions.

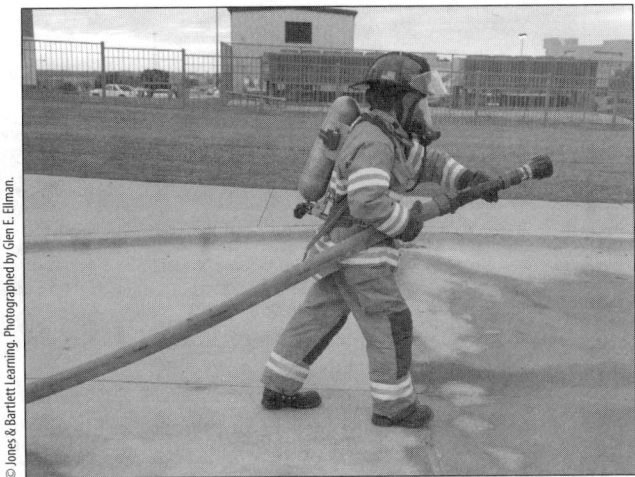

Don all PPE and SCBA. Select the correct handline for the task at hand. _____ the hose line from the fire apparatus into position.

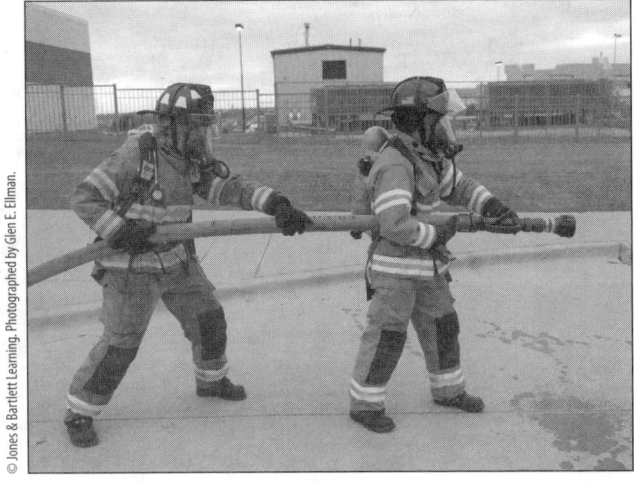

Signal that you are ready for water, and open the nozzle a _____ amount to allow air to escape and to ensure water is flowing. Advance the hose line as needed.

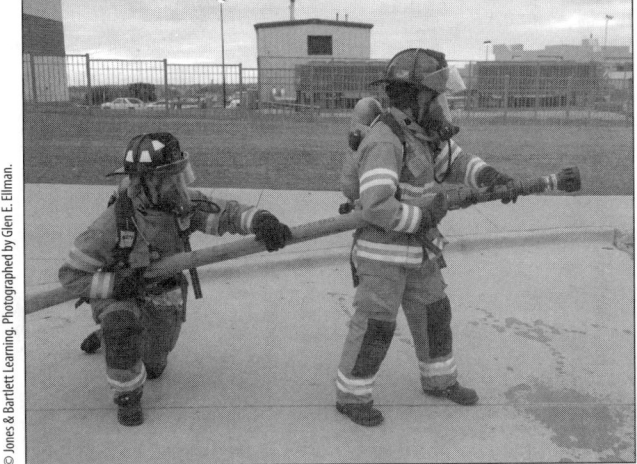

Before attacking the fire, the fire fighter on the nozzle should _____ the hose on his or her hip while grasping the nozzle with one hand and supporting the hose with the other hand. The second fire fighter should stay 3 ft (0.9 m) behind him or her and grasp the hose, securing it with two hands.

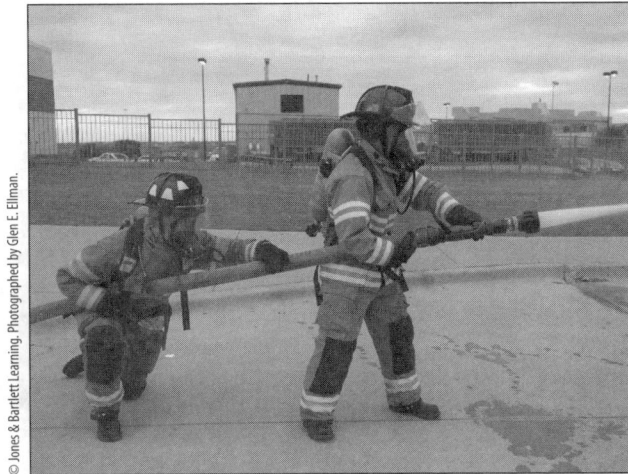

Open the nozzle in a _____ fashion, and direct water onto the fire or designated exposure.

Skill Drill 17-7: Operating a Deck Gun Fire Fighter I, NFPA 1001:4.3.8
Test your knowledge of this skill drill by filling in the correct words in the photo captions.

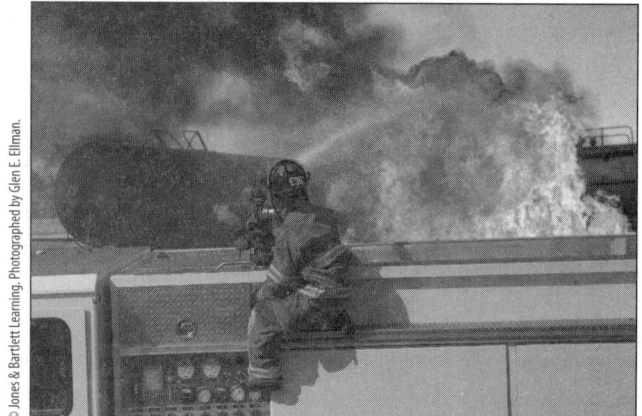

Make sure that all firefighting personnel are _____ of the structure. Place the deck gun in the correct position. Aim the deck gun at the fire or at the target exposure. Signal the pump driver/operator that you are ready for water.

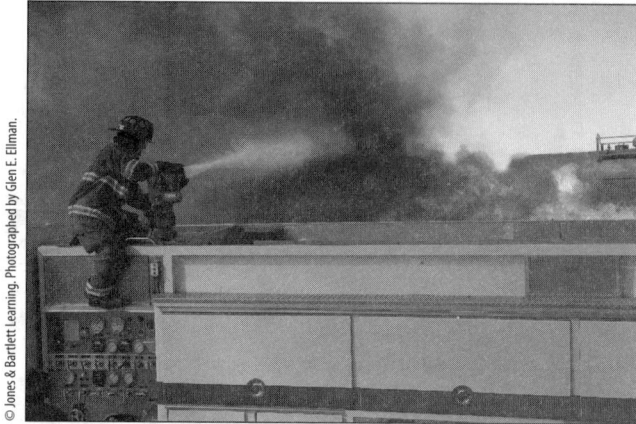

Once water is flowing, adjust the _____, aim, or water flow as necessary.

Skill Drill 17-9: Locating and Suppressing Concealed-Space Fires Fire Fighter I, NFPA 1001:4.3.8
Test your knowledge of this skill drill by filling in the correct words in the photo captions.

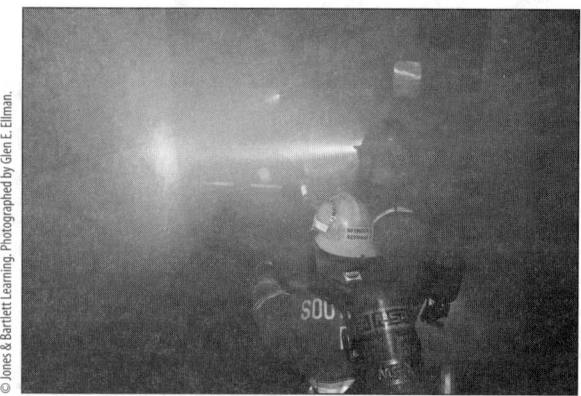

Locate the area of the building where a hidden fire is believed to exist. Look for signs of fire such as smoke coming from cracks or openings in walls, charred areas with no outward evidence of fire, and peeling or bubbled paint or wallpaper. Listen for cracks and pops or hissing steam. Use a _____ _____ _____ to look for areas of heat that may indicate a hidden fire. Use the back of your hand to feel for heat coming from a wall or floor.

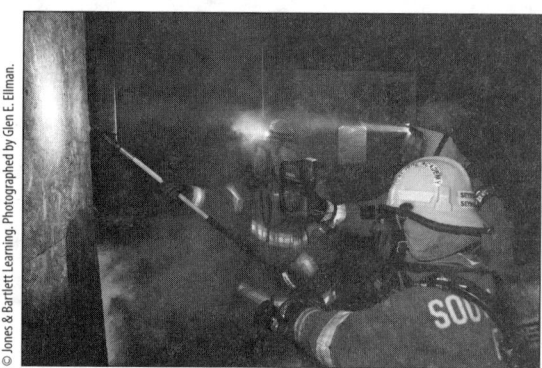

If a hidden fire is suspected, use a tool such as an axe or _____ tool to remove the building material over the area. If fire is found, expose the area as much as possible without causing unnecessary damage, and extinguish the fire using conventional firefighting methods.

Skill Drill 17-10: Extinguishing an Outside Class A Fire: Fire Fighter I, NFPA 1001: 4.3.8

Test your knowledge of this skill drill by placing the photos below in the correct order. Number the first step with a "1," the second step with a "2," and so on.

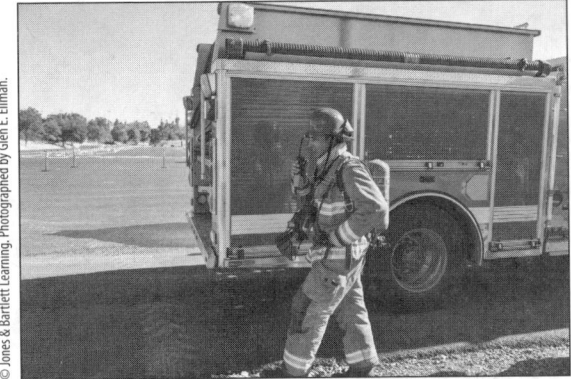

_____ Don full PPE, including SCBA; enter the personnel accountability system; and work as a team. Perform size-up, and give an arrival report. Call for additional resources if needed. Ensure that apparatus is positioned uphill and upwind of the fire and that it protects the scene from traffic.

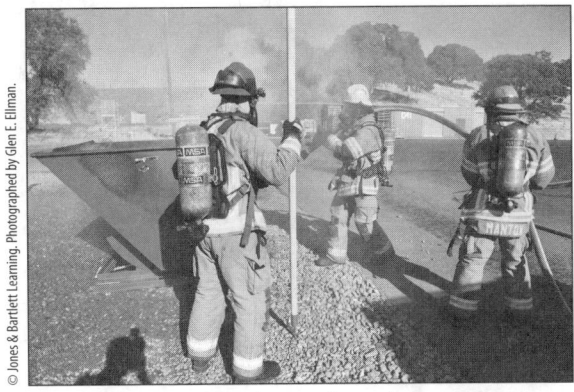

_____ Overhaul the fire, and notify command when the fire is under control. Identify obvious signs of the origin and cause of the fire. Preserve any evidence of arson. Return the equipment and crew to service.

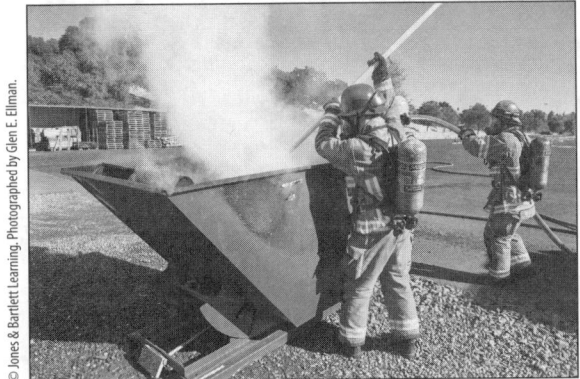

_____ Break up compact materials with hand tools or hose streams.

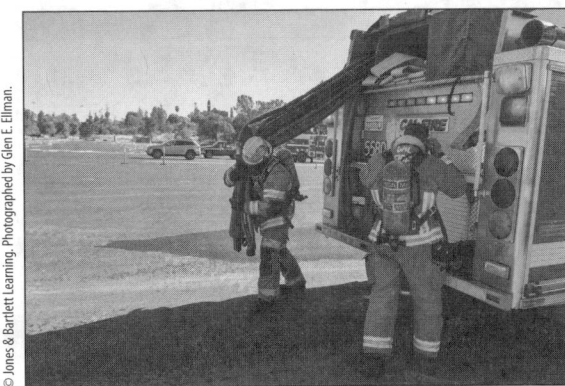

_____ Deploy an appropriate attack line (at least 1½ in. [38 mm] in diameter).

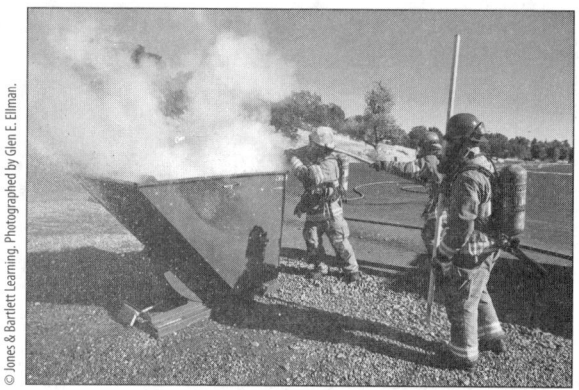

_____ Direct the crew to attack the fire in a safe manner—uphill and upwind from the fire.

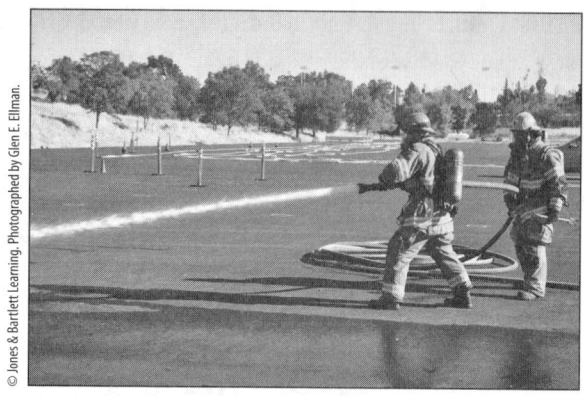

_____ Open the nozzle to purge air from the system, and make sure water is flowing. If using an adjustable nozzle, ensure that it is set to the proper nozzle pattern. Shut down the nozzle until you are in a position to apply water.

Skill Drill 17-11: Extinguishing a Vehicle Fire: Fire Fighter I, NFPA 1001: 4.3.7
Test your knowledge of this skill drill by placing the photos below in the correct order. Number the first step with a "1," the second step with a "2," and so on.

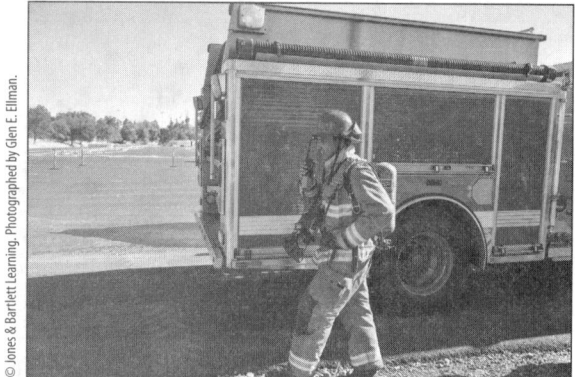

_____ Don full PPE, including SCBA; enter the personnel accountability system; and work as a team. Perform size-up, and give an arrival report. Call for additional resources if needed. Ensure that apparatus is positioned uphill and upwind of the fire and that it protects the scene from traffic.

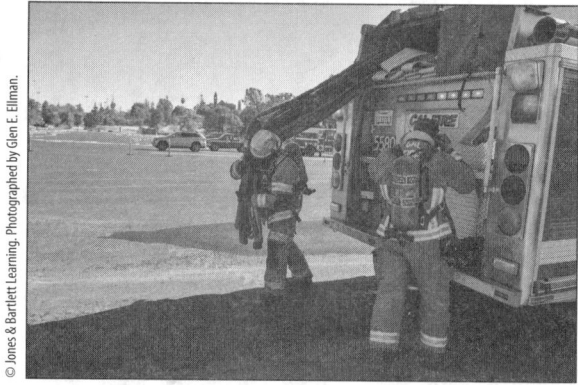

_____ Deploy an appropriate attack line (at least 1½ in. [38-mm] in diameter).

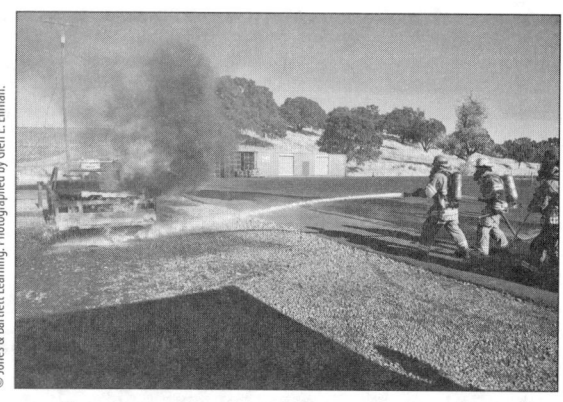

_____ Direct the crew to attack the fire in a safe manner. Attack from uphill and upwind of the fire and at a 45-degree angle, and extinguish any fire under the vehicle.

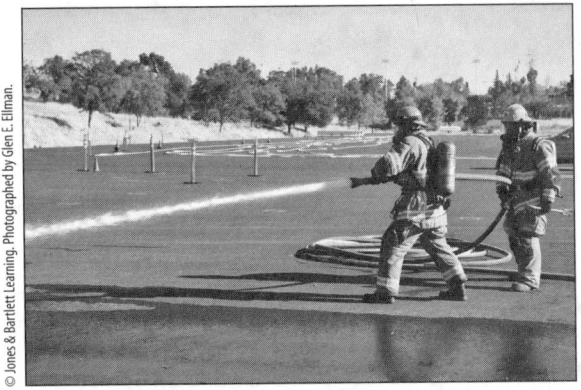

_____ Open the nozzle to purge air from the system, and make sure water is flowing. If using an adjustable nozzle, ensure that it is set to the proper nozzle pattern. Shut down the nozzle until you are in a position to apply water.

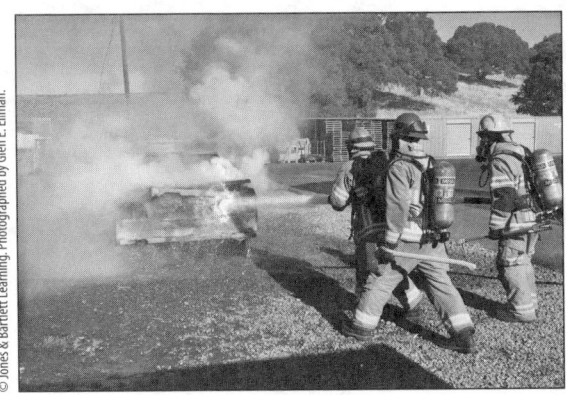

_____ Carefully approach the vehicle, and completely suppress the fire.

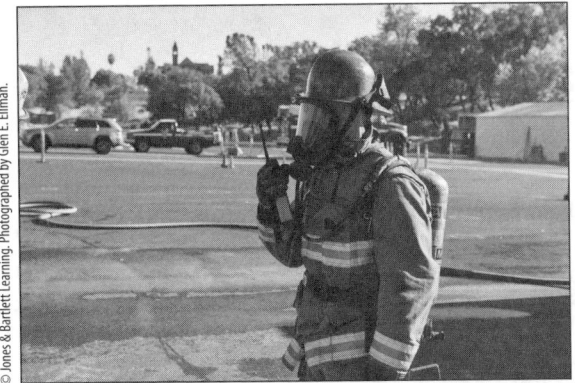

_____ Notify command when the fire is under control. Identify obvious signs of the origin and cause of the fire. Preserve any evidence of arson. Return the equipment and crew to service.

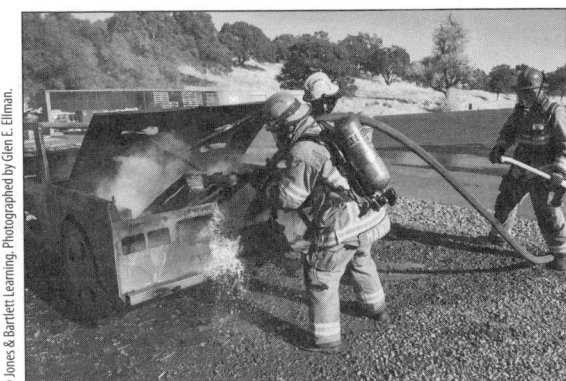

_____ Overhaul all areas of the vehicle, including the passenger compartment, engine compartment, and cargo area (trunk).

Fire Fighter Survival

Workbook Activities

The following activities have been designed to help you. Your instructor may require you to complete some or all of these activities as a regular part of your fire fighter training program. You are encouraged to complete any activity your instructor does not assign you, as a way to enhance your learning in the classroom.

Chapter Review

The following exercises provide an opportunity to refresh your knowledge of this chapter.

Matching

Match each of the terms in the left column to the appropriate definition in the right column.

_____ 1. Hazardous conditions
_____ 2. Guideline
_____ 3. SOPs
_____ 4. Safe location
_____ 5. Self-rescue
_____ 6. Hazard recognition
_____ 7. Rehabilitation
_____ 8. Risk–benefit analysis
_____ 9. RIC
_____ 10. Mayday

A. Indicates a fire fighter is in trouble and requires immediate assistance
B. A rope used for orientation when inside a structure when there is low or no visibility
C. Defines the manner in which a fire department conducts operations at an emergency incident
D. An extension of the two-in/two-out rule
E. Becomes easier through study and experience
F. May not be evident by simple observation
G. A temporary place of refuge in which to await rescue
H. Weighs the positive results that can be achieved against the probability and severity of potential negative consequences
I. Escaping or exiting a hazardous area under one's own power
J. Reduces the effects of fatigue during an emergency operation

Multiple Choice

Read each item carefully, and then select the best response.

_____ 1. When a fire fighter needs immediate assistance, the incident commander should immediately deploy
  A. the SOP.
  B. the PASS.
  C. the RIC.
  D. the radio.

_____ 2. Fire fighters will accept a higher level of risk in exchange for
  A. the possibility of saving lives.
  B. the possibility of saving property.
  C. property that is lost.
  D. persons who are already lost.

CHAPTER 18

_____ 3. When initiating a mayday,
   A. give a weather report.
   B. give a LUNAR report.
   C. give a CISD report.
   D. give a PASS report.

_____ 4. Upon reaching a downed fire fighter, what is the most critical decision for the rescuers?
   A. How much time and effort will be needed to remove the fire fighter
   B. The treatment of the fire fighter's injuries
   C. The location of the fire fighter and rescuers
   D. How to exit the structure

_____ 5. Which of the following must be learned and practiced before they can be implemented?
   A. CISMs
   B. SOPs
   C. GOPs
   D. DUIs

_____ 6. The time rating for how long a SCBA cylinder will last is based on
   A. the standard consumption rate plus 10 minutes.
   B. the standard consumption rate under high-exertion conditions.
   C. the standard consumption rate under low-exertion conditions.
   D. an increased consumption rate based on average fire conditions.

_____ 7. Observable factors that might indicate a hazard include
   A. building construction.
   B. weather conditions.
   C. occupancy.
   D. All of the above.

_____ 8. What does the NFPA 704 diamond indicate?
   A. PARs are present.
   B. RICs are present.
   C. Ventilation is necessary.
   D. Hazardous materials are present.

_____ 9. A strap or harness type component attached to a fire fighter's protective coat is known as a (an)
   A. Firefighter Safety Device.
   B. Emergency Escape Strap.
   C. Firefighter Drag Harness.
   D. Drag Rescue Device.

_____ 10. What is the most important outcome in any fire department operation?
   A. Fire fighter survival
   B. No rekindle
   C. Effective ICS
   D. Reduced water damage

_____ 11. Comparing potential positive results to potential negative consequences is called
   A. causative factors.
   B. management factors.
   C. risk–benefit analysis.
   D. standard operating procedures.

_____ 12. To stay oriented when inside a burning structure, the fire fighter should use a hose line or a
   A. team member.
   B. radio.
   C. guideline.
   D. structure wall.

_____ 13. A roll call taken by each supervisor at an emergency incident is known as a(n)
   A. team roll call.
   B. incident report.
   C. personnel accountability report.
   D. incident roll.

_____ 14. While awaiting rescue, a fire fighter may find a temporary location that provides refuge. What is this location called?
   A. Safety point
   B. Safe location
   C. Rescue point
   D. Landmark

_____ 15. What is the first step of self-rescue?
   A. Manually set off your PASS alarm.
   B. Initiate a mayday.
   C. Exit the structure.
   D. Orient yourself within the structure.

_____ 16. During an incident, if fire fighters observe an increase in risk of their operations, they must report it to the
   A. company officer.
   B. sector officer.
   C. safety officer.
   D. incident commander.

_____ 17. The manner in which a fire department conducts operations at an emergency incident is defined by
   A. general operating guidelines.
   B. the incident commander.
   C. department policies.
   D. standard operating procedures.

_____ 18. The standard radio terminology used to report an imminent hazardous condition or situation is
   A. "Emergency traffic."
   B. "Mayday."
   C. "Halt operations."
   D. "Retreat."

_____ 19. A crew that is assigned to stand by fully dressed, be equipped for action, and be ready to be deployed at an incident scene is called a(n)
   A. technical rescue crew.
   B. EMS team.
   C. special recovery team.
   D. rapid intervention crew.

_____ 20. A systematic way to keep track of the location and function of all personnel operating at the scene of an incident is
   A. a team inventory.
   B. a personnel accountability system.
   C. the chain of command.
   D. the two-in/two-out rule.

Vocabulary

Define the following terms using the space provided.

1. Personnel Accountability Report:

   _____
   _____
   _____

2. Safe location:

   _____
   _____
   _____

3. Air management:

   _____
   _____
   _____

4. Self-rescue:

   _____
   _____
   _____

5. Rapid intervention company/crew (RIC):

   _____
   _____
   _____

Fill-In

Read each item carefully, and then complete the statement by filling in the missing word(s).

1. Hazardous conditions may or may not be evident by _____ _____.

2. The word _____ is used to indicate that a firefighter is in trouble and requires immediate assistance.

3. During an incident, company officers and safety officers are involved in risk analysis on a(n) _____ basis.

4. Air _____ is important to all fire fighters and relates to the basic fact that air equals time.

5. The assessment of the risks and benefits and the decision to commit crews to the interior of a burning structure is the responsibility of the _____.

6. The only way to become proficient at a skill is through _____.

7. The purpose of _____ is to reduce the effects of fatigue during an emergency operation.

8. Team _____ means that a company arrives at a fire together, works together, and leaves together.

9. Safety and survival inside a fire building can be directly related to remaining _____ within the building.

10. A _____ _____ _____ is a portable air supply intended for use by an RIC.

True/False

If you believe the statement to be more true than false, write the letter "T" in the space provided. If you believe the statement to be more false than true, write the letter "F."

1. _____ Teamwork and communication are critical parts of all emergency operations.
2. _____ The activation of the low-pressure alarm on a SCBA indicates that it is time to leave the structure.
3. _____ A room with a door and a window could be used as a safe location.
4. _____ Fire fighters must be capable of working in environments that include a wide range of hazards.
5. _____ A hose coupling can be used to indicate the direction out of a structure.
6. _____ Rapid intervention crews/companies should be in place at any incident where fire fighters are in operation.
7. _____ When you reach a downed fire fighter, the first step is to assess if their SCBA is functioning.
8. _____ The best method to remain oriented within an involved structure is to stay in contact with a team member.
9. _____ The members of a company should always be oriented to one another's location, activities, and condition.
10. _____ It is permissible to risk the life of a fire fighter only in a situation where there is a reasonable and realistic possibility of saving a life.

Short Answer

Complete this section with short written answers using the space provided.

1. List five of the rules of engagement for fire fighter survival.

   _____
   _____
   _____
   _____

2. Identify a simply stated risk–benefit philosophy for a fire department.

   _____
   _____
   _____
   _____

3. List five of the components of the concept of team integrity.

___

Fire Alarms

The following real case scenarios will give you an opportunity to explore the concerns associated with fire fighter survival. Read each scenario, and then answer each question in detail.

1. While performing a search in a commercial structure, you crawl into a portion of fallen suspended ceiling and become entangled in electric wire and communication cables. What steps should you take to remove yourself from the wires and cables?

___

2. You have become confused and disoriented during a primary search of a second-floor apartment. You decide to attempt to locate a window to call for assistance or to exit the building. How should you proceed?

___

Skill Drills

Skill Drill 18-1: Initiating a Mayday Call for Emergency Assistance Fire Fighter I, NFPA 1001: 4.2.4

Test your knowledge of this skill drill by filling in the correct words in the photo captions.

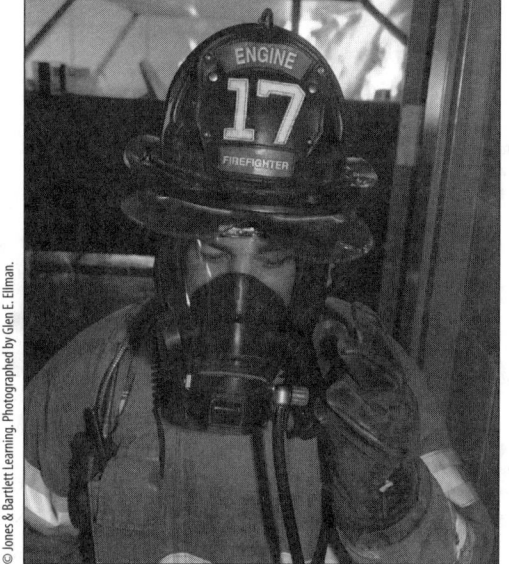

1. Use your radio to call "MAYDAY, MAYDAY, MAYDAY." Give a _____ report (your location, unit number, name, air or assignment, and resources needed) or report who, what, where.

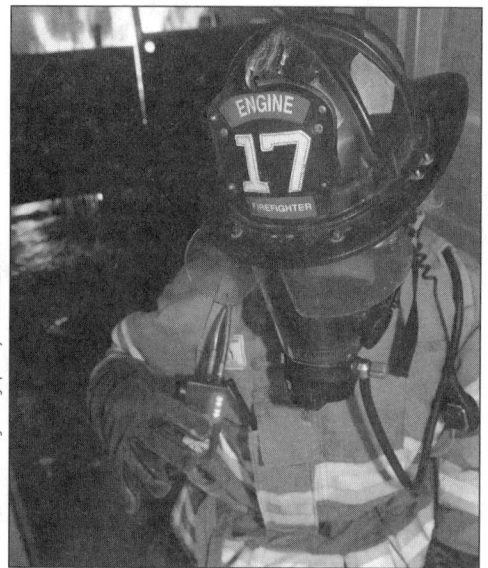

2. Activate your _____ device. Attempt self-rescue. If you are able to move, identify a safe location where you can await rescue.

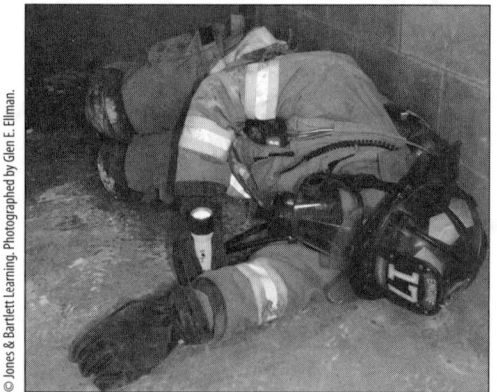

3. If unable to self-rescue, lie on your side in a _____ position with your _____ device pointing out so it can be heard.

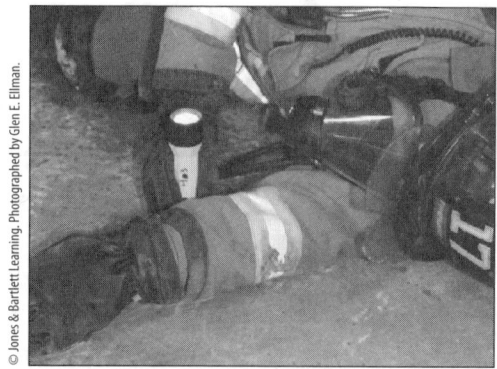

4. Point your _____ toward the ceiling. Slow your breathing as much as possible to conserve your air supply.

Skill Drill 18-2: Performing Self-Rescue Using a Hose Line Fire Fighter I, NFPA 1001: 4.3.5
Test your knowledge of this skill drill by filling in the correct words in the photo captions.

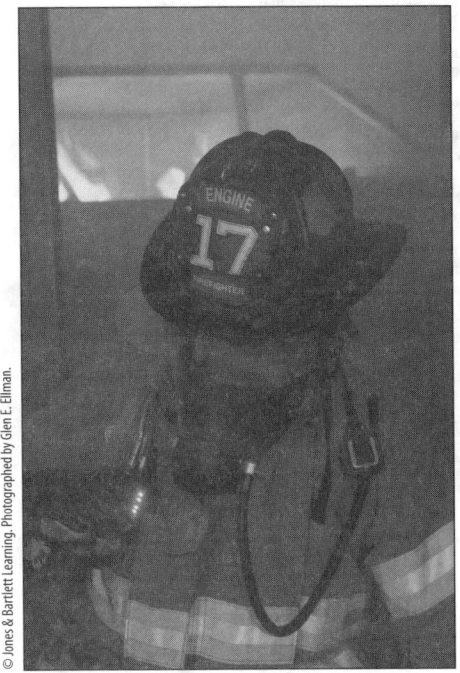

1. Initiate a _____. Stay calm, and control your breathing.

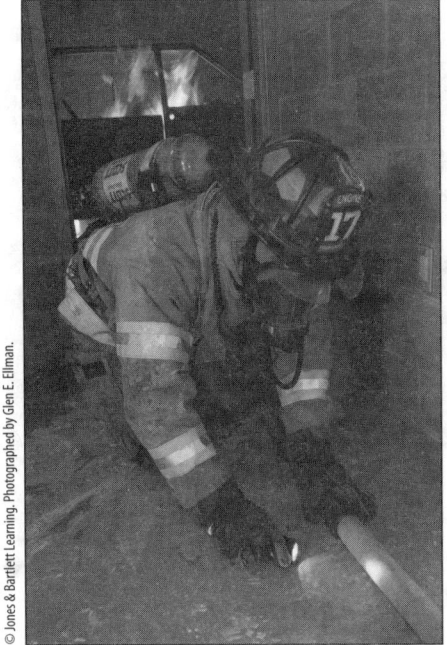

2. Systematically search the room to locate a hose line. Follow the hose line to a hose coupling. Identify the male and female ends of the coupling. Move from the _____ coupling to the male coupling.

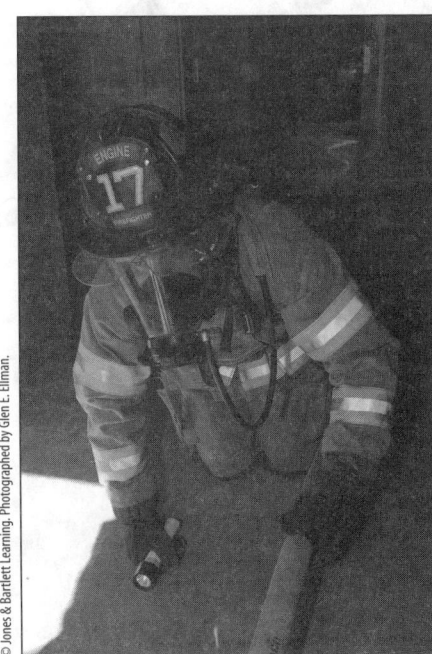

3. Follow the _____ out. Exit the hazard area. Notify command of your location.

Skill Drill 18-3: Locating a Door or Window for Emergency Exit Fire Fighter I, NFPA 1001: 4.3.5

Test your knowledge of this skill drill by placing the photos below in the correct order. Number the first step with a "1," the second step with a "2," and so on.

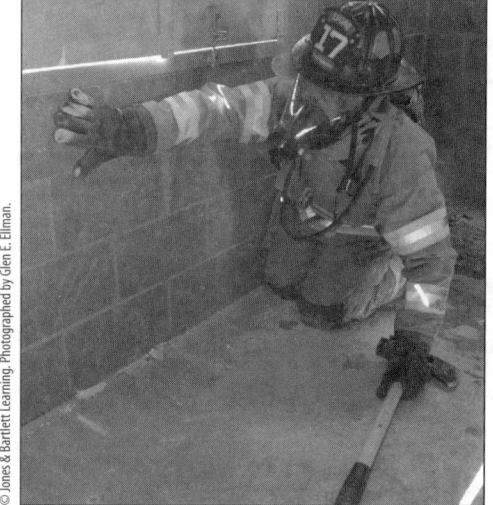

_____ Use a sweeping motion on the wall to locate an alternative exit. Identify the opening as a window, interior door, or external door. Beware of closets, bathrooms, and other openings without egress.

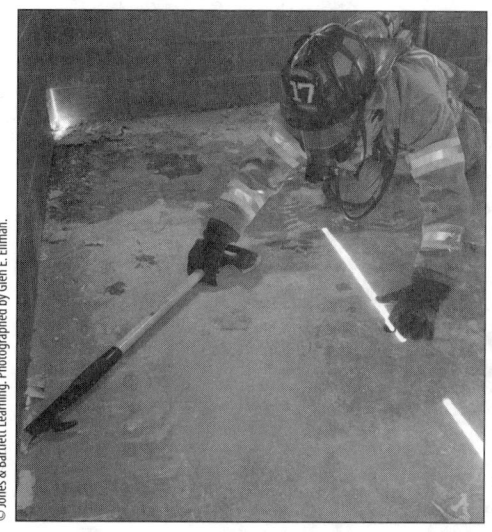

_____ Systematically locate a wall.

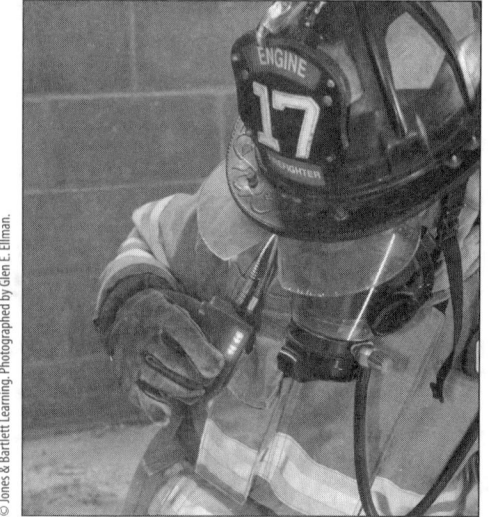

_____ Initiate a mayday. Stay calm, and control your breathing.

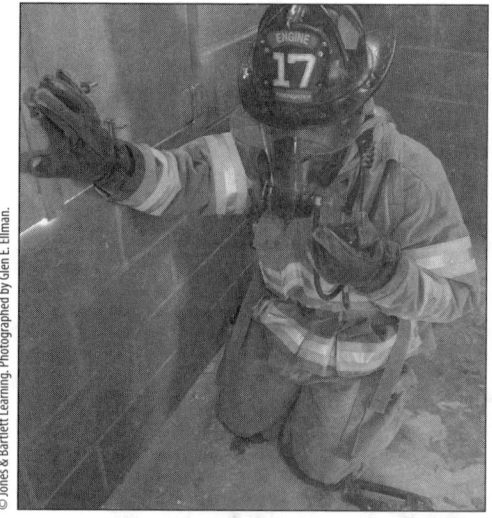

_____ If the first opening identified is not adequate for an exit, continue to search. Maintain your orientation, and stay low. Exit the room safely if possible. If unable to exit, assume the downed fire fighter position by lying on your stomach or side on the floor in a safe location, or find refuge. Keep command informed of your situation.

Skill Drill 18-4: Using the Backhanded Swim Technique to Escape Through a Wall Fire Fighter I, NFPA 1001: 4.3.5

Test your knowledge of this skill drill by filling in the correct words in the photo captions.

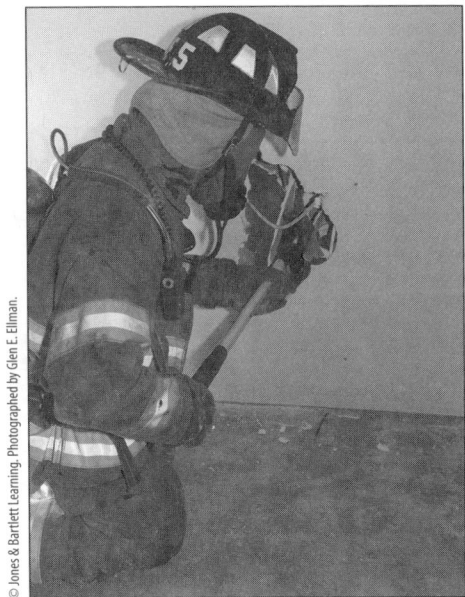

1. Identify _____ conditions that require exiting through a wall. Initiate a mayday. Use a hand tool or your feet to open a hole in the wall between two studs. If using a hand tool, drive the tool completely through the wall to check for _____ on the other side.

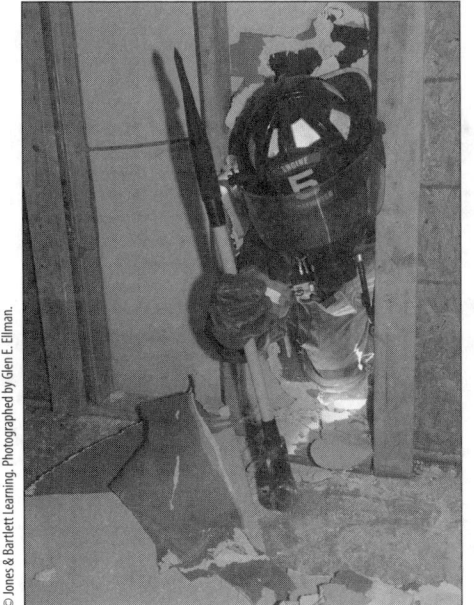

2. Enlarge the hole. Enter the hole _____ first to check the floor and fire conditions on the other side of the wall.

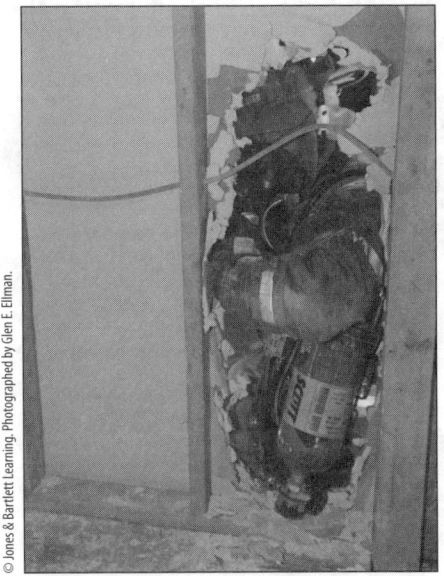

3. Loosen the _____ waist strap, and remove one shoulder strap. Sling the _____ to one side to reduce your profile.

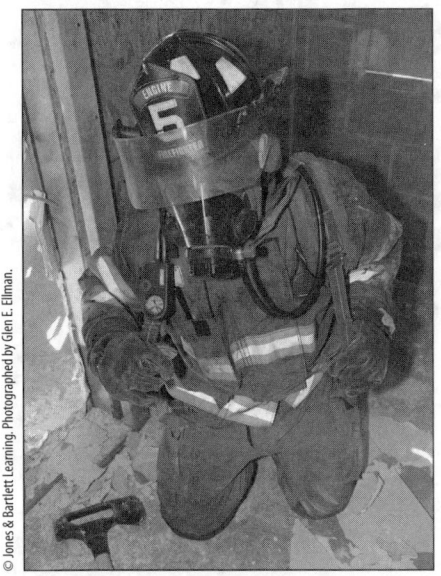

4. Escape through the opening in the wall. Adjust the _____ straps to their normal position.

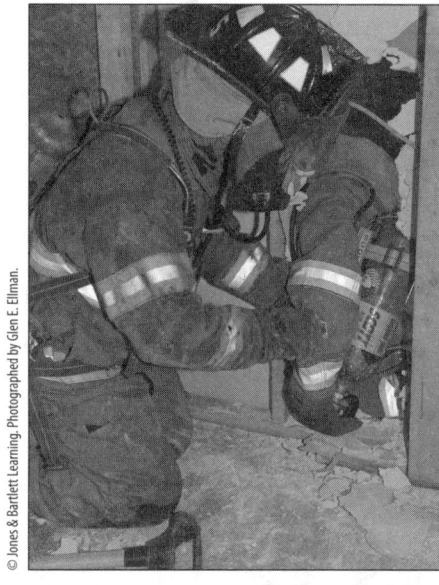

5. Assist others through the opening in the wall. Report your _____ to command.

Skill Drill 18-5: Using the Forward Swim Technique to Escape Through a Wall Fire Fighter I, NFPA 1001: 4.3.5

Test your knowledge of this skill drill by placing the photos below in the correct order. Number the first step with a "1," the second step with a "2," and so on.

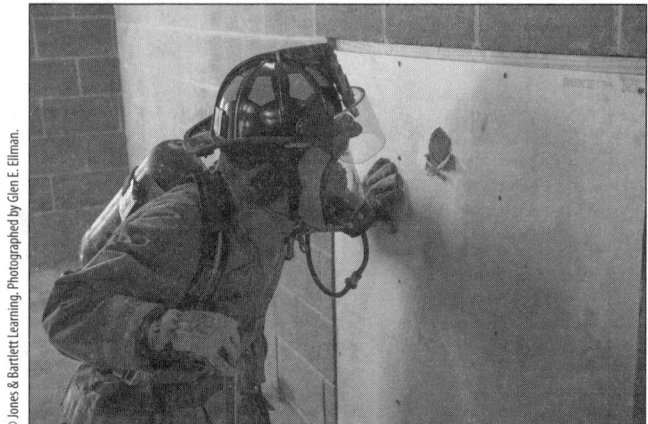

_____ Enlarge the hole. Check the floor and fire conditions on the other side of the wall. Loosen the SCBA shoulder straps if necessary, but do not remove them.

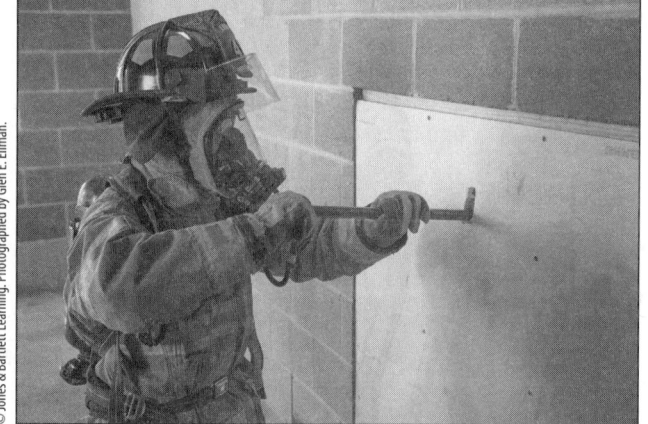

_____ Identify deteriorating conditions that require exiting through a wall. Initiate a mayday. Use a hand tool or your feet to open a hole in the wall between two studs. If using a hand tool, drive the tool completely through the wall to check for obstacles on the other side.

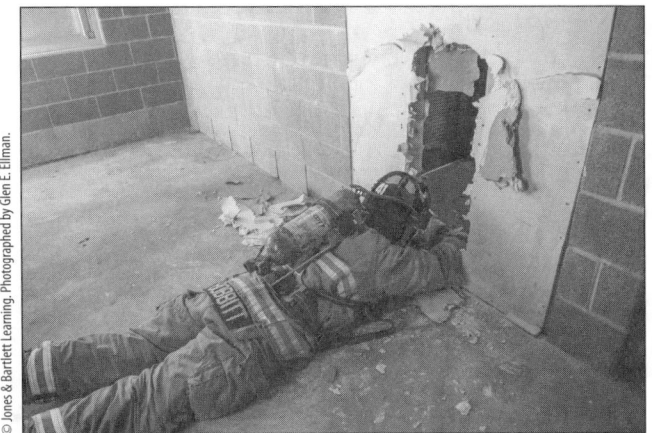

_____ Lie prone, with your stomach flat on the ground and your head pointed toward the wall opening. Stretch your arms toward your head and attempt to touch your ears with your upper arms to reduce your profile.

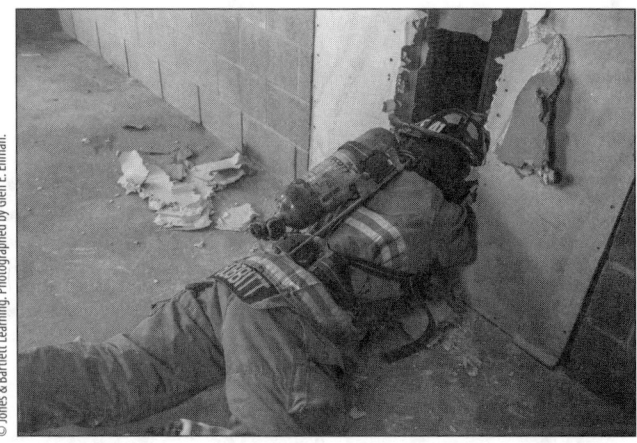

_____ Extend your arms, and head into the wall opening first.

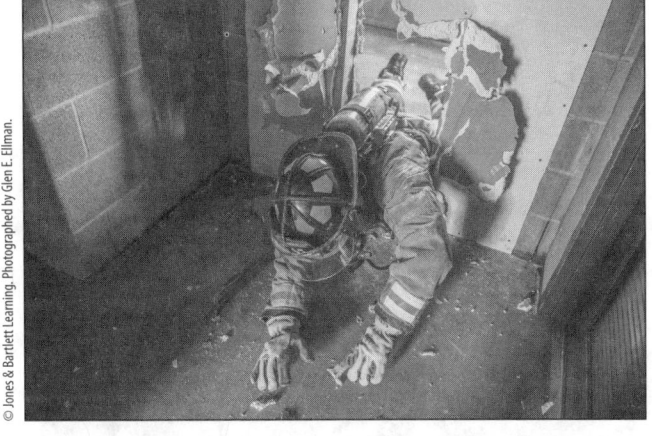

_____ Rotate your shoulders, SCBA, and waist as necessary to escape through the opening. Do not lift yourself up on your elbows, as this will raise your profile. Assist others through the opening in the wall. Report your status to command.

Skill Drill 18-6: Escaping from an Entanglement Fire Fighter I, NFPA 1001: 4.3.5

Test your knowledge of this skill drill by placing the photos below in the correct order. Number the first step with a "1," the second step with a "2," and so on.

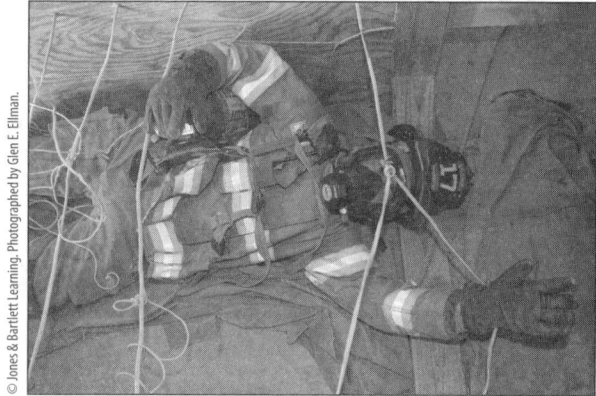

_____ Loosen the SCBA straps, remove one arm, and slide the air pack to the front of your body to try to free the SCBA.

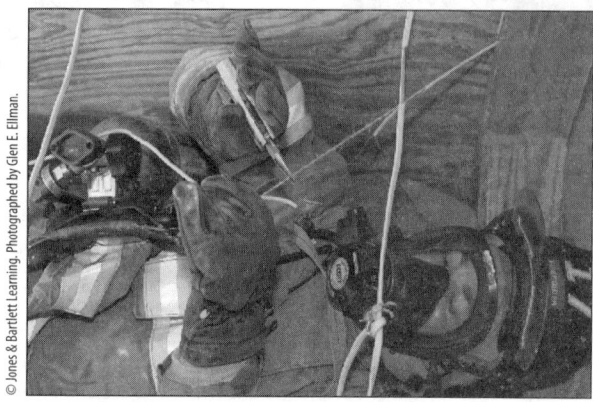

_____ Cut the wires or cables causing the entanglement. Be aware of any possible electrocution risk. If you are unable to disentangle yourself, notify command of your situation. If you are able to exit, notify command that you are out of danger.

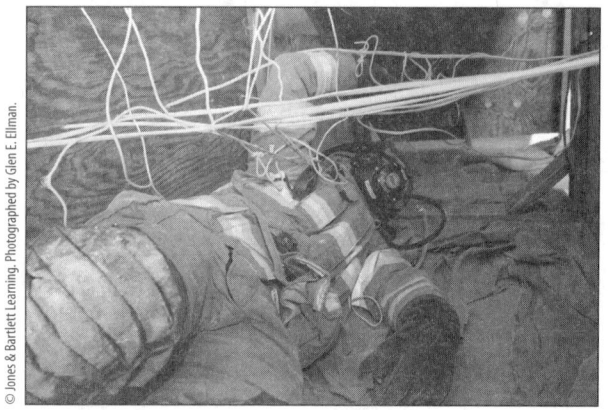

_____ Use the swimmer stroke to try to free yourself.

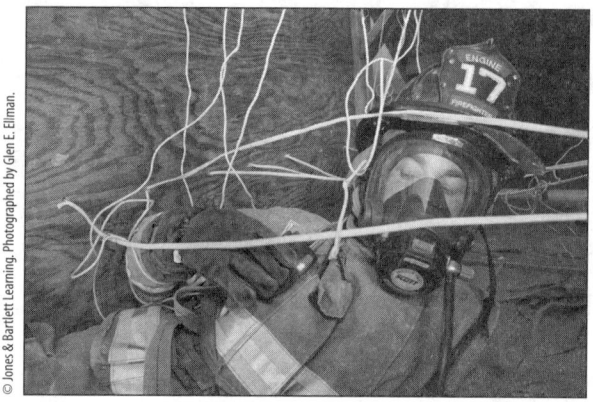

_____ Initiate a mayday. Stay calm, and control your breathing.

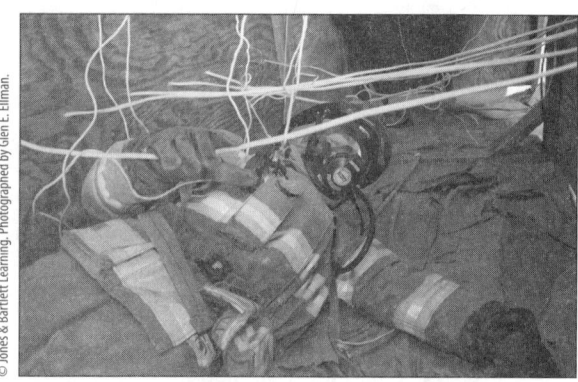

_____ Change your position—back up and turn on your side to try to free yourself.

Skill Drill 18-7: Rescuing a Downed Fire Fighter Using SCBA Straps as a Rescue Harness Fire Fighter I, NFPA 1001: 4.3.5
Test your knowledge of the skill drill by filling in the correct words in the photo captions.

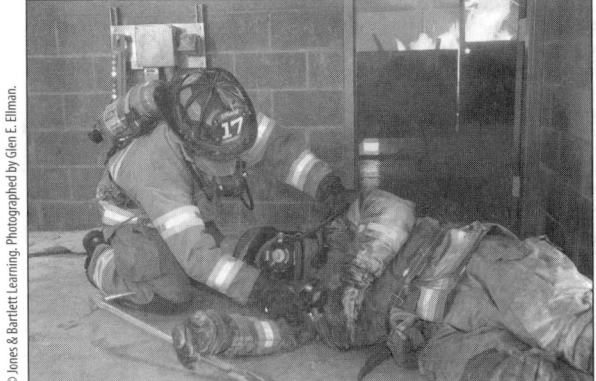

1. Locate the downed fire fighter. Activate the _____ procedure, if that step has not already been taken. Quickly assess the condition of the downed fire fighter and the situation. Shut off the _____ device as needed to aid in communication.

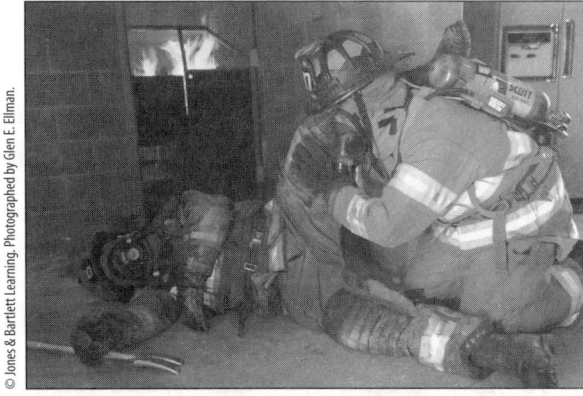

2. Position yourself at the _____ of the downed fire fighter. Lift one leg of the downed fire fighter up onto your _____.

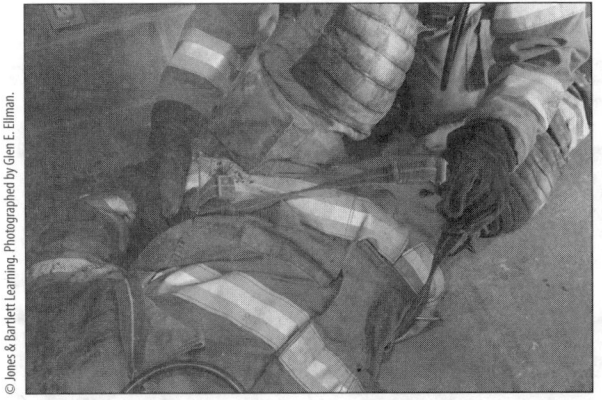

3. Locate and loosen the _____ straps and _____ straps (if needed) of the downed fire fighter's SCBA harness.

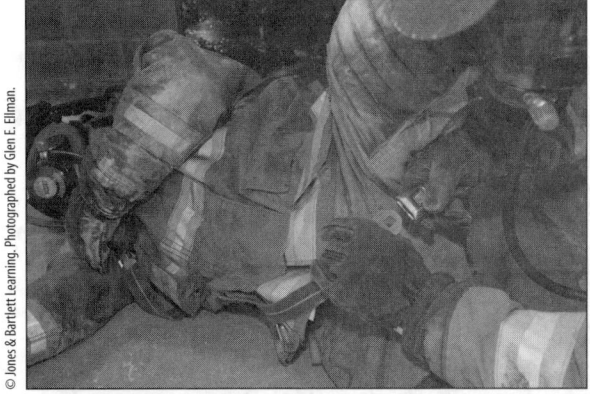

4. Unbuckle the downed fire fighter's _____ strap, and buckle the _____ strap under the lifted leg. Tighten the straps. Remove the downed fire fighter from the hazard area to a safe area.

Skill Drill 18-9: Rescuing a Downed Fire Fighter as a Two-Person Team Fire Fighter I, NFPA 1001:4.3.9
Test your knowledge of this skill drill by filling in the correct words in the photo captions.

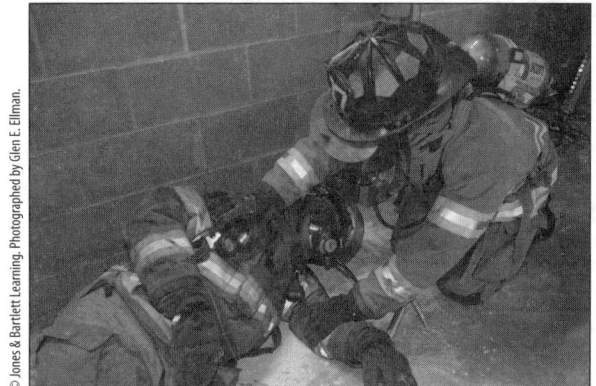

1. Locate the downed fire fighter. Activate the mayday procedure, if that step has not already been taken. Shut off the PASS device to aid in communication. Assess the situation and the condition of the downed fire fighter. Use the _____ _____ to fill the downed fire fighter's air supply cylinder, if needed.

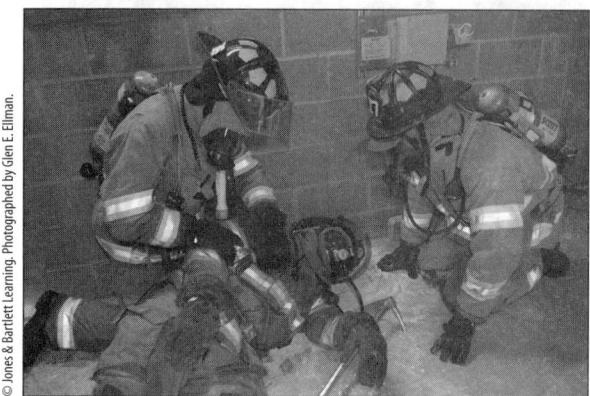

2. The second fire fighter converts the downed fire fighter's SCBA harness into a _____ _____.

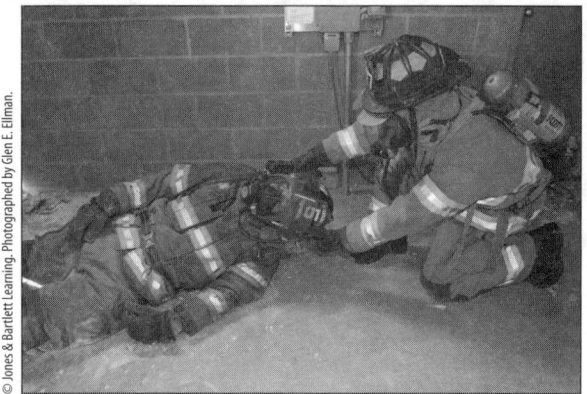

3. The first fire fighter grabs the shoulder straps or uses the _____ to create a handle to pull the downed fire fighter.

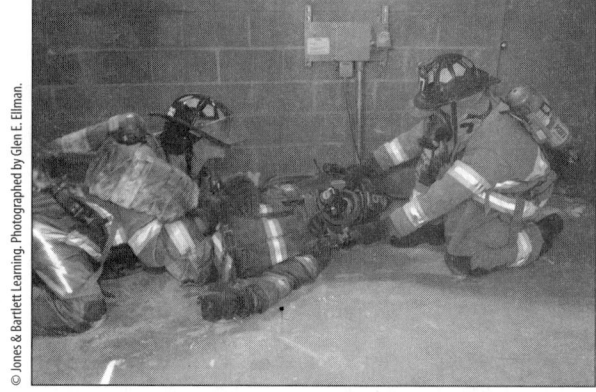

4. The second fire fighter stays at the downed fire fighter's _____ and supports the _____ of the downed fire fighter.

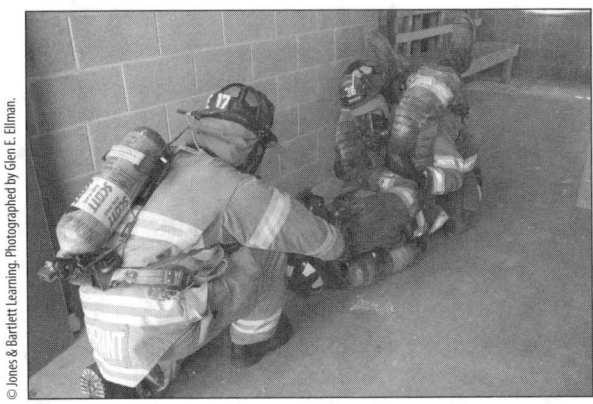

5. Remove the downed fire fighter from the _____ area to a _____ area.

Skill Drill 18-10: Supplying Air to a Downed Fire Fighter Using the Low-Pressure Hose from a Rapid Intervention Pack Fire Fighter I, NFPA 1001:4.3.9
Test your knowledge of this skill drill by placing the photos below in the correct order. Number the first step with a "1," the second step with a "2," and so on.

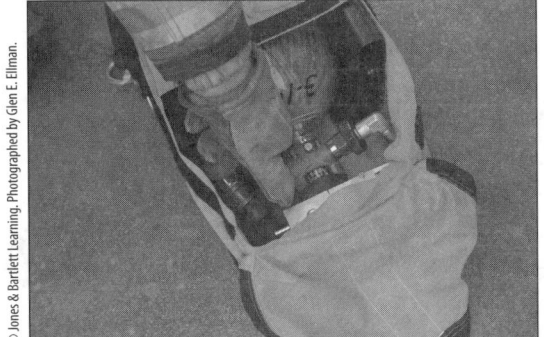

_____ Inspect the rapid intervention pack for proper operation, and make sure that the air cylinder is full. Turn on the air cylinder valve.

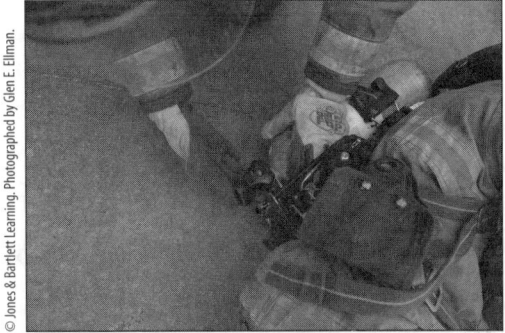

_____ Check the downed fire fighter's SCBA to determine which parts of the fire fighter's SCBA are not operating properly.

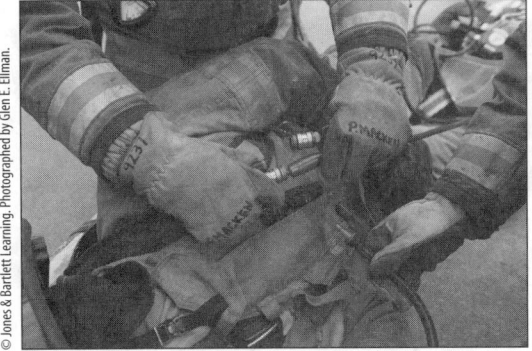

_____ If the problem is that there is no air being supplied to the fire fighter's low-pressure SCBA hose, and the rest of the SCBA is operational, detach the low-pressure hose from the fire fighter's SCBA regulator, and attach the low-pressure hose from the rapid intervention pack to the SCBA regulator.

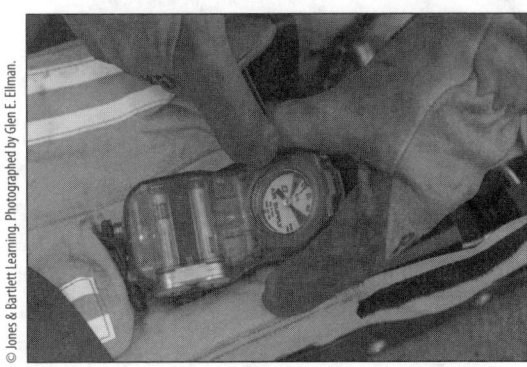

_____ Continue to monitor the air pressure and operation of the downed fire fighter's SCBA and the pressure in the rapid intervention pack air cylinder.

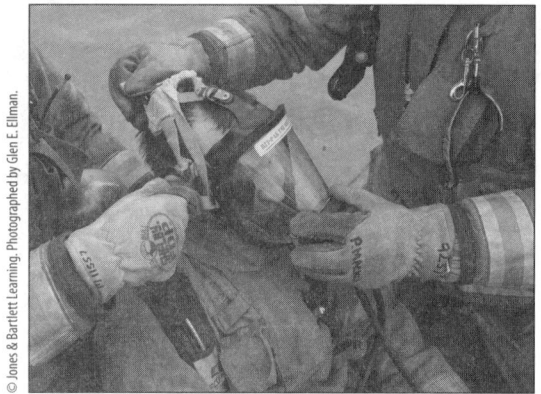

_____ If the problem is that the fire fighter's face piece has been displaced, is missing, or is damaged, remove the fire fighter's helmet, hood, and face piece. Place the emergency face piece from the rapid intervention pack on the fire fighter, and attach the rapid intervention pack regulator and low-pressure hose to the emergency face piece.

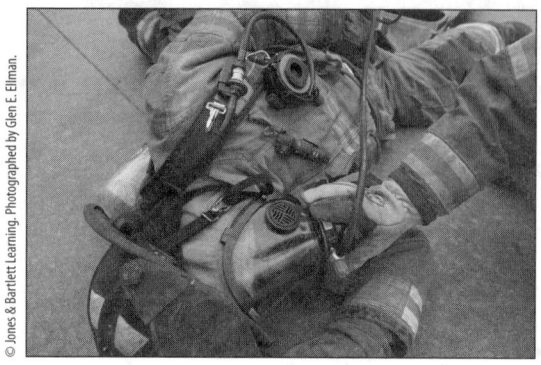

_____ If the problem is that the fire fighter's SCBA regulator is not operating properly, attach the low-pressure hose of the rapid intervention pack to the pack's regulator. Detach the fire fighter's SCBA regulator, and attach the rapid intervention pack regulator and low-pressure hose.

Skill Drill 18-11: Supplying Air to a Downed Fire Fighter Using the High-Pressure Hose from a Rapid Intervention Pack Fire Fighter I, NFPA 1001:4.3.9

Test your knowledge of this skill drill by placing the photos below in the correct order. Number the first step with a "1," the second step with a "2," and so on.

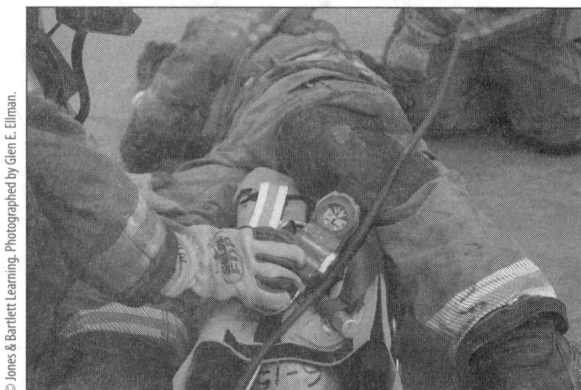

_____ Disconnect the high-pressure hose from the RIC UAC, and monitor the air pressure and operation of the downed fire fighter's SCBA.

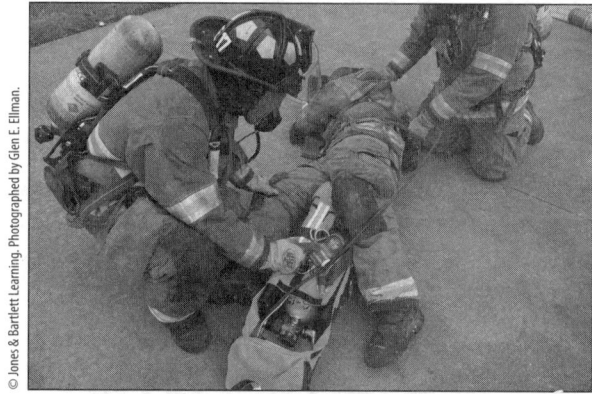

_____ Attach the rapid intervention pack high-pressure hose to the RIC UAC of the fire fighter's SCBA, and leave it in place until the pressure is equalized between the two air cylinders.

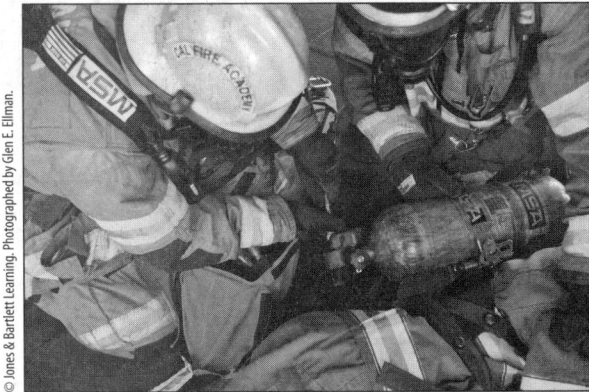 _____ Check the rapid intervention pack to ensure that the air cylinder is full and the high-pressure hose is in proper condition. Turn on the air cylinder valve.

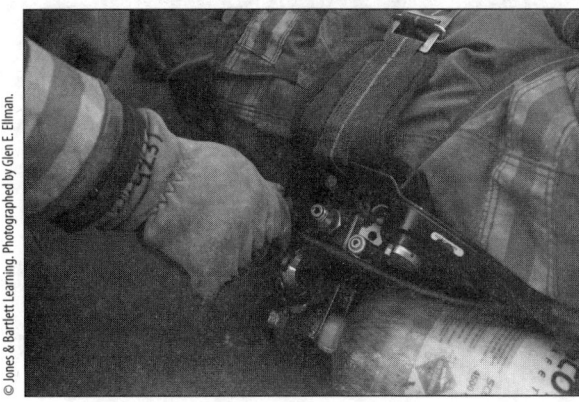 _____ Remove the high-pressure hose from the rapid intervention pack, and inspect the fire fighter's RIC UAC to ensure it is clean and undamaged.

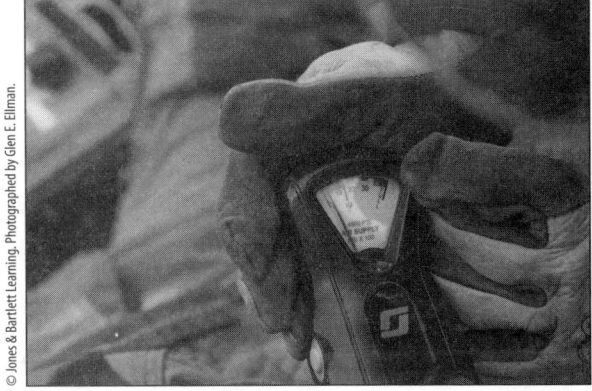 _____ Check the downed fire fighter's SCBA to be sure it is operating properly, that the face piece and regulator are attached, and that the air supply is low.

Salvage and Overhaul

Workbook Activities

The following activities have been designed to help you. Your instructor may require you to complete some or all of these activities as a regular part of your fire fighter training program. You are encouraged to complete any activity your instructor does not assign to you, as a way to enhance your learning in the classroom.

Chapter Review

The following exercises provide an opportunity to refresh your knowledge of this chapter.

Matching

Match each of the terms in the left column to the appropriate definition in the right column.

_____ 1. Rekindle	A. Protect property and belongings from damage, particularly from the effects of smoke and water

_____ 2. Floodlight	B. Catches dripping water and directs it toward a drain or to the outside

_____ 3. Carryall	C. A light designed to project a narrow, concentrated beam of light

_____ 4. Water chute	D. Causes more property damage to occur, and the fire department could be held responsible for the additional losses

_____ 5. Salvage	E. Projects a more diffuse light over a wide area

_____ 6. Spotlight	F. A piece of equipment capable of providing electricity for portable lighting

_____ 7. Salvage covers	G. Large square or rectangular sheets of heavy canvas or plastic material that are used to protect furniture and other items from water runoff, falling debris, soot, and particulate matter in smoke residue

_____ 8. Water catch-all	H. A device used as a mobile power outlet

_____ 9. Generator	I. A temporary pond that holds dripping water in one location

_____ 10. Junction box	J. Heavy canvas with handles used to carry debris

Multiple Choice

Read each item carefully, and then select the best response.

_____ 1. Before a fire fighter can work without a self-contained breathing apparatus (SCBA), the atmosphere must be tested and determined safe by the
   A. safety officer.
   B. incident commander.
   C. RIC leader.
   D. department captain.

_____ **2.** The building's construction, its contents, and the size of the fire are factors in determining
   A. salvage operations.
   B. the area that needs to be overhauled.
   C. who the incident commander is.
   D. the placement of the rapid intervention company/crew.

_____ **3.** Sprinklers should not be shut down until the IC declares the fire
   A. is completely out.
   B. is under control.
   C. has spread to other rooms of the structure.
   D. is being ventilated.

_____ **4.** Fire damage to the building's structural components may potentially lead to
   A. atmospheric contamination.
   B. reignition.
   C. rekindling.
   D. structural collapse.

_____ **5.** Which type of device catches dripping water and directs it toward a drain or to the outside?
   A. Water chute
   B. Water catch-all
   C. Drain
   D. Fire-fighter-made opening

_____ **6.** What is the best way to prevent water damage at a fire scene?
   A. Increase the number of ventilation sites
   B. Use higher flow rates
   C. Use the building sprinkler system
   D. Limit the amount of water used

_____ **7.** Which type of lights are most often used during the first few critical minutes of an incident?
   A. 1500-watt portable lights
   B. Battery-powered lights
   C. 300-watt quartz lights
   D. 1000-watt halogen lights

_____ **8.** The main control for a sprinkler system is usually a(n)
   A. sprinkler box.
   B. scupper.
   C. OS&Y valve or PIV.
   D. water valve.

_____ **9.** A long section of protective material used to cover a section of carpet is called a
   A. floor cover.
   B. floor runner.
   C. carpet tarp.
   D. drop tarp.

_____ 10. Mobile power outlets, which are placed in convenient locations for cords to be attached, are also known as
   A. junction boxes.
   B. generators.
   C. inverters.
   D. extension outlets.

_____ 11. To stop the flow from a sprinkler, insert a
   A. hand tool.
   B. sprinkler wedge.
   C. sprinkler key.
   D. cloth.

_____ 12. During salvage operations, smaller pictures and valuable objects should be placed in
   A. the pockets of the fire fighter's PPE.
   B. smaller tarps.
   C. drawers.
   D. the corner.

_____ 13. Fire can extend directly from the basement to the attic, without obvious signs of fire, in a
   A. balloon-frame building.
   B. platform-frame building.
   C. Type I building.
   D. remodeled building.

_____ 14. Efforts to protect property and belongings from damage are called
   A. overhaul.
   B. salvage.
   C. rescue.
   D. recovery.

_____ 15. The most common method of protecting building contents is to cover them with
   A. heat-reflective blankets.
   B. salvage covers.
   C. overhaul tarps.
   D. salvage tarps.

_____ 16. Fire fighters' salvage efforts at residential fires often focus on protecting
   A. expensive items or property.
   B. isolated property.
   C. personal property.
   D. market items.

_____ 17. The most efficient way to protect a room's contents is to move all the furniture to
   A. the center of the room.
   B. the wall farthest from the flames.
   C. the walls nearest the window(s) used for ventilation and fire suppression.
   D. the front of the room.

_____ 18. How much does a gallon (4 liters) of water weigh?
   A. 2.24 pounds (1 kg)
   B. 4.5 pounds (2 kg)
   C. 6 pounds (2.7 kg)
   D. 8.3 pounds (3.8 kg)

Vocabulary

Define the following terms using the space provided.

1. Salvage cover:
   _____
   _____
   _____

2. Sprinkler wedge:
   _____
   _____
   _____

3. Floor runner:
   _____
   _____
   _____

4. Overhaul:
   _____
   _____
   _____

5. Sprinkler stop:
   _____
   _____
   _____

6. Balloon-frame construction:
   _____
   _____
   _____

Fill-In

Read each item carefully, and then complete the statement by filling in the missing word(s).

1. A(n) _____ _____ should always be present during overhaul operations to note any hazards and ensure that operations are conducted safely.

2. _____ teams remain at the fire scene and watch for signs of rekindling.

3. A(n) _____ vacuum is a special piece of equipment used to suck up water during salvage operations.

4. Buckets, tubs, wheelbarrows, and _____ can be used to remove debris from a building.

5. Salvage and overhaul have a(n) _____ priority than search and rescue.

Fundamentals of Fire Fighter Skills

6. A(n) _____ _____ _____ can distinguish between objects or areas with different temperatures.

7. _____ ensures that a fire is completely extinguished.

8. During salvage and overhaul efforts, fire fighters must attempt to preserve _____ related to the cause of the fire, particularly when arson is expected.

9. Look, listen, and _____ to detect signs of potential burning.

10. Salvage efforts are usually aimed at preventing or limiting _____ _____ that result from smoke and water damage.

11. Sprinkler heads that have been activated must be _____ before they can be restored to normal operations.

12. Generators should have _____-_____ _____ (_____) to prevent a fire fighter from receiving a potentially fatal electric shock.

True/False

If you believe the statement to be more true than false, write the letter "T" in the space provided. If you believe the statement to be more false than true, write the letter "F."

1. _____ The entire area around a fire building should be illuminated.
2. _____ When entering an area for salvage operations, fire fighters should roll a floor runner ahead of themselves.
3. _____ The damage caused to property by smoke and water is usually much less costly to repair or replace than the property that is burned.
4. _____ The cause of the fire can also indicate the extent of overhaul necessary.
5. _____ Pike poles are used to pull down sections of ceiling.
6. _____ Salvage efforts can be done during fire suppression.
7. _____ Sprinkler control valves should always be locked in the closed position.
8. _____ The IC may order hydraulic or standard overhaul procedures.
9. _____ Water used in fire suppression can create potential hazards for fire fighters.
10. _____ Salvage crews begin on the floor of the fire to prevent water damage to room contents.

Short Answer

Complete this section with short written answers using the space provided.

1. List four potential hazards present during overhaul operations.

_____
_____
_____
_____

2. Identify five tools used in salvage operations.

___

3. List five tools used in overhaul operations.

___

4. List five indicators of possible structural collapse.

___

Fire Alarms

The following real case scenarios will give you an opportunity to explore the concerns associated with salvage and overhaul. Read each scenario, and then answer each question in detail.

You are assigned to the second ladder company arriving at a third-floor apartment fire in a multistory residential structure. The IC has ordered your company to the floor below the fire for salvage operations. Water is running from the ceiling into a second-floor apartment, causing much water damage. Your company officer orders you to protect the contents of the family room and then build a water chute to divert water to an outside window.

1. Which actions will you take to protect the family room contents?

___

2. After you return from the fire described in question 1, your company officer instructs you to clean and check the salvage covers for wear. What is the proper method for cleaning and inspecting salvage covers?

___

Skill Drills

Skill Drill 19-3: Using a Sprinkler Stop Fire Fighter I, NFPA 1001:4.3.14
Test your knowledge of this skill drill by filling in the correct words in the photo captions.

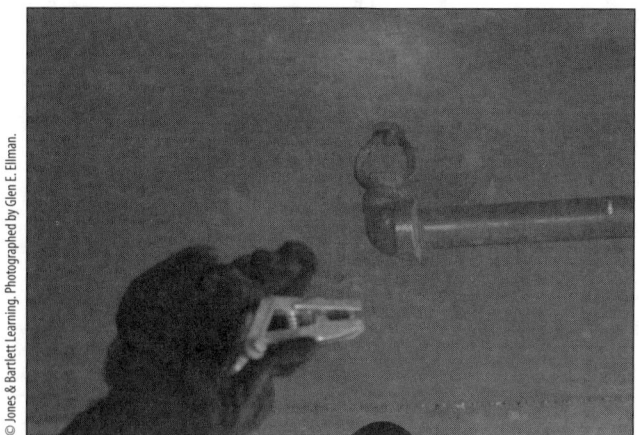

1. Have a _____ in hand.

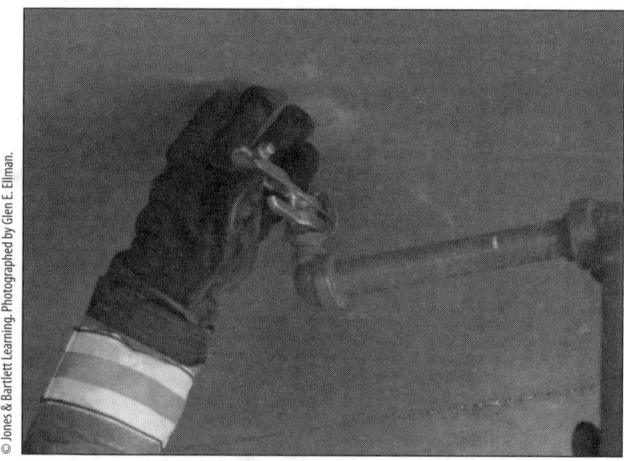

2. Place the _____ - _____ part of the sprinkler stop over the sprinkler orifice and between the frame of the sprinkler.

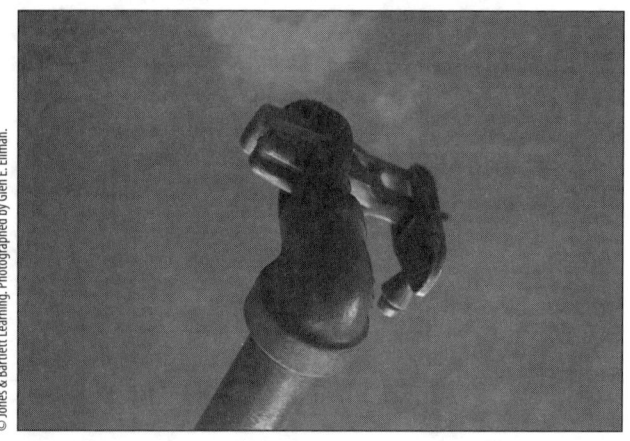

3. Push the _____ to expand the sprinkler stop until it snaps into position.

Skill Drill 19-4: Closing and Reopening a Main OS&Y Valve Fire Fighter I, NFPA 1001: 4.3.14
Test your knowledge of this skill drill by filling in the correct words in the photo captions.

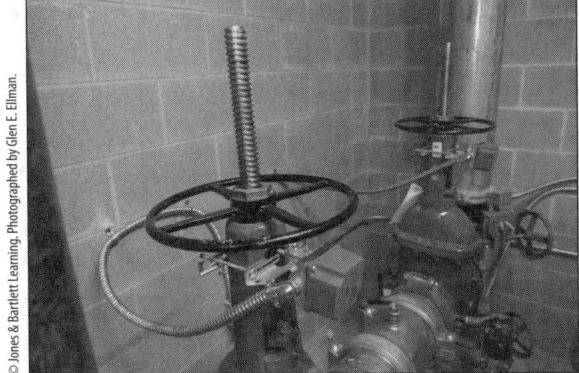

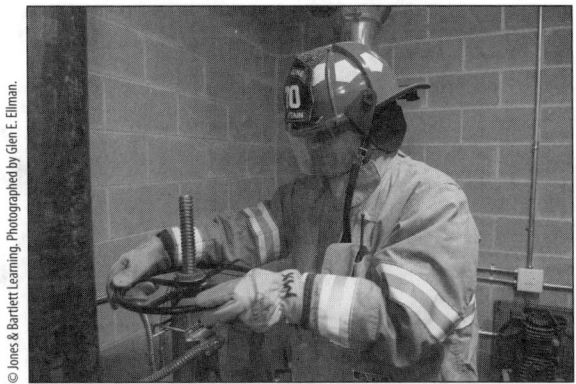

1. Locate the _____ valve as indicated on the preincident plan. Identify the valve that controls sprinklers in the fire area. If the valve is locked in the open position with a chain and padlock, and the key is readily available, unlock and remove the chain. If no key is available, cut the lock or the chain with a pair of bolt cutters. Cut a _____ close to the padlock so the chain can be _____.

2. Turn the valve handle _____ to close the valve. Keep turning until resistance is strong and little of the valve stem is visible.

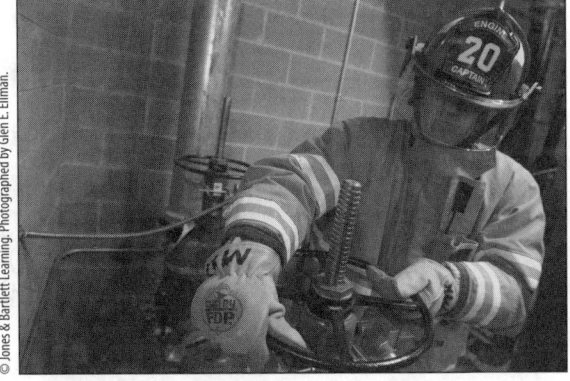

3. To reopen the OS&Y valve, turn the handle _____ until resistance is strong and the valve stem is visible again. Lock the _____ in the open position.

Skill Drill 19-5: Closing and Reopening a Main Post Indicator Valve Fire Fighter I, NFPA 1001: 4.3.14
Test your knowledge of this skill drill by filling in the correct words in the photo captions.

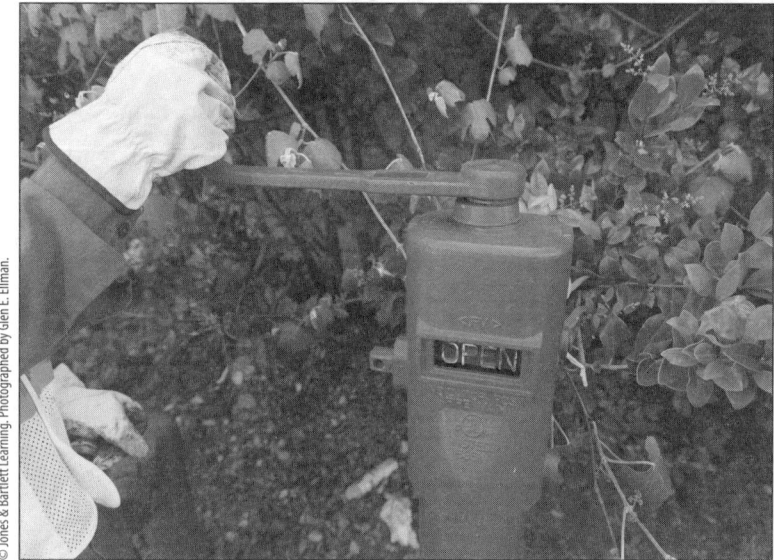

1. Locate the PIV as indicated in the preincident plan. Unlock the padlock with a key, or cut the lock with a pair of _____ .
2. Remove the handle from its storage position on the PIV, and place it on top of the valve, similar to the use of a _____ . Turn the valve stem in the direction indicated on top of the valve to close the valve. Keep turning until resistance is strong and the visual indicator changes from "Open" to "Shut."
3. To reopen the PIV, turn the valve stem in the _____ direction until resistance is strong and the indicator changes back to "Open." Lock the valve in the open position.

Skill Drill 19-6: Constructing a Water Chute Fire Fighter I, NFPA 1001: 4.3.14
Test your knowledge of this skill drill by placing the photos below in the correct order. Number the first step with a "1," the second step with a "2," and so on.

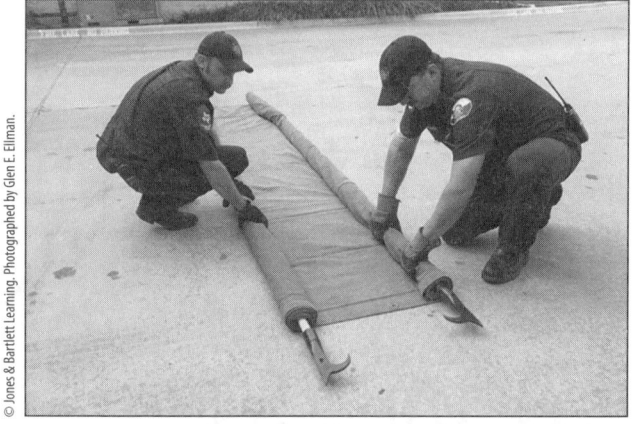

_____ Repeat the actions in Step 2 on the opposite edge of the cover, rolling the opposite edge tightly toward the middle until the two rolls are 1 to 3 ft (30 to 91 cm) apart.

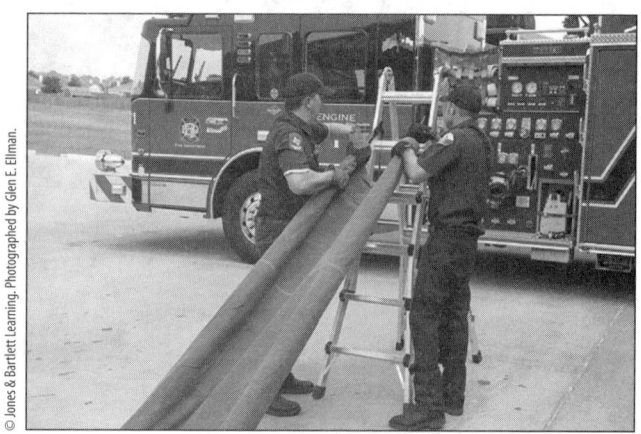

_____ Use a stepladder or other tall object to support chutes constructed with pike poles.

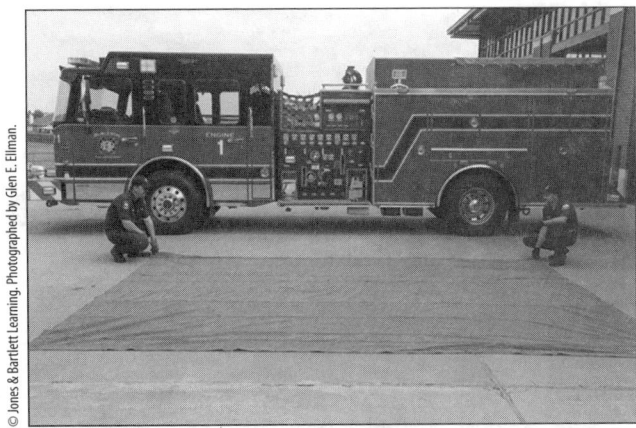

_____ Fully open a large salvage cover flat on the ground.

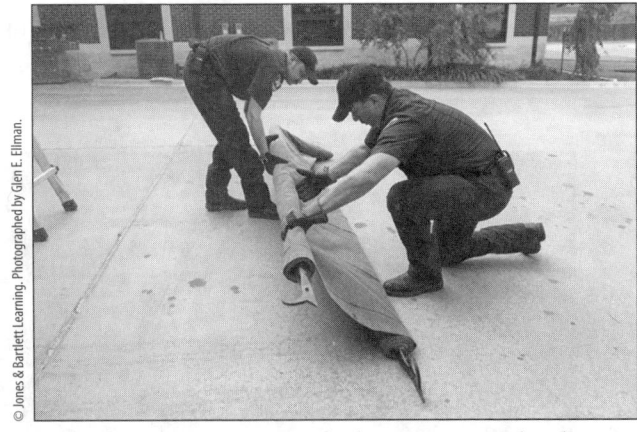

_____ Turn the cover upside down. Position the chute so that it collects dripping water and channels it toward a drain or outside opening. Place the chute on the floor, with one end propped up by a chair or other object.

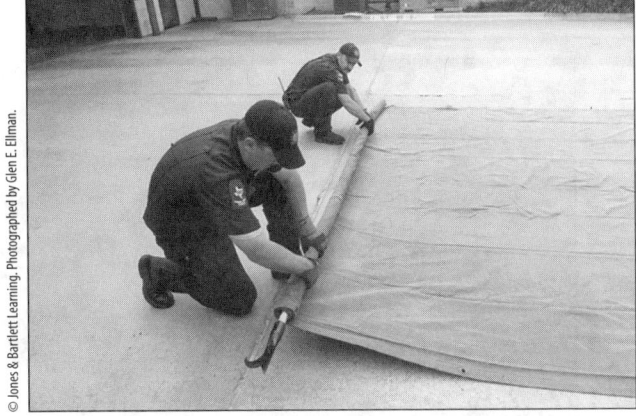

_____ If using pike poles, lay one pole on one edge of the cover, and roll the cover around the handle. Roll the cover tightly toward the middle.

266 FUNDAMENTALS OF FIRE FIGHTER SKILLS

Skill Drill 19-7: Constructing a Water Catch-All Fire Fighter I, NFPA 1001: 4.3.14
Test your knowledge of this skill drill by filling in the correct words in the photo captions.

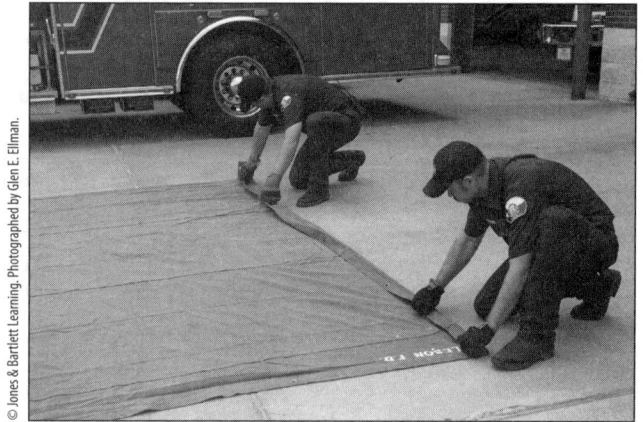

1. Open a large _____ on the ground, and roll each edge of the cover toward the opposite side.

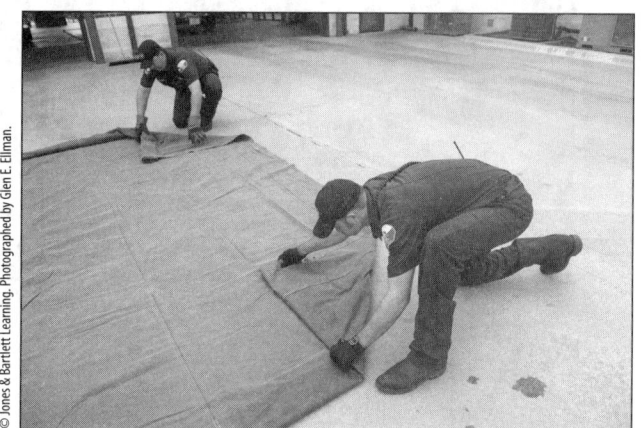

2. Fold each corner over at a _____ -degree angle, starting each fold approximately 3 ft (91 cm) in from the edge.

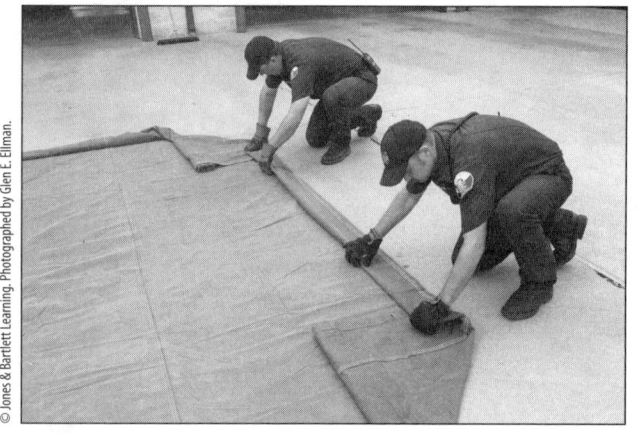

3. Roll the remaining two edges _____ approximately 2 ft (61 cm).

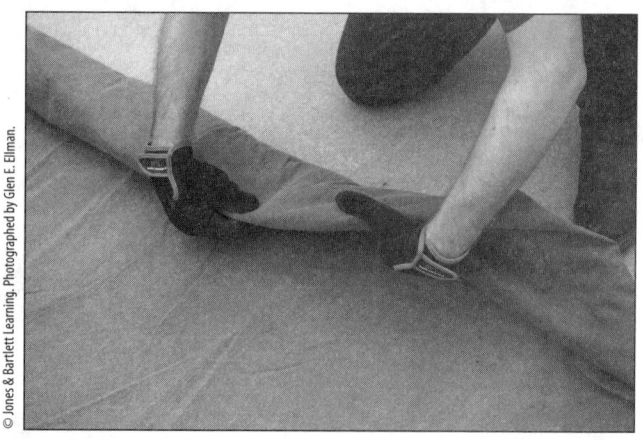

4. Lift the rolled edge over the _____, and tuck it in under the flaps to lock the corners in place.

Skill Drill 19-9: Performing a Salvage Cover Fold for Two-Fire Fighter Deployment Fire Fighter I, NFPA 1001: 4.3.14

Test your knowledge of this skill drill by placing the photos below in the correct order. Number the first step with a "1," the second step with a "2," and so on.

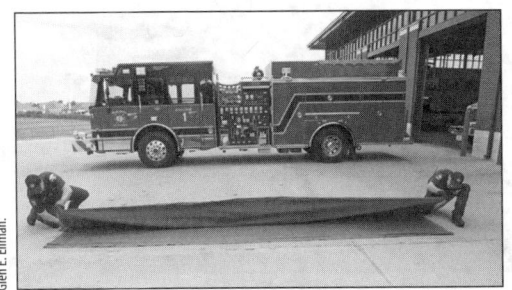

_____ Together, grasp the unfolded edge, and fold the cover in half again. Flatten the salvage cover to remove any trapped air.

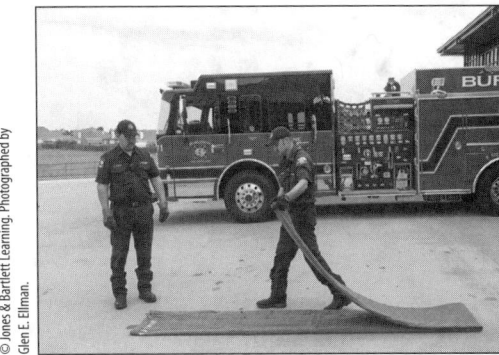

_____ Move to the newly created narrow ends of the salvage cover, and fold the salvage cover in half lengthwise.

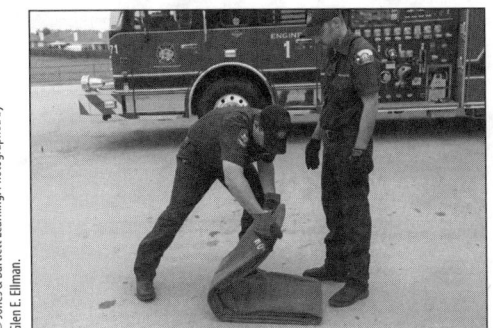

_____ Fold the cover in half a third time.

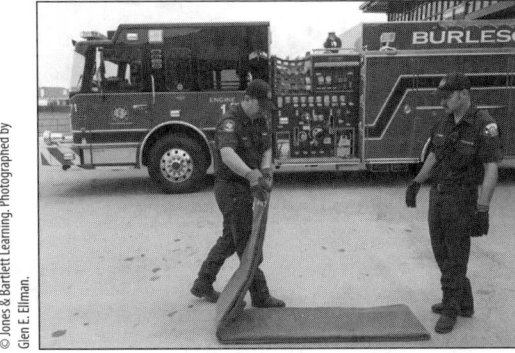

_____ Fold the salvage cover in half lengthwise again. Make certain that the open end is on top.

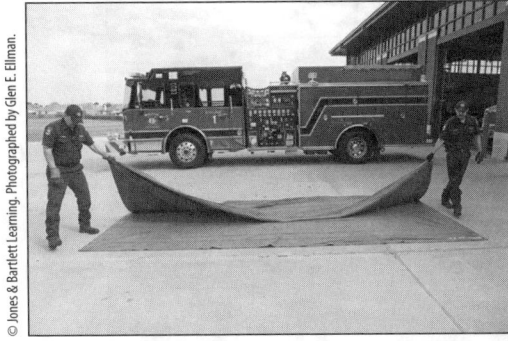

_____ Spread the salvage cover flat on the ground with a partner facing you. Together, fold the cover in half.

Skill Drill 19-10: Folding and Rolling a Salvage Cover Fire Fighter I, NFPA 1001: 4.3.14

Test your knowledge of this skill drill by filling in the correct words in the photo captions.

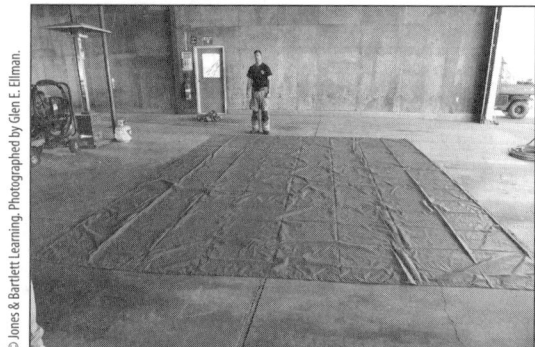

1. Spread the salvage cover flat on the ground with a partner _____ you.

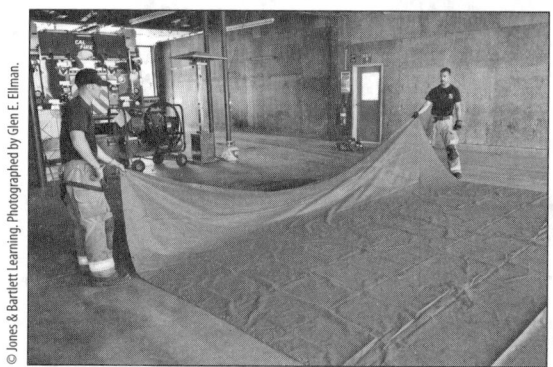

2. Together, fold the outside edge in to the middle of the cover, creating a fold at the _____.

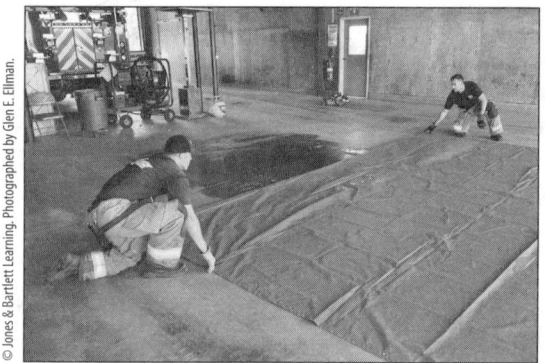

3. Fold the outside fold in to the _____ of the cover, creating a second fold.

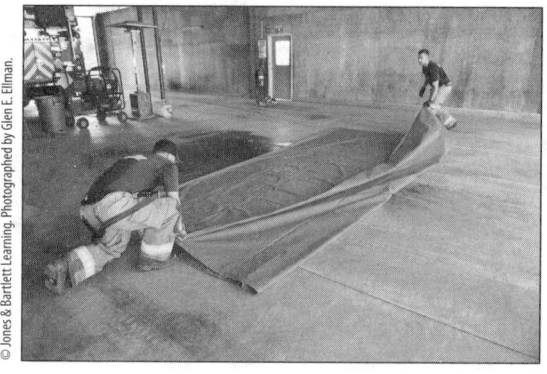

4. Repeat Step 2 from the _____ side of the cover.

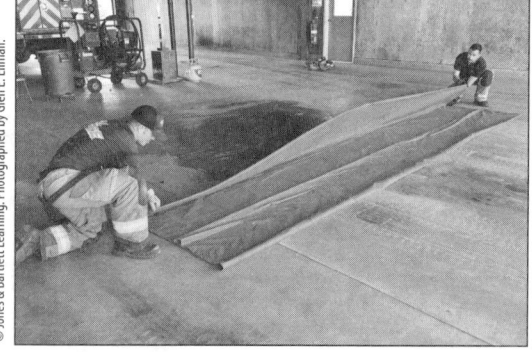

5. Repeat Step 3 from the opposite side of the cover so the folded edges meet at the middle of the cover, with the folds touching but not _____.

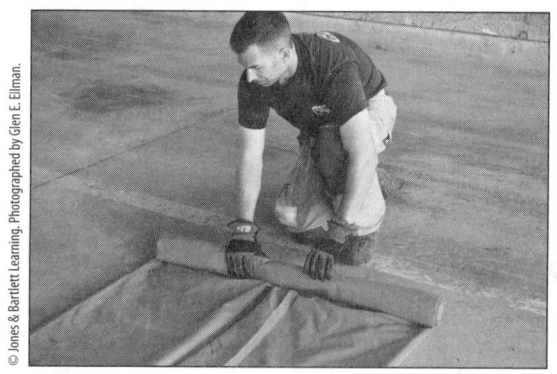

6. Tightly roll up the folded salvage cover from the _____.

Skill Drill 19-14: Using a Multi-gas Meter Fire Fighter I, NFPA 1001: 4.3.21

Test your knowledge of this skill drill by placing the photos below in the correct order. Number the first step with a "1," the second step with a "2," and so on.

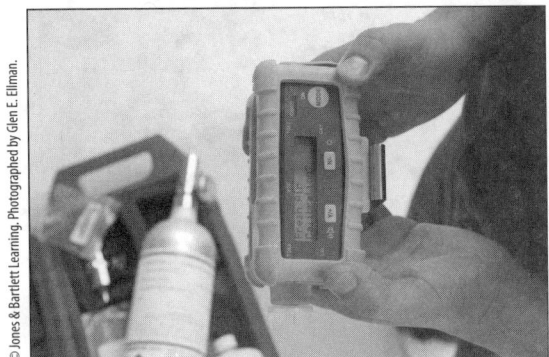

_____ Perform a fresh air calibration, and "zero" the unit.

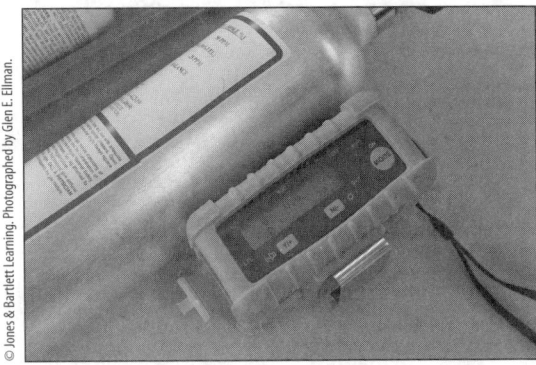

_____ Allow the device to reset, or return to fresh air calibration state, then review the alarm levels and resetting procedures for addressing sensors that become saturated, or exposed to too much gas or vapor.

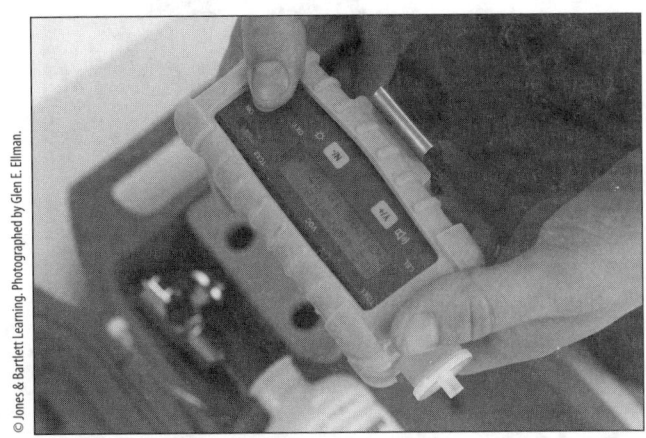

_____ Turn the unit on and let it warm up (usually 5 minutes is sufficient) in a well-ventilated area, away from the fire scene and any vehicles. Ensure the battery has sufficient life for the operational period. Identify the installed sensors (e.g., oxygen, flammability, hydrogen sulfide, carbon monoxide), and verify that the sensors are not expired. Review alarm limits and the audio and visual alarm notifications associated with those limits. Review and understand the types of gases and vapors that could harm or destroy the sensors. Use other methods to check for those substances (e.g., pH paper) to ensure they are not present in the atmosphere to be sampled. Care must be taken to avoid pulling liquids into the device—it is designed to sample air, not liquid!

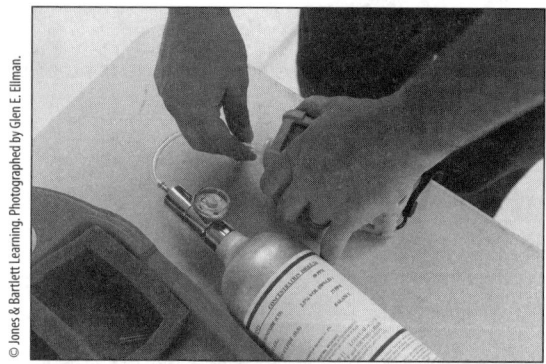

_____ Ensure the meter is operating correctly by exposing the unit to a substance or substances that the unit should detect and react to accordingly. In essence, you are making sure the unit will "see" what it is supposed to see before it is called upon to see it in a real situation.

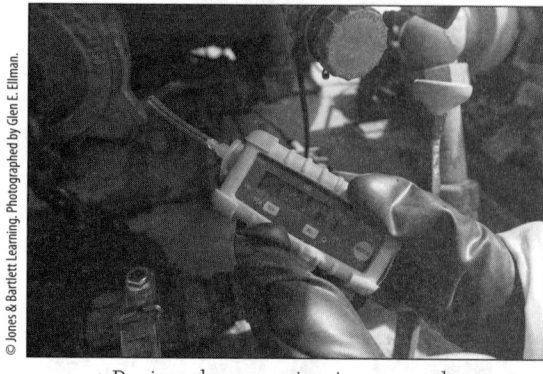

_____ Review decontamination procedures. Carry out monitoring and detection per the device manufacturer's instructions. If the high- or low-level alarm activates, follow the standard operating procedures established by the authority having jurisdiction.

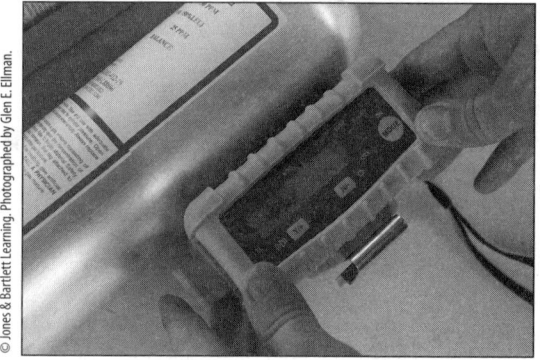

_____ Perform a test on the pump by occluding the inlet and ensuring the appropriate alarm sounds.

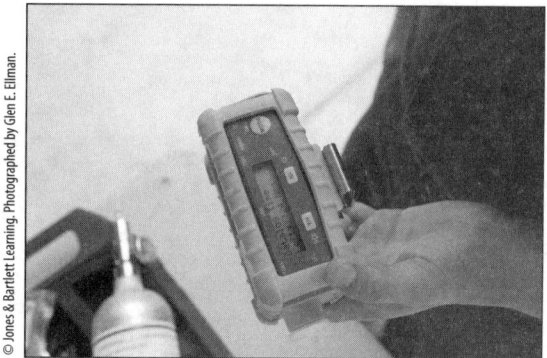

_____ Review other device functions such as screen illumination, data logging (if available), and low-battery alarm.

Skill Drill 19-16: Opening an Interior Wall Fire Fighter I, NFPA 1001: 4.3.13
Test your knowledge of this skill drill by placing the photos below in the correct order. Number the first step with a "1," the second step with a "2," and so on.

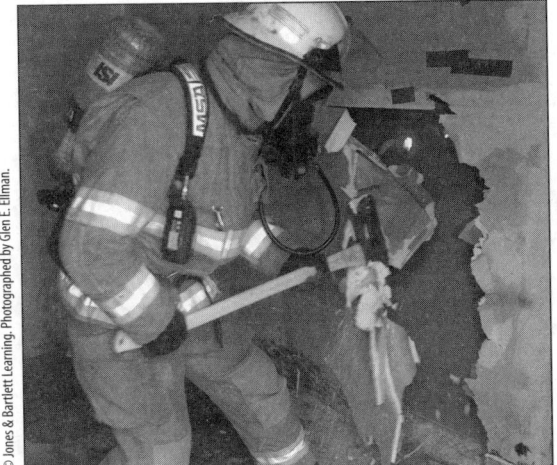

_____ Make two vertical cuts, using the pick end of the axe to pull the wall material away from the studs and open the wall. Work from top to bottom. Remove items such as baseboards or window and door trim with a Halligan tool or axe.

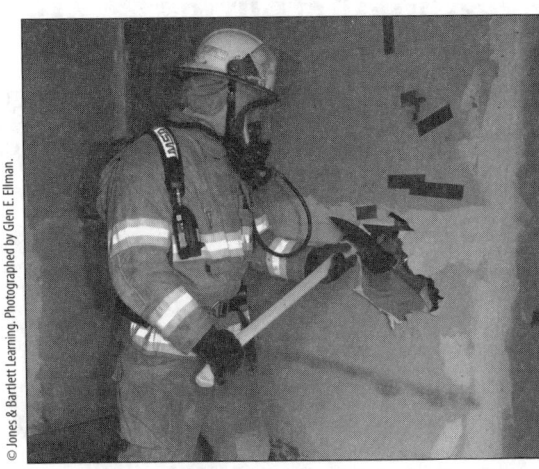

_____ Determine which area of the wall will be opened. Open those areas most heavily damaged by the fire first, followed by the surrounding areas.

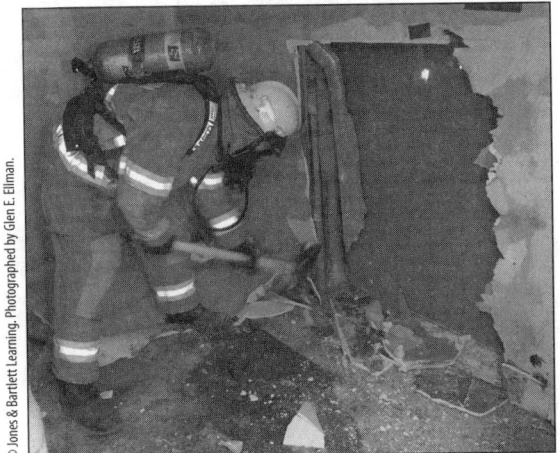

_____ Continue opening additional sections of the wall until the desired area is open. Pull out any insulation, such as fiberglass, found behind the wall.

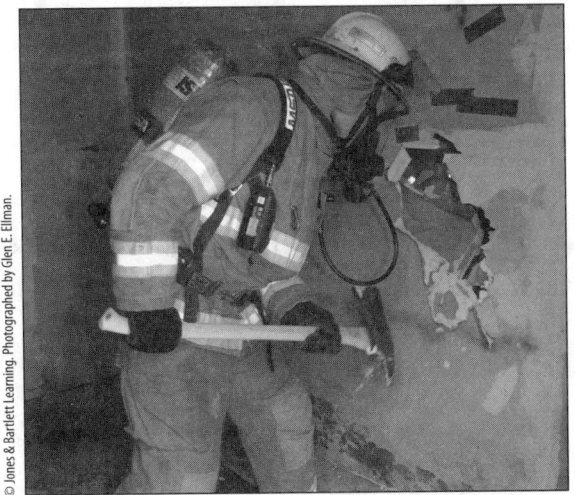

_____ Use the axe blade to begin cutting near the top of the wall. Cut downward between wall studs. Be alert for electrical switches or receptacles, as they indicate the presence of electrical wires behind the wall.

Fire Fighter Rehabilitation

Workbook Activities

The following activities have been designed to help you. Your instructor may require you to complete some or all of these activities as a regular part of your fire fighter training program. You are encouraged to complete any activity your instructor does not assign to you, as a way to enhance your learning in the classroom.

Chapter Review

The following exercises provide an opportunity to refresh your knowledge of this chapter.

Matching

Match each of the terms in the left column to the appropriate definition in the right column.

_____ 1. Electrolytes

_____ 2. Rehabilitate

_____ 3. Frostbite

_____ 4. Fully encapsulated suits

_____ 5. Emergency incident rehabilitation

_____ 6. Glucose

_____ 7. Dehydration

_____ 8. Personal protective equipment (PPE)

_____ 9. Hypothermia

_____ 10. Rehydrating

A. A protective suit that completely covers the fire fighter, including the breathing apparatus

B. Damage to tissue resulting from exposure to cold

C. Part of the overall emergency effort

D. A condition in which the body temperature falls below 95°F (35°C)

E. Certain salts and other chemicals that are dissolved in body fluids and cells

F. A state in which fluid losses are greater than fluid intake into the body

G. To restore to a condition of health or to a state of useful and constructive activity

H. More complicated than just drinking a lot of fluids

I. Protective clothing and breathing apparatus used by fire fighters to reduce and prevent injuries

J. Needed to burn fat efficiently and release energy

CHAPTER 20

Multiple Choice
Read each item carefully, and then select the best response.

_____ 1. Which of the following is *not* a function of an emergency incident rehabilitation center?
   A. Relief from climatic conditions
   B. Medical monitoring
   C. Rehydration
   D. Staging

_____ 2. Which of the following is the best rehabilitation food source during a short duration incident?
   A. Water and a high-protein sports bar
   B. Coffee or tea and a high-protein sports bar
   C. Fruit juice and pasta
   D. A complete meal that includes complex carbohydrates

_____ 3. Conditioning plays a significant role in
   A. endurance.
   B. glucose intake.
   C. intensity.
   D. reassignment.

_____ 4. Which of the following is the only fuel that the body can readily use during high-intensity physical activity?
   A. Carbohydrates
   B. Fats
   C. Proteins
   D. Electrolytes

_____ 5. The best way to prepare for physical work is to do activities that match
   A. the type of work.
   B. the duration of work.
   C. the intensity of work.
   D. All of the above.

_____ 6. A fire fighter must stay at the rehabilitation center until his or her body temperature returns to
   A. a range consistent with the environment.
   B. a temperature above pre-entry levels.
   C. a normal range.
   D. below pre-entry levels.

_____ 7. Which of the following may require rehabilitation?
   A. Training exercises
   B. Athletic events
   C. Standby assignments
   D. All of the above.

_____ 8. What is a benefit of proper nutrition?
   A. Stress reduction
   B. Health improvements
   C. Increased energy
   D. All of the above.

_____ 9. Rehabilitation enables fire fighters to
   A. perform more safely and effectively.
   B. review personal protective equipment items.
   C. discuss emergency response strategies.
   D. observe and assess response tactics.

_____ 10. During a high-rise fire, a department may assign three companies to do the work that is normally done by one company because
   A. there is a larger structure to protect.
   B. the higher the structure, the more distance to the ground.
   C. there is more equipment to carry.
   D. it enables the companies to rotate duties.

Vocabulary
Define the following terms using the space provided.

1. Rehabilitate:

   _____
   _____
   _____

2. Dehydration:

   _____
   _____
   _____

3. Hypothermia:

   _____
   _____
   _____

4. Frostbite:

   _____
   _____
   _____

5. Emergency incident rehabilitation:

   _____
   _____
   _____

Fill-In

Read each item carefully, and then complete the statement by filling in the missing word(s).

1. Blood sugar, or _____, is the fuel the body uses for energy.

2. When a fire fighter has abnormal vital signs, is suffering pain, or is injured, he or she needs to have further medical _____ and _____.

3. _____ can actually cause a swing in energy levels because it stimulates the production of insulin.

4. _____ is a critical factor in maintaining health and well-being.

5. _____ happens only when a fire fighter is rested, rehydrated, refueled, and fit to return to active duty.

6. _____ is caused by drinking too much too quickly.

7. The amount of rest needed to recover from physical exertion is directly related to the _____ of the work performed.

8. The stomach can absorb and can lose up to _____ quart(s) of fluid per hour.

9. _____ occurs when body tissues are damaged due to prolonged exposure to the cold.

10. _____ are a major source of fuel for the body and can be found in grains, vegetables, and fruits.

True/False

If you believe the statement to be more true than false, write the letter "T" in the space provided. If you believe the statement to be more false than true, write the letter "F."

1. _____ Fats are used for energy and for breaking down some vitamins.
2. _____ Regular rehabilitation enables fire fighters to accomplish more work during a major incident.
3. _____ Rehabilitation helps improve the quality of decision making.
4. _____ Taking short breaks, replacing fluids, ingesting healthy food, and cooling or rewarming are all measures that reduce the risk of injury and illness.
5. _____ Rehabilitation enables fire fighters to perform more safely and effectively at an emergency scene.
6. _____ Thirst is a reliable indicator of dehydration.
7. _____ On a cold day, coffee or hot chocolate are appropriate beverages to rehabilitate fire fighters.
8. _____ Rest should begin as soon as you arrive for rehabilitation.
9. _____ Carbohydrates are fattening and should generally be avoided.
10. _____ A crew should rest at least 20 minutes after the use of two 30-minute SCBA cylinders.

Short Answer

Complete this section with short written answers using the space provided.

1. Describe the types of meals a fire fighter should eat during rehabilitation for short and extended incidents.

_____
_____
_____
_____

2. Identify the personal responsibilities of each fire fighter during rehabilitation.

_____
_____
_____
_____

3. Why are caffeinated and sugar-rich beverages not recommended for rehabilitation?

_____
_____
_____
_____

4. What are the basic concepts of field reduction of contamination?

_____
_____
_____
_____

Fire Alarms

The following real case scenarios will give you an opportunity to explore the concerns associated with fire fighter rehabilitation. Read each scenario, and then answer each question in detail.

1. After fighting a winter-time (temperature 15°F) defensive fire for 2 hours, your partner comments that he has been wet for the last hour, and his feet and hands are hurting and causing a great deal of pain. How should you help him?

_____
_____
_____
_____
_____
_____

2. You have just finished clearing brush and shrubs from the path of a wildland fire. It is a warm, 85°F summer day with no breeze. You begin to feel warm, plus you are exhausted, sweating profusely, and feeling lightheaded. What should you do?

_____
_____
_____
_____
_____

Wildland and Ground Cover Fires

Workbook Activities

The following activities have been designed to help you. Your instructor may require you to complete some or all of these activities as a regular part of your fire fighter training program. You are encouraged to complete any activity your instructor does not assign to you, as a way to enhance your learning in the classroom.

Chapter Review

The following exercises provide an opportunity to refresh your knowledge of this chapter.

Matching

Match each of the terms in the left column to the appropriate definition in the right column.

_____ 1. Slash
_____ 2. Heel of the fire
_____ 3. Head of the fire
_____ 4. Spot fire
_____ 5. Black
_____ 6. Pocket
_____ 7. Island
_____ 8. Backfiring
_____ 9. Wildland
_____ 10. Fine fuel
_____ 11. Fuel volume

A. Fuel that ignites and burns easily
B. A new fire that starts outside the perimeter of the main fire
C. An area that has already been burned
D. The traveling edge of a fire
E. The leftovers of a logging and land-clearing operation
F. A planned operation to remove fuel by burning out large selected areas
G. The amount of fuel present in a given area
H. An unburned area surrounded by burned land
I. The area close to the area of origin
J. Land in an uncultivated natural state that is covered by timber, woodland, brush, or grass
K. The unburned area between a finger and the main body of the fire

Multiple Choice

Read each item carefully, and then select the best response.

_____ 1. The changes of elevation in the land, as well as the positions of natural and human-made features, is
   A. geography.
   B. geology.
   C. physiology.
   D. topography.

CHAPTER 21

_____ 2. A firefighting attack that involves building a fire line along natural fuel breaks, along favorable breaks in topography, or at a considerable distance from the fire and burning out the intervening fuel is called a(n)
   A. mounted attack.
   B. indirect attack.
   C. direct attack.
   D. counter attack.

_____ 3. The technique used to remove fuel by burning is called
   A. adze.
   B. backfiring.
   C. direct attack.
   D. flanking.

_____ 4. A firefighting attack that requires only one team of fire fighters is called a(n)
   A. pincer attack.
   B. backfiring attack.
   C. flanking attack.
   D. indirect attack.

_____ 5. How much water do small apparatus used for fighting wildland fires typically carry?
   A. 800 gallons (3028 liters)
   B. 200–300 gallons (757–1136 liters)
   C. 2000 gallons (7571 liters)
   D. 50–100 gallons (189–379 liters)

_____ 6. Which combination tool is used to create a fire line?
   A. McLeod fire tool
   B. Adze
   C. Pulaski axe
   D. Halligan tool

_____ 7. What is the top priority in a wildland fire attack?
   A. Containment
   B. Extinguishment
   C. Minimization of damage
   D. Safety

_____ 8. A firefighting attack that requires two teams of fire fighters attacking both flanks of a wildland fire is called a(n)
   A. pinch attack.
   B. backfiring attack.
   C. flanking attack.
   D. counter attack.

_____ 9. Which term describes wildland fuels that have uninterrupted connections?
   A. Fuel compactness
   B. Fuel continuity
   C. Fuel volume
   D. Fuel moisture

_____ 10. The firefighting attack most often used for large wildland and ground fires that are too dangerous for a direct attack is the
   A. pincer attack.
   B. backfiring attack.
   C. flanking attack.
   D. indirect attack.

_____ 11. An unburned area between a finger and the traveling (main body) edge of the fire is called a(n)
   A. island.
   B. lapse.
   C. pocket.
   D. spot fire.

_____ 12. Unplanned and uncontrolled fires burning in vegetative fuels that sometimes include structures are called
   A. ground cover fires.
   B. aerial fires.
   C. wildland fires.
   D. urban fires.

_____ 13. As wildland and ground fires grow and reach into areas with new fuel, the traveling edge of the fire is called the
   A. heel of the fire.
   B. head of the fire.
   C. rear of the fire.
   D. arm of the fire.

_____ 14. The partly decomposed organic material on a forest floor is called
   A. ground duff.
   B. slash.
   C. medium fuel.
   D. heavy fuel.

_____ 15. The three causes of wildland fires are natural, accidental, and
   A. intentional fires.
   B. occupational fires.
   C. combustion fires.
   D. mechanical fires.

_____ 16. Fuels that are located close to the surface of the ground are considered
   A. aerial fuels.
   B. subsurface fuels.
   C. super surface fuels.
   D. surface fuels.

Vocabulary

Define the following terms using the space provided.

1. Heavy fuels:

   _____
   _____
   _____

2. Fuel continuity:

   _____
   _____
   _____

3. Backpack pump extinguisher:
_____
_____
_____

4. Topography:
_____
_____
_____

5. Aerial fuels:
_____
_____
_____

Fill-In
Read each item carefully, and then complete the statement by filling in the missing word(s).

1. For small fires with a light fuel load, _____ _____ _____ may be an effective firefighting tactic.

2. The relative _____ is the ratio of the amount of water vapor present in the air compared to the maximum amount the air can hold at a given temperature.

3. The second side of the fire triangle is _____.

4. The location where a wildland or ground fire begins is called the _____.

5. Vegetative fuels can be located _____, _____, or _____ the ground.

6. A(n) _____ fire is a new fire that starts outside the perimeter of the main fire.

7. _____-wing aircraft can take on a load of water from a lake and apply it to the fire.

8. _____ conditions have a major impact on the behavior of wildland fires.

9. _____ and _____ fires can advance and change directions quickly.

10. Fires spread more _____ in fine fuels than in heavy timber and brush.

True/False
If you believe the statement to be more true than false, write the letter "T" in the space provided. If you believe the statement to be more false than true, write the letter "F."

1. _____ The two most critical weather conditions that influence a wildland fire are moisture and wind.

2. _____ Fire shelters can be carried in a protective pouch on a fire fighter's belt.

3. _____ The amount of moisture in a fuel is related to the season of the year.

4. _____ A direct attack on a wildland fire is made by attacking the left flank of the main body.

5. _____ Roots, moss, duff, and decomposed stumps are examples of heavy fuels.
6. _____ The rising of heated air in a wildland fire will preheat the fuels above the main body of the fire.
7. _____ The fire triangle consists of three elements: fuel, oxygen, and heat.
8. _____ Wildland fires are unplanned and uncontrolled fires burning in vegetative fuel that sometimes includes structures.
9. _____ Fine fuels have a small surface area relative to their volume.
10. _____ When relative humidity is high, the moisture from the air is absorbed by vegetative fuels, making them less susceptible to ignition.

Short Answer

Complete this section with a short written answer using the space provided.

1. List three hazards of wildland fires.

   _____
   _____
   _____
   _____

Fire Alarms

The following real case scenarios will give you an opportunity to explore the concerns associated with wildland and ground fires. Read each scenario, and then answer each question in detail.

1. Your company is assigned to assist in fighting a wildland fire by using a flanking attack. How should you proceed?

   _____
   _____
   _____
   _____
   _____
   _____

2. Your company is assigned to begin triaging a group of homes that are in the path of an approaching wildland fire. What are some considerations you should use in triaging these structures?

   _____
   _____
   _____
   _____
   _____
   _____

Skill Drills

Skill Drill 21-1: Suppressing a Ground Cover Fire, Fire Fighter I, NFPA 1001: 4.3.19
Test your knowledge of this skill drill by filling in the correct words in the photo captions.

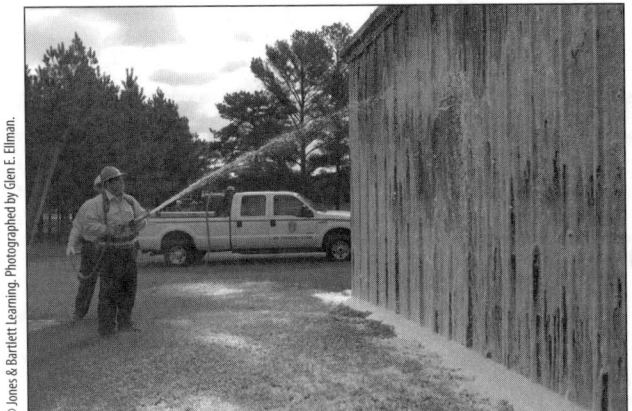

1. Don appropriate personal protective equipment (PPE). Identify safety and _____. Protect exposures if necessary.

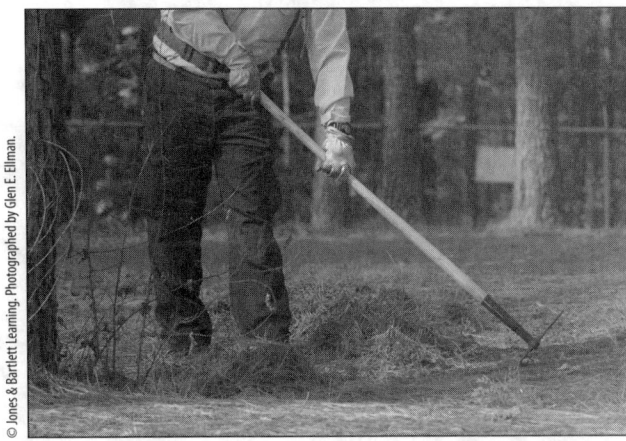

2. Construct a fire _____ by removing fuel with hand tools.

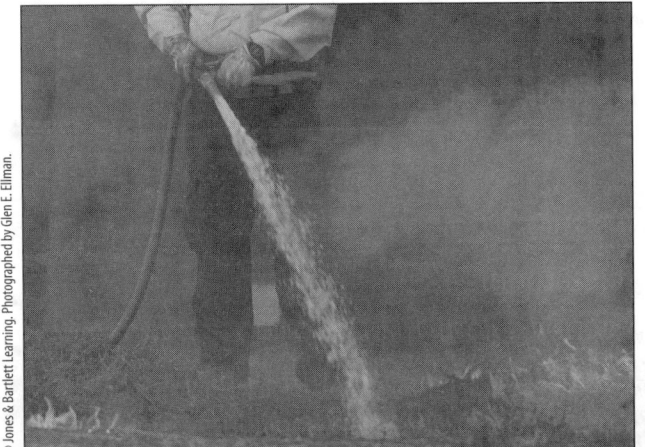

3. As an alternative to Step 2, extinguish the fire with a backpack pump extinguisher or a _____.

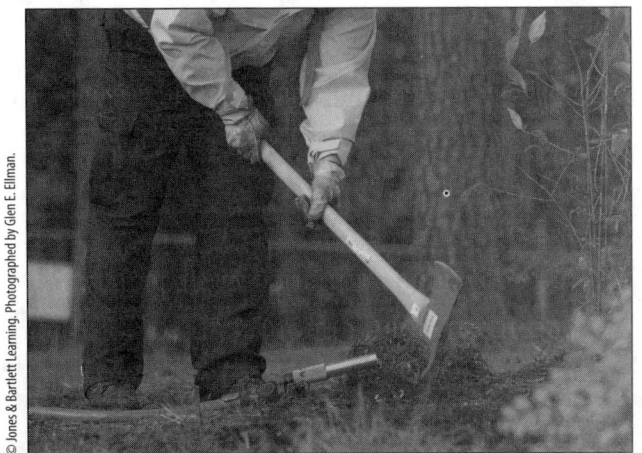

4. Overhaul the area _____ to ensure complete extinguishment of the ground cover fire.

Skill Drill 21-2: Using a Fire Shelter, Fire Fighter I, NFPA 1001: 4.3.19

Test your knowledge of this skill drill by placing the photos below in the correct order. Number the first step with a "1," the second step with a "2," and so on.

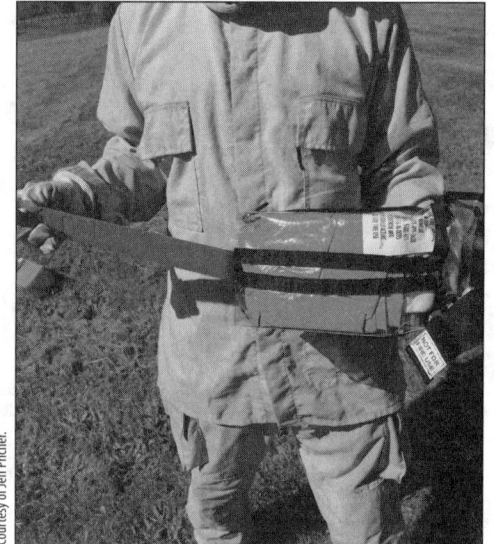

_____ Pull the red ring to tear off the plastic bag covering the shelter.

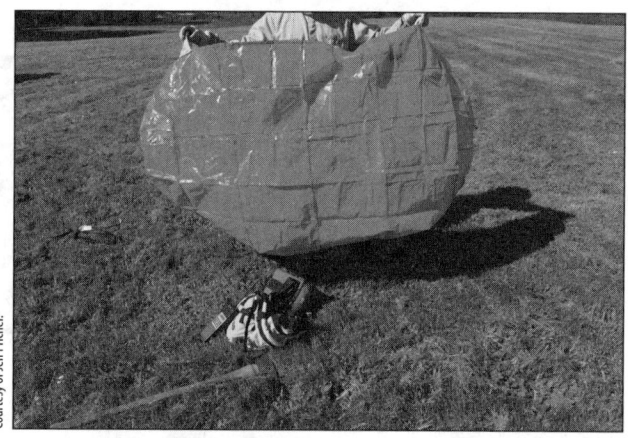

_____ Shake the shelter until it is unfolded. If it is windy, lie on the ground to unfold the shelter.

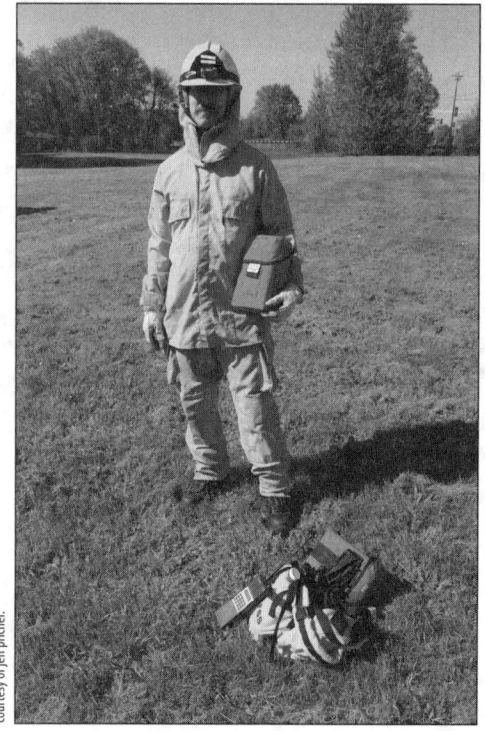

_____ Pick the largest available clearing. Wear gloves and a hard hat, and cover your face and neck if possible. Scrape away flammable litter if you have time.

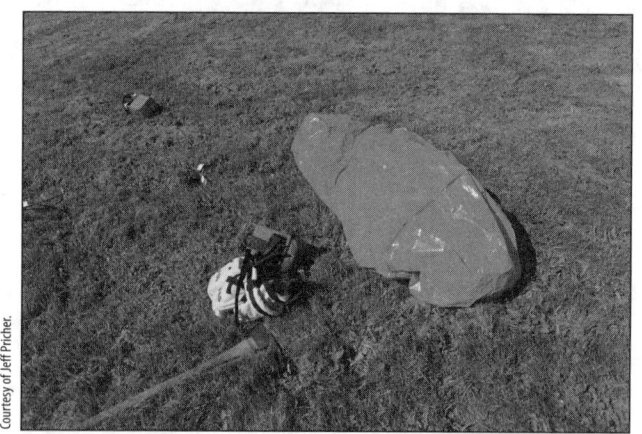

_____ Lie down in the shelter with your feet toward the oncoming fire. Push the sides out for more protection, and keep your mouth near the ground.

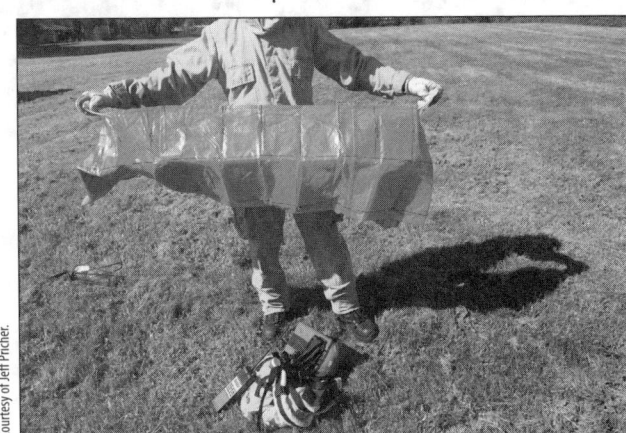

_____ Grasp the handle labeled "Left Hand" in your left hand and the handle labeled "Right Hand" in your right hand.

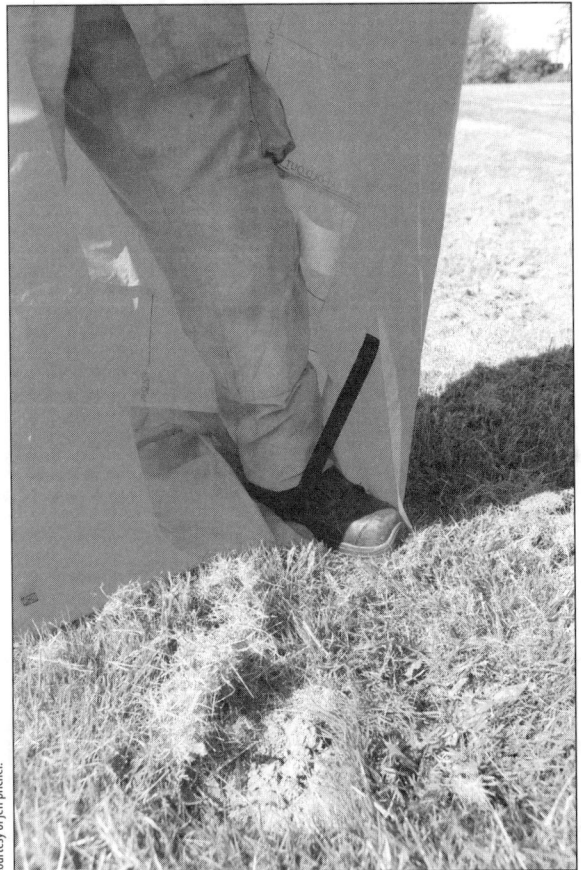

_____ Slip your feet through the hold-down straps.

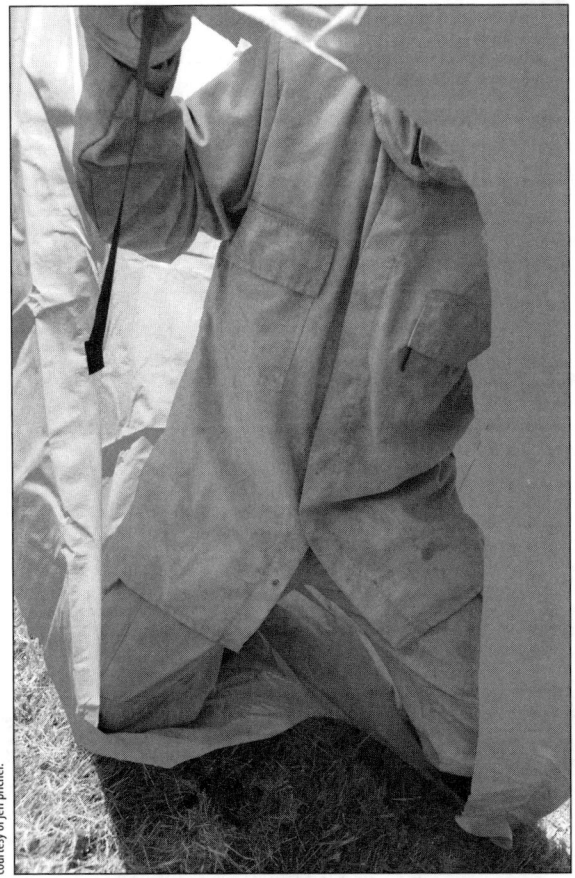

_____ Slip your arms through the hold-down straps.

Establishing and Transferring Command

Workbook Activities

The following activities have been designed to help you. Your instructor may require you to complete some or all of these activities as a regular part of your fire fighter training program. You are encouraged to complete any activity your instructor does not assign you, as a way to enhance your learning in the classroom.

Chapter Review

The following exercises provide an opportunity to refresh your knowledge of this chapter. All questions in this chapter are Fire Fighter II level.

Matching

Match each of the terms in the left column to the appropriate definition in the right column.

_____ 1. Staging area 　A. Usually refers to companies and/or crews working in the same geographic area

_____ 2. Task force 　B. A supervisory level established to manage the span of control above the division, or group, level

_____ 3. Size-up 　C. A location close to the incident scene where a number of units can be held in reserve, ready to be assigned if needed

_____ 4. Branch 　D. An organized group of fire fighters, working without an apparatus, under the leadership of a company officer

_____ 5. Transfer of command 　E. The officer in charge of a fire department company

_____ 6. Single command 　F. Includes two to five single resources, such as different types of units assembled to accomplish a specific task

_____ 7. Division 　G. Usually refers to companies and/or crews working on the same task or function

_____ 8. Crew 　H. The process of initially evaluating an emergency situation

_____ 9. Company officer 　I. The most traditional perception of the Command function; the genesis of the term *incident commander*

_____ 10. Group 　J. Occurs when one person relinquishes command to another individual

CHAPTER 22

Multiple Choice

Read each item carefully, and then select the best response.

_____ 1. The incident commander's (IC's) representative and the position responsible for exchanging information with outside agencies or directing people to the proper authority is the
   A. liaison officer.
   B. safety officer.
   C. public information officer.
   D. Planning Section Chief.

_____ 2. The exterior sides of a building are generally known as sides
   A. north, east, south, and west.
   B. A, B, C, and D.
   C. one, two, three, and four.
   D. right, left, top, and bottom.

_____ 3. If an incident requires more resources than the local community can provide, most departments have
   A. auxiliary or relief workers.
   B. state-level response plans.
   C. mutual aid agreements.
   D. support response teams.

_____ 4. A standard system of assigning and keeping track of the resources involved in the incident is the
   A. incident resources system.
   B. resource management system.
   C. unified resources system.
   D. operational resources system.

_____ 5. An ICS developed in the 1970s for day-to-day fire department incidents was the
   A. Unified Command System.
   B. FIRESCOPE.
   C. Fire-ground Command System.
   D. Task Force System.

_____ 6. When fire fighters advance into the fire building with hose lines to overpower the fire, they are part of a (an)
   A. defensive attack.
   B. defensive response.
   C. offensive attack.
   D. rapid intervention team.

_____ 7. The section of the ICS that is responsible for providing supplies, services, facilities, and materials during the incident is the
   A. Operations Section.
   B. Planning Section.
   C. Logistics Section.
   D. Administration Section.

_____ 8. Which position is established when the first-arriving unit arrives on the scene?
   A. Command
   B. Division supervisor
   C. Operations Section Chief
   D. ICS director

_____ 9. The number of subordinates who report to one supervisor at any level within the organization is the
   A. integrated communications.
   B. unified command.
   C. unity of command.
   D. span of control.

_____ 10. To track all fire fighters, there should be a(n) _____ at every incident scene.
   A. incident commander
   B. personnel accountability system
   C. incident management system
   D. accountability officer

_____ 11. The section of the ICS that is responsible for the collection, evaluation, dissemination, and use of information relevant to the incident is the
   A. Operations Section.
   B. Planning Section.
   C. Logistics Section.
   D. Administration Section.

_____ 12. The initial size-up of an incident is conducted by
   A. the second arriving unit on the scene.
   B. the first arriving Chief officer on the scene.
   C. the first arriving unit on the scene.
   D. reviewing the preincident plan.

_____ 13. The section of the ICS that is responsible for the management of all actions that are directly related to controlling the incident is the
   A. Operations Section.
   B. Planning Section.
   C. Logistics Section.
   D. Administration Section.

_____ 14. The section of the ICS that is responsible for any legal issues that may arise during an incident is the
   A. Operations Section.
   B. Planning Section.
   C. Logistics Section.
   D. Finance/Administration Section.

_____ 15. What is the management concept in which each person has only one direct supervisor?
   A. Integrated communications
   B. Unified command
   C. Unity of command
   D. Span of control

_____ 16. What is the first consideration at any emergency incident?
   A. Protecting property
   B. Protecting lives
   C. Controlling traffic
   D. Conducting a complete size-up

_____ 17. When multiple agencies with overlapping jurisdictions and legal responsibilities respond to the same incident, ICS may employ a(n)
   A. incident command system.
   B. unity of command.
   C. fire-ground command system.
   D. unified command.

_____ 18. Companies or crews working in the same geographic area are termed
   A. divisions.
   B. groups.
   C. sectors.
   D. teams.

_____ 19. The safety officer, liaison officer, and public information officer are always part of the
   A. command staff.
   B. rapid intervention team.
   C. Operations Section.
   D. ICS general staff.

_____ 20. A fire department's basic resources are
   A. its personnel and apparatus.
   B. its preincident plans and trained personnel.
   C. its specialized equipment and apparatus.
   D. its specially trained personnel.

_____ 21. Which officer has the authority to stop or suspend operations when unsafe situations occur?
   A. Health officer
   B. Liaison officer
   C. Operations officer
   D. Safety officer

_____ 22. The officer responsible for gathering and releasing incident information to the news media is the
   A. liaison officer.
   B. public information officer.
   C. Operations Section Chief.
   D. Public Relations Chief.

_____ 23. A crew is a group of fire fighters who are working
   A. on their own.
   B. as ICS Section Chiefs.
   C. without apparatus.
   D. outside the ICS.

_____ 24. An individual vehicle and its assigned personnel are considered a
   A. single resource.
   B. crew.
   C. branch.
   D. division.

Fundamentals of Fire Fighter Skills

Labeling
Label the following diagram with the correct terms.

1. Creating branches within the operations section is one way to manage the span of control during a large incident.

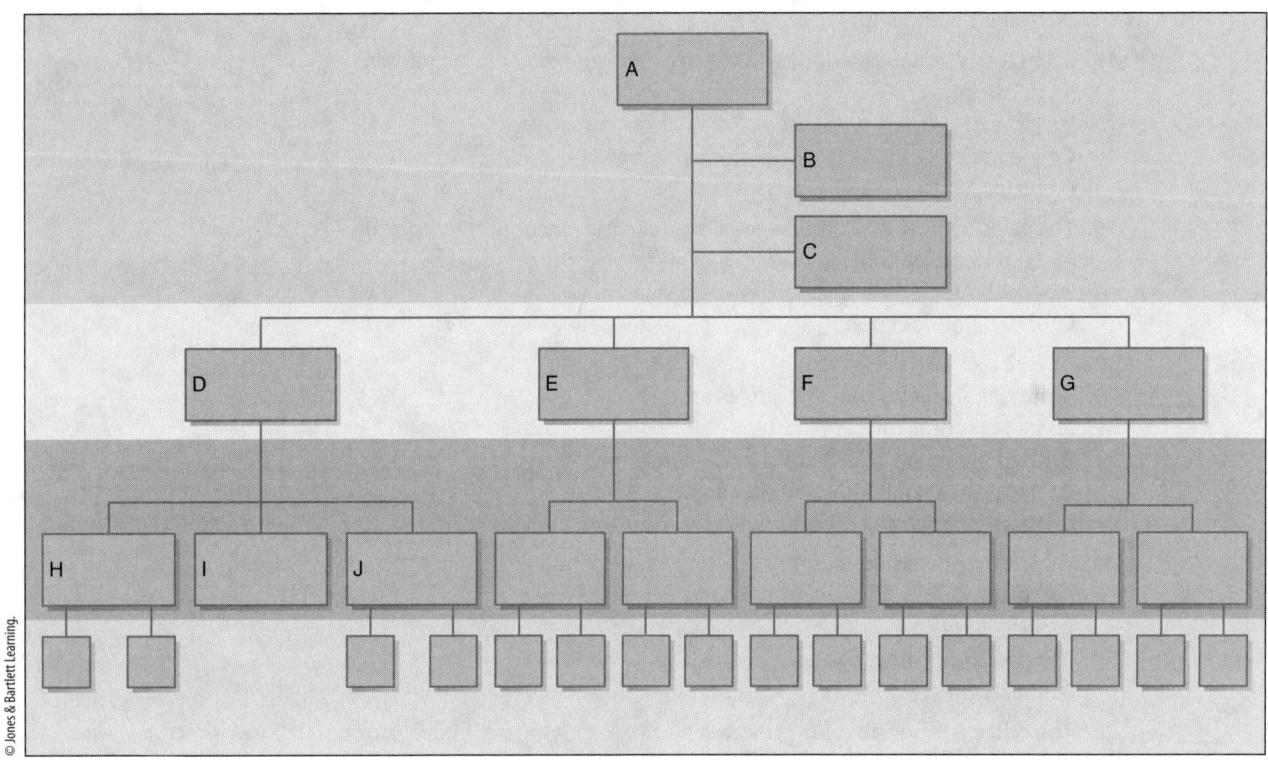

A. _____

B. _____

C. _____

D. _____

E. _____

F. _____

G. _____

H. _____

I. _____

J. _____

2. Location designators in ICS.

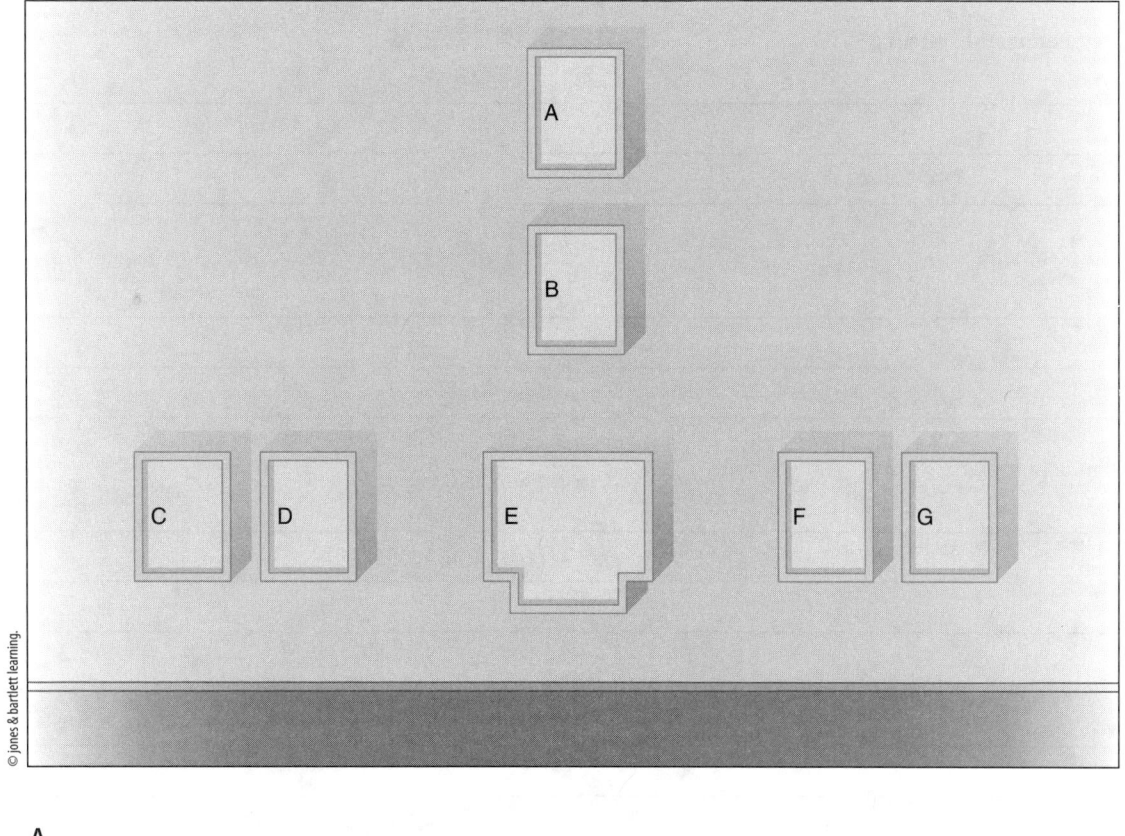

A. _____
B. _____
C. _____
D. _____
E. _____
F. _____
G. _____

Vocabulary

Define the following terms using the space provided.

1. Incident command system:

2. Unified command:

3. Incident action plan:

4. National Incident Management System:

5. Command staff:

6. Division:

7. Resource management:

8. Size-up:

9. Freelancing:

_____
_____
_____

10. Crew Resource Management (CRM):

_____
_____
_____

Fill-In
Read each item carefully, and then complete the statement by filling in the missing word(s).

1. In the ICS structure, _____ is ultimately responsible for managing an incident and has the authority to direct all activities.

2. _____ are events that can be predicted or anticipated, based on facts, observations, and previous experiences.

3. A(n) _____ _____ is an individual vehicle and its assigned personnel.

4. The primary reason for establishing divisions and groups is to maintain a(n) effective _____ _____ _____.

5. Planning, supervision, and _____ are key components of an ICS.

6. Standard _____ is a strength of the ICS. Understanding this is the first step in understanding the system.

7. The modular design of ICS allows the _____ to expand based on the needs of the incident.

8. The size-up process requires a(n) _____ approach to managing information.

9. The staff of the four sections within the ICS are known as the ICS _____ _____.

10. The IC who adopts a(n) _____ strategy has determined that there is no lives or property left to save or that the potential for saving lives or property does not justify the risk to fire fighters.

True/False
If you believe the statement to be more true than false, write the letter "T" in the space provided. If you believe the statement to be more false than true, write the letter "F."

1. _____ The Logistics Section Chief reports directly to the Planning Section Chief.
2. _____ Defensive strategies are used to protect exposed properties because defensive strategies are ineffective in extinguishing fires.
3. _____ An engine and its crew are considered to be a single resource.
4. _____ Prior to the ICS, the organization established to direct operations often varied based on the chief on duty.
5. _____ Freelancing is dangerous.

6. _____ The Operations Section is responsible for updating the incident action plan.
7. _____ An ICS provides a standard, professional, organized approach to managing emergency incidents.
8. _____ The issues addressed by the Finance/Administration Section are usually addressed after the incident.
9. _____ The incident action plan outlines the overall strategy for an emergency incident.
10. _____ The different components of the ICS have different goals and objectives.

Short Answer
Complete this section with short written answers using the space provided.

1. Identify the four major functional components within the ICS.

2. When an officer relinquishes command, he or she needs to give the new IC a situation status report that includes which six pieces of information?

3. Identify 5 of the 11 important characteristics of an ICS.

4. List the components of the acronym SLICE-RS.

Fire Alarms

The following real case scenarios will give you an opportunity to explore the concerns associated with ICS. Read each scenario, and then answer each question in detail.

1. You are the team leader for an exposure crew on a fire in an apartment complex under construction. You are assigned to Division C, and your task is to protect an adjacent apartment building labeled exposure C. The Division D supervisor directs your crew to move your line and protect exposure D. How should you proceed?

   _____
   _____
   _____
   _____
   _____
   _____

2. Your engine company is dispatched to a commercial structure fire in a large pizza restaurant. The building is a wood-frame construction with a lightweight truss. The building is 75 percent involved with fire in the attic area. You are the acting officer and need to decide the overall strategy. How will you proceed?

   _____
   _____
   _____
   _____
   _____
   _____

Skill Drills

Skill Drill 22-1: Operating Within the ICS Fire Fighter II, NFPA 1001: 5.1.2
Test your knowledge of this skill drill by placing the steps below in the correct order. Number the first step with a "1," the second step with a "2," and so on.

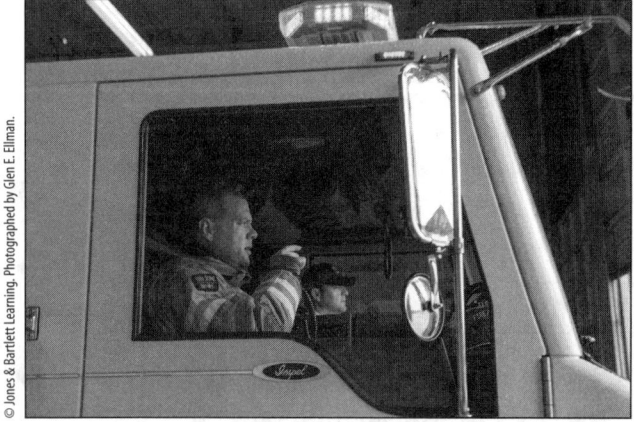

_____ Account for yourself and for other team members.

_____ Assess the scene, hazards, equipment, and PPE to ensure your safety.

_____ Provide personnel accountability reports as necessary.

_____ When given an assignment, repeat that information over the radio to verify it.

_____ Report completion of each assignment to your supervising officer.

_____ Verify that the ICS is in use.

_____ Update your supervising officer regularly.

Skill Drill 22-2: Establishing Command Fire Fighter II, NFPA 1001: 5.1.2
Test your knowledge of this skill drill by filling in the correct words in the steps below.

The initial report to establish command should include the following information:

A _____-_____ report

_____ _____ (and location of the ICP, for larger incidents)

The unit or individual who is _____ command

An _____ situation report

The initial _____ being taken

Skill Drill 22-3: Transferring Command Fire Fighter II, NFPA 1001: 5.1.2

Test your knowledge of this skill drill by placing the steps below in the correct order. Number the first step with a "1," the second step with a "2," and so on.

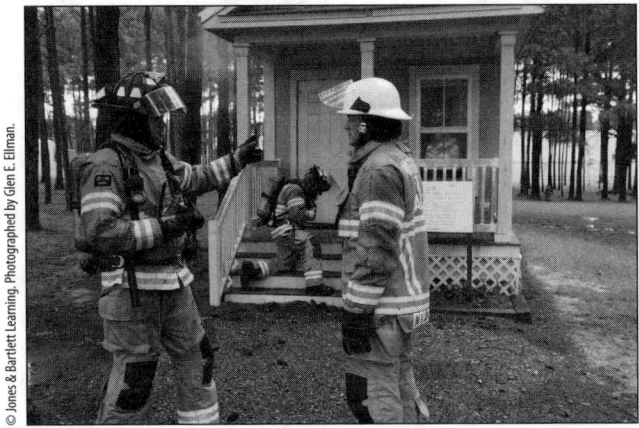

_____ Communicate to the incoming command officer the tactical priorities, action plans, hazardous conditions, potentially hazardous conditions, accomplishments, effectiveness of operations, status of resources, and need for additional resources.

_____ Follow departmental procedures for transferring command.

_____ Formally announce the transfer of command over the radio.

_____ Transfer command in a face-to-face meeting, if possible. If not possible, transfer command over the radio.

_____ Establish the ICS.

Advanced Fire Suppression

Workbook Activities

The following activities have been designed to help you. Your instructor may require you to complete some or all of these activities as a regular part of your fire fighter training program. You are encouraged to complete any activity your instructor does not assign you, as a way to enhance your learning in the classroom.

Chapter Review

The following exercises provide an opportunity to refresh your knowledge of this chapter.

Matching

Match each of the terms in the left column to the appropriate definition in the right column.

_____ 1. Master stream device   A. Foam concentrate mixed with water

_____ 2. Indirect attack   B. Device used to apply large quantities of water to a fire

_____ 3. Combination attack   C. Foam used for fires in ordinary combustibles

_____ 4. Batch mix   D. Foam concentrate poured directly into apparatus booster tank

_____ 5. Eductor   E. Type of fire attack used to quickly remove heat from fire

_____ 6. S.L.I.C.E.-R.S.   F. Explosion that occurs in a pressurized container

_____ 7. Foam injector   G. Acronym developed to assist with scene size-up

_____ 8. Foam solution   H. Adds foam concentrate to the water stream under pressure

_____ 9. BLEVE   I. Attack that uses both indirect and direct attack

_____ 10. Class A foam   J. Draws foam concentrate into a moving stream of water or hose line

Multiple Choice

Read each item carefully, and then select the best response.

_____ 1. Which foam application method uses an object to deflect the foam stream down onto the fire?
   A. Overhead method
   B. Bounce-off method
   C. Bank shot method
   D. Rain-down method

_____ 2. What is the initial objective in a defensive operation?
   A. To ensure the least amount of property damage
   B. To provide a safe environment for the fire fighter
   C. To prevent the fire from spreading
   D. To prepare the fire fighter for offensive attacks

CHAPTER 23

_____ 3. Which type of foam is used to fight fires involving ordinary combustible materials?
   A. Class A foam
   B. Class B foam
   C. Protein foam
   D. Fluoroprotein foam

_____ 4. An offensive fire attack initiated by an exterior, indirect handline operation is known as a
   A. master stream attack.
   B. cellar nozzle attack.
   C. transition attack.
   D. deluge attack.

_____ 5. Which device mixes the foam concentrate into the fire stream?
   A. Foam eductor
   B. Foam injector
   C. Foam regulator
   D. Foam Proportioner

_____ 6. The decision about which type of fire attack to implement is made by the
   A. fire fighter.
   B. Captain.
   C. Incident Commander.
   D. Fire Chief.

_____ 7. Which of the following is a correct foam application technique?
   A. Sweep
   B. Bankshot
   C. Rain-down
   D. All of the above

_____ 8. When fire fighters begin with an indirect attack and then continue with a direct attack, which type of attack are they utilizing?
   A. Aggressive
   B. Combination
   C. Flow path
   D. Multiple

_____ 9. Which device adds foam concentrate to the water stream under pressure?
   A. Foam injectors
   B. Aerator
   C. Bresnan nozzle
   D. Pick-up tube

_____ 10. In situations where the temperature is increasing and it appears that the room or space is ready to experience flashover, fire fighters should use a(n)
   A. indirect attack.
   B. exterior attack.
   C. master stream attack.
   D. ceiling attack.

_____ 11. Once a foam blanket has been applied
   A. you may walk through the spill.
   B. keep a fog spray on the foam surface.
   C. it must not be disturbed.
   D. the fuel under the foam cannot produce flammable vapors.

_____ 12. To prevent explosions in possible overheating situations, propane tanks are equipped with
   A. relief valves.
   B. release valves.
   C. connection valves.
   D. vapor space.

_____ 13. Many newer homes use lightweight engineered structural materials to support large, open floor spaces. These large areas may suddenly collapse, especially if the fire is
   A. in the flow path.
   B. in the attic space.
   C. in the exterior walls.
   D. in the basement.

_____ 14. The NFPA standard that specifies the minimum number of fire fighters needed for safe and effective interior firefighting operations for volunteer fire departments is NFPA
   A. 1500.
   B. 1705.
   C. 1720.
   D. 1901.

_____ 15. The acronym S.L.I.C.E.-R.S. was developed as a tool to assist fire fighters and officers during _____.
   A. response
   B. interior fire attack
   C. incident command
   D. size-up

_____ 16. A situation in which a burning liquid fuel is dripping, spraying, or flowing over the edges of a container is known as a
   A. hazardous materials fire.
   B. spill-over fire.
   C. two-dimensional fire.
   D. three-dimensional fire.

_____ 17. Each length of fire hose should be tested
   A. after each use.
   B. annually.
   C. every 2 years unless damage is suspected.
   D. when purchased and every 5 years.

_____ 18. Compressed air foam has excellent surface-adherence properties, so it can be a good choice for
   A. application on three-dimensional flammable liquid spills.
   B. spills that cover a large area.
   C. preventative application on exposure buildings.
   D. fires involving combustible metals.

_____ 19. What type of synthetic-based foam is particularly suitable for spill-related fires involving gasoline and light hydrocarbons?
   A. Protein foam
   B. Fluoroprotein foam
   C. Aqueous film-forming foam (AFFF)
   D. Compressed air foam

_____ 20. Storing propane as a liquid is very efficient because it has an expansion ratio of
   A. 212:1.
   B. 270:1.
   C. 300:1.
   D. 500:1.

Vocabulary

Define the following terms using the space provided.

1. BLEVE:

    _____
    _____
    _____

2. Rain-down:

    _____
    _____
    _____

3. Transitional attack:

    _____
    _____
    _____

4. Eductor:

    _____
    _____
    _____

5. Combination attack:

    _____
    _____
    _____

Fill-In

Read each item carefully, and then complete the statement by filling in the missing word(s).

1. Directing water onto a fire from a safe distance is a (n) _____ operation.

2. Because many structure fires are ventilation-limited fires, it is important that _____ _____ _____ be in place before ventilation is initiated.

3. An initial interior attack can be started using water from the _____ on the apparatus even before a permanent water supply has been established.

4. A comprehensive size-up identifies critical life-safety issues that should impact the development of the _____ _____ _____.

5. _____ foams are made from animal by-products.

6. A(n) _____ attack uses a straight or solid hose stream to deliver water onto the base of the fire.

7. Most liquid fuel fires can be extinguished using _____ or foam.

8. A _____-dimensional fire refers to a spill, pool, or open container of liquid that is burning only on the top surface.

9. _____ is increasingly being used as an alternative fuel for vehicles, and it is often stored to power emergency electrical generators.

10. Smoke explosions, backdrafts, and flashover are known as _____ fire events.

True/False

If you believe the statement to be more true than false, write the letter "T" in the space provided. If you believe the statement to be more false than true, write the letter "F."

1. _____ One of the most crucial decisions made by the IC is whether to initiate a defensive or offensive fire attack.
2. _____ Foam can be applied with a wide range of expansion rates, depending on the amount of air that is mixed into the stream and the size of the bubbles produced.
3. _____ Exterior fire operations are generally more dangerous than interior operations.
4. _____ When attempting to use foam to extinguish a flammable-liquid fire, it is not necessary to cover the spill completely.
5. _____ Although it is nontoxic, propane can cause asphyxiation.
6. _____ When used as a protective layer on an exposure building, drier foam is more appropriate.
7. _____ High-expansion foam is used in fixed fire protection systems to provide a thick layer of foam.
8. _____ "Softening the target" is a term used to describe defensive fire operations.
9. _____ If a flammable gas fire is extinguished and the fuel continues to leak, there is a high probability that it will reignite explosively.
10. _____ Many fire fighters have been injured or killed while working outside of burning buildings.

Short Answer

Complete this section with short written answers using the space provided.

1. Describe how foam suppresses fire.

   _____
   _____
   _____
   _____

2. Identify five of the indicators of a possible building collapse.

   _____
   _____
   _____
   _____

3. Describe the characteristics of Class A foam.

   _____
   _____
   _____
   _____

4. List the components of the acronym S.L.I.C.E.-R.S.

5. List the five major categories of Class B foam.

Fire Alarms

The following real case scenarios will give you an opportunity to explore the concerns associated with water supply. Read each scenario, and then answer each question in detail.

1. You are the company officer on an engine company that is dispatched to a fire involving a horizontal LPG tank. Upon arrival, the IC assigns you to deploy protective fire streams and shut off the discharge valve on the tank. He has assigned another engine company to assist you. How should you proceed?

2. You are a fire fighter on an engine company that is dispatched to a flammable liquid spill at a local gas station. Upon arrival, your company officer completes the size-up and determines that approximately 10 gallons of gasoline have been spilled on open ground. After setting up for a foam operation, she instructs you to use the roll-in method to apply the foam. How should you proceed?

Skill Drills

Skill Drill 23-1: Coordinating an Interior Attack Fire Fighter II, NFPA 1001: 5.3.2

Test your knowledge of this skill drill by placing the photos below in the correct order. Number the first step with a "1," the second step with a "2," and so on.

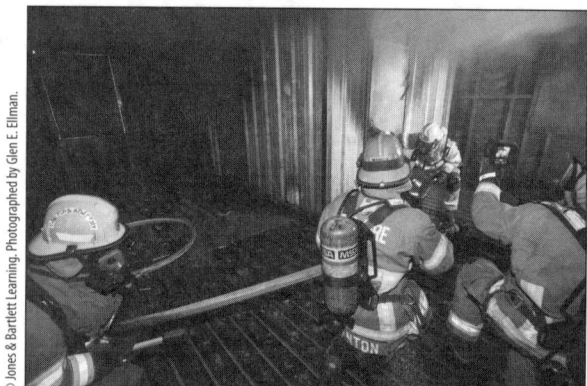

_____ Coordinate fire attack, ventilation, and search and rescue operations.

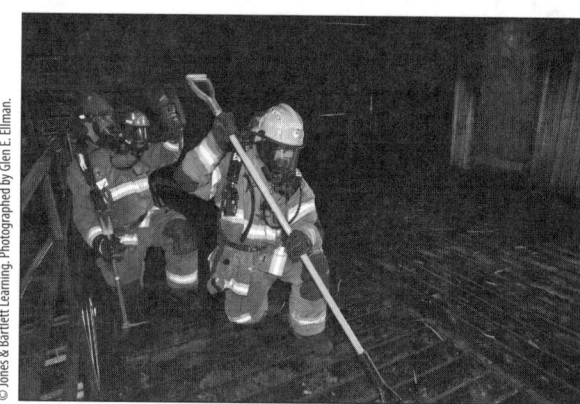

_____ Ensure complete extinguishment of the fire during overhaul. Exit the hazard area, account for all members of the team, and report to incident command.

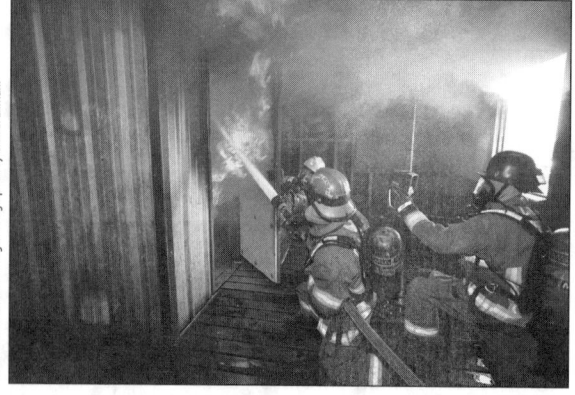

_____ Maintain constant crew integrity at all times. Monitor air supply, and notify command of changing fire or smoke conditions.

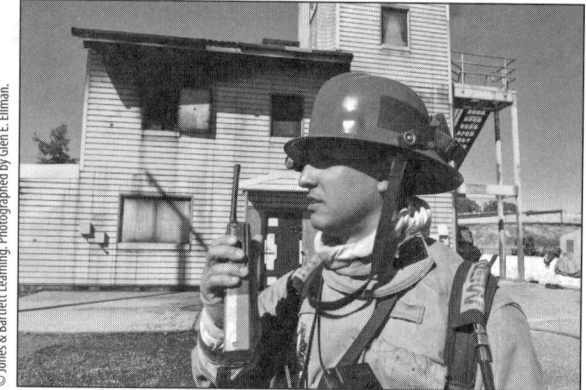

_____ Don full personal protective equipment (PPE), including self-contained breathing apparatus (SCBA). Report to the IC, check into the personnel accountability system, and proceed to work as a team. Perform size-up, and give an arrival report. Call for additional resources if needed.

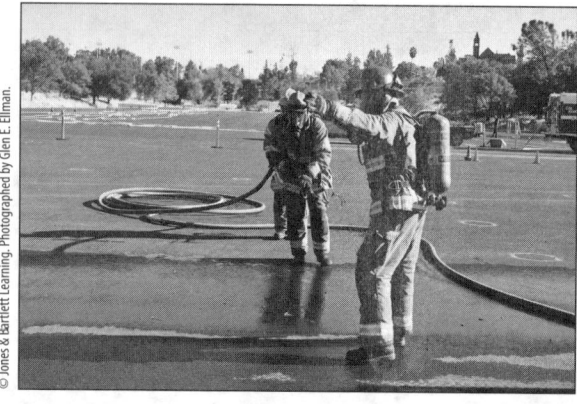

_____ Ensure that an adequate water supply and appropriate backup resources are available. Select the appropriate attack technique. Communicate the attack technique to the team.

Skill Drill 23-2: Suppressing a Flammable Gas Cylinder Fire: Fire Fighter II, NFPA 1001: 5.3.3

Test your knowledge of this skill drill by placing the photos below in the correct order. Number the first step with a "1," the second step with a "2," and so on.

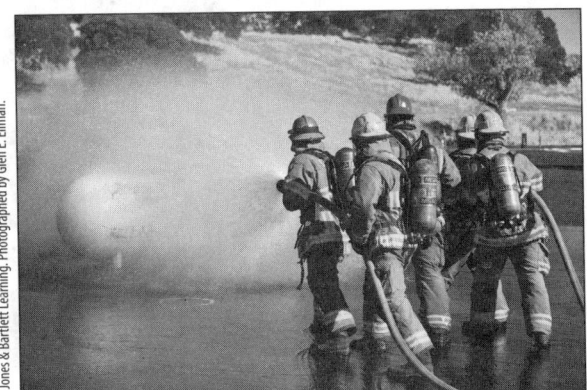

_____ Wearing full PPE, two teams of fire fighters, using a minimum of two 1¾-in. (45-mm) hose lines, advance toward the side of the tank. Do not approach the tank from either end. The team leader should be located between the two nozzle persons. The leader coordinates the advance toward the cylinder.

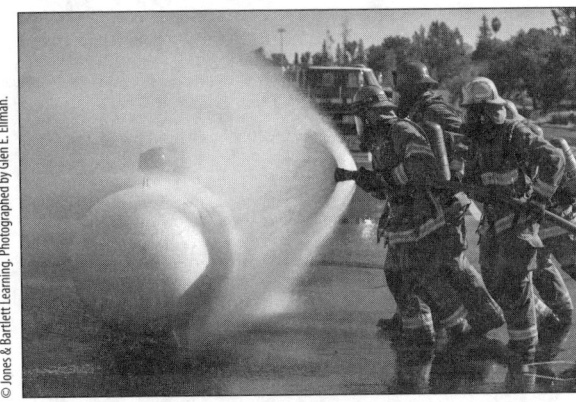

_____ Gradually adjust the nozzles to a wide fog pattern as you approach the side of the tank. Make sure the fog streams overlap as you reach the tank.

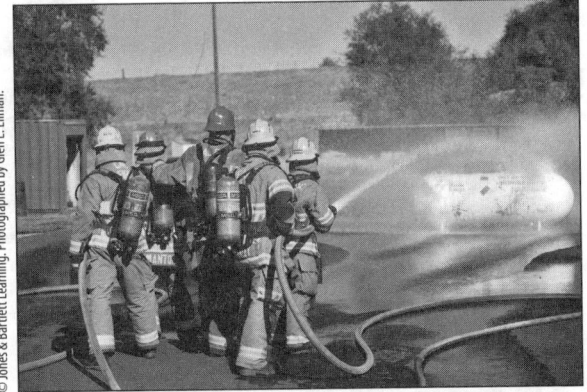

_____ Using a straight stream, cool the tank from as far away as possible until the pressure relief valve resets.

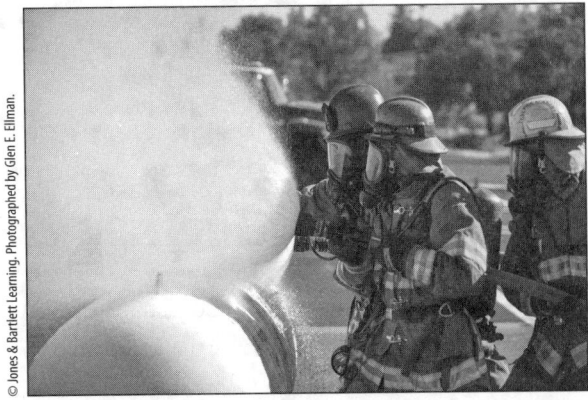

_____ When the cylinder is reached, the two nozzle teams isolate the discharge valve from the fire with their fog streams while the leader closes the discharge valve, eliminating the fuel source.

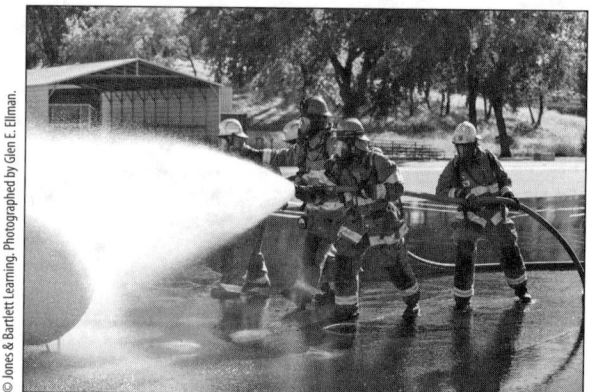
_____ As cooling continues, fire fighters slowly back away from the cylinder while adjusting the nozzles to a straight stream as they retreat.

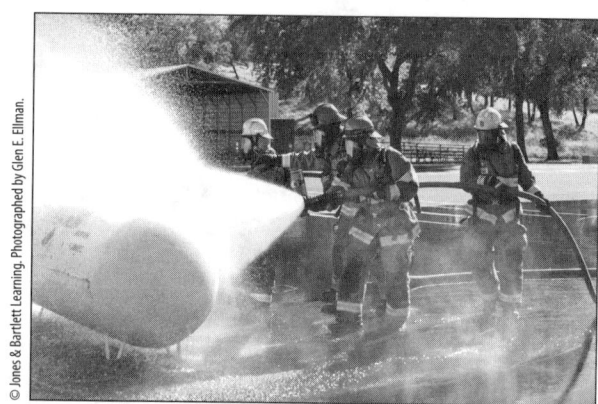
_____ After the burning gas is extinguished, the fire fighters continue to apply water to the cylinder to cool the metal, with the goal of preventing tank failure and a subsequent BLEVE.

Skill Drill 23-3: Operating an In-Line Foam Eductor Fire Fighter II, NFPA 1001: 5.3.1
Test your knowledge of this skill drill by filling in the correct words in the photo captions.

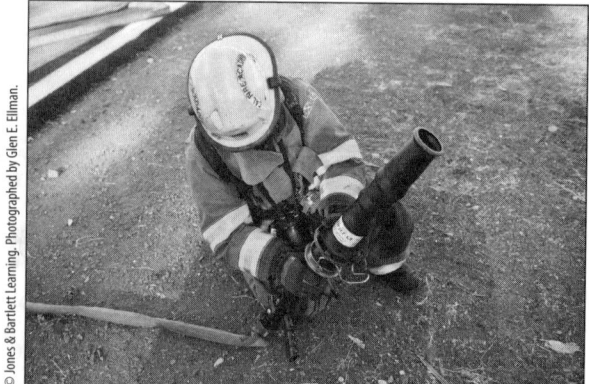

Don all PPE. Make sure all necessary equipment is available, including an in-line foam eductor and the correct nozzle. Ensure that enough foam concentrate is available to suppress the fire. Deploy an _____ _____ line, remove the nozzle, and replace it with the foam nozzle.

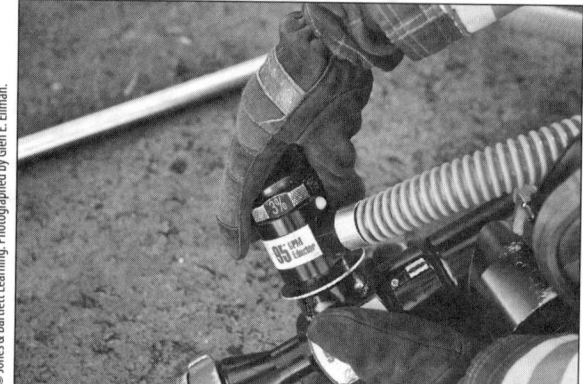

Place the foam concentrate container next to the eductor, check the percentage at which the foam concentrate should be used (found on _____ _____), and set the metering device on the eductor accordingly.

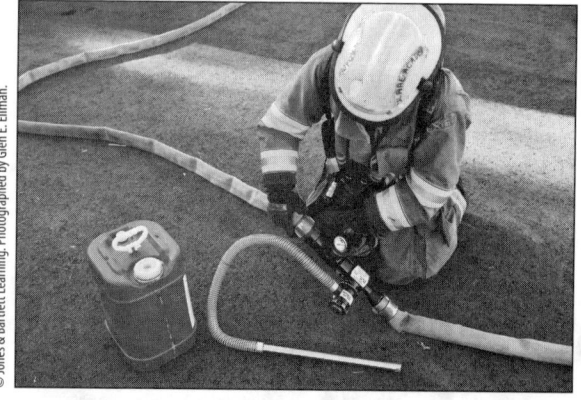

Place the in-line eductor in the hose line according to the manufacturer's instructions and your department's _____.

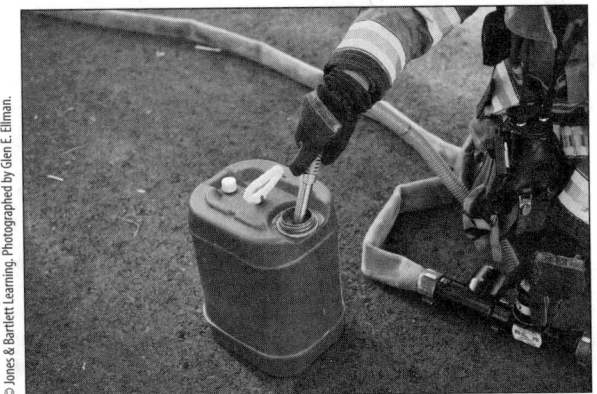
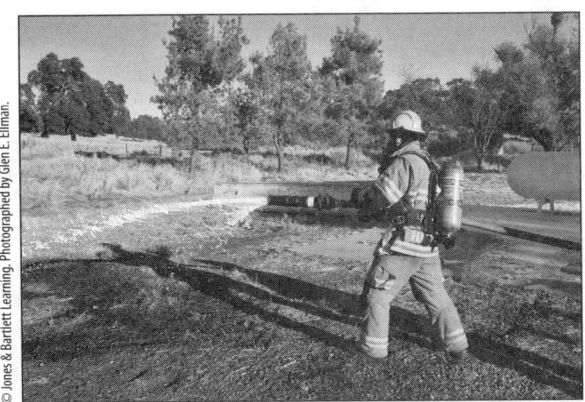

Place the _____ _____ from the eductor into the foam concentrate, keeping both items at similar elevations to ensure sufficient induction of foam concentrate. Charge the hose line with water per your department SOPs or as directed by the manufacturer.

Flow water through the hose line until foam starts to come out of the nozzle. The hose line is now ready to be _____ onto the fuel. Apply foam using one of the three application methods (roll-in method, bounce-off method, or rain-down method) depending on the situation.

Skill Drill 23-4: Performing the Rain-Down Method of Applying Foam Fire Fighter II, NFPA 1001: 5.3.1
Test your knowledge of this skill drill by placing the photos below in the correct order. Number the first step with a "1," the second step with a "2," and so on.

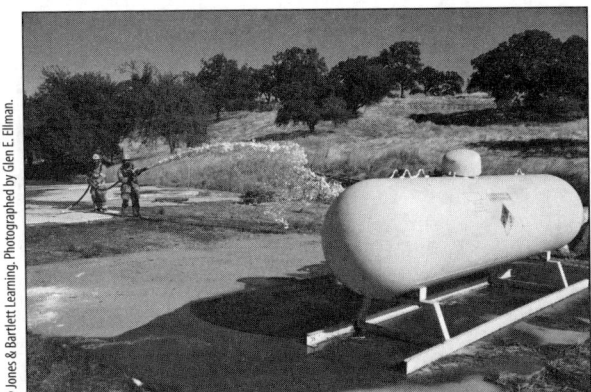
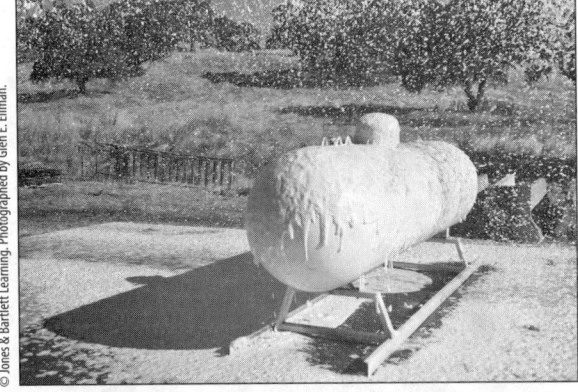

_____ Move within a safe range of the fuel product or tank, and open the nozzle.

_____ Allow the foam to flow across the surface of the fuel product or tank until it is completely covered.

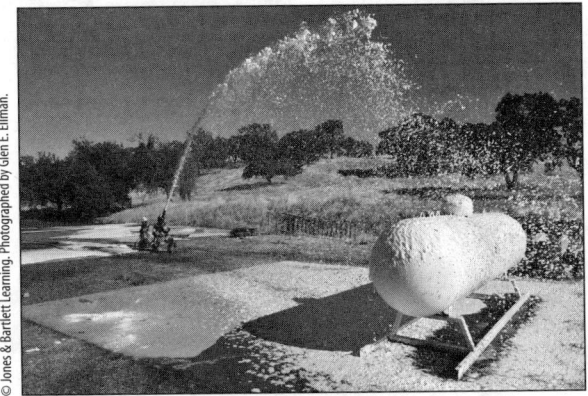
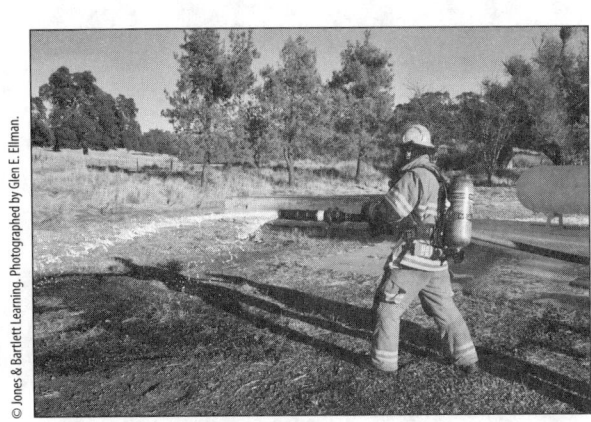

_____ Direct the stream of foam into the air so that the foam gently falls onto the surface of the fuel product or tank.

_____ Open the nozzle and test to ensure that foam is being produced.

Skill Drill 23-5: Performing the Roll-In Method of Applying Foam Fire Fighter II, NFPA 1001: 5.3.1

Test your knowledge of this skill drill by filling in the correct words in the photo captions.

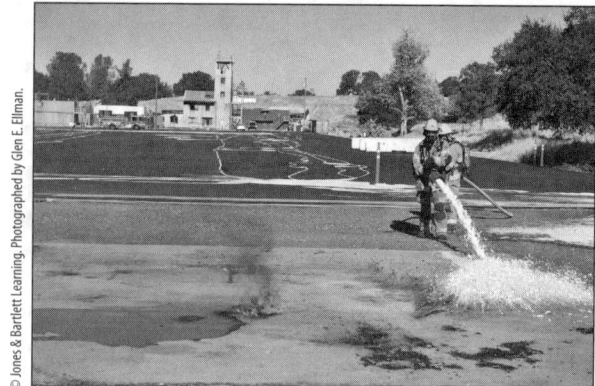

Open the nozzle and test it to ensure that foam is being produced. Move within a safe range of the fuel product or tank, and open the nozzle. Direct the stream of foam onto the ground just in front of the _____ of the product.

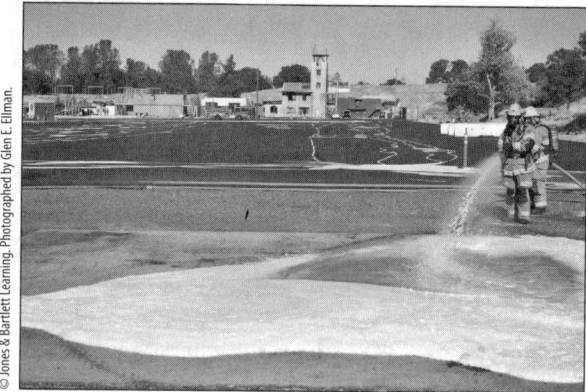

Allow the foam to _____ across the top of the pool of the fuel product or tank until it is completely covered.

Skill Drill 23-6: Performing the Bounce-Off Method of Applying Foam Fire Fighter II, NFPA 1001: 5.3.1

Test your knowledge of this skill drill by filling in the correct words in the photo captions.

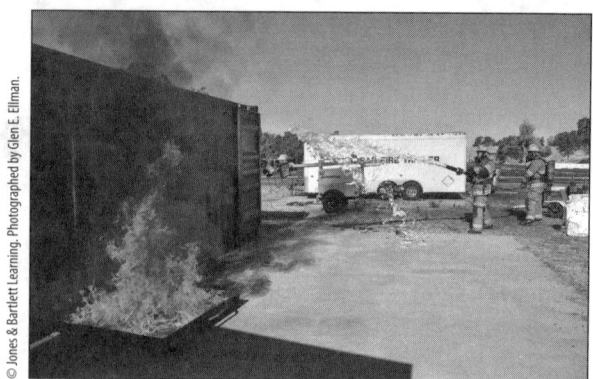

Open the nozzle and test it to ensure that _____ is being produced.

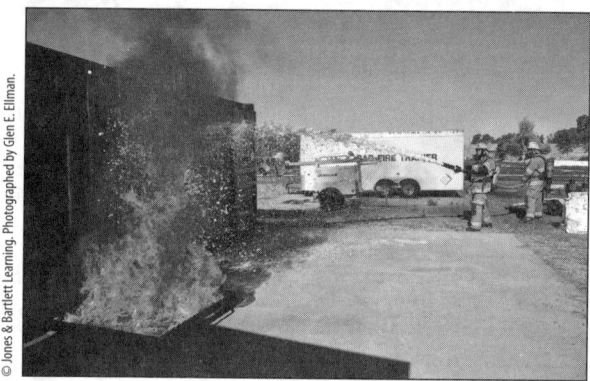

Move to within a safe range of the fuel product or tank, and open the nozzle. Direct the _____ of foam onto a solid structure such as a wall or metal tank so that the foam is directed off the object and onto the pool of the product or tank.

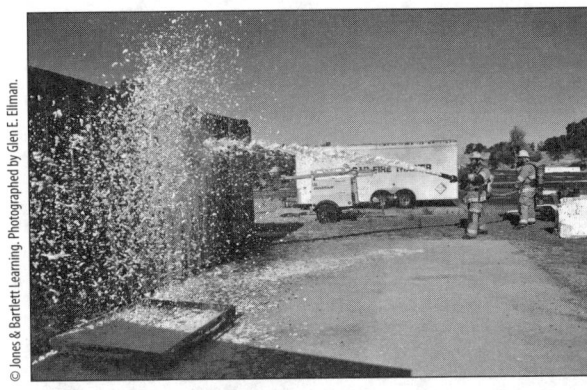

Allow the foam to flow across the top of the pool of the product or tank until it is completely _____. Be aware that the foam may need to be bounced off several areas of the solid object to extinguish the burning product.

Skill Drill 23-7: Performing an Annual Service Test on a Fire Hose Fire Fighter II, NFPA 1001: 5.5.5

Test your knowledge of this skill drill by placing the photos below in the correct order. Number the first step with a "1," the second step with a "2," and so on.

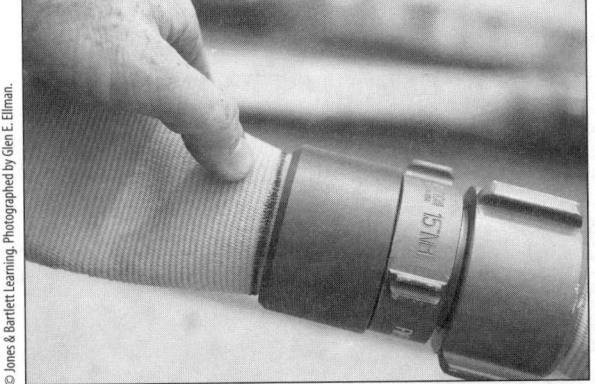

_____ Inspect the marks placed on the hose jacket near the couplings to determine whether slippage occurred.

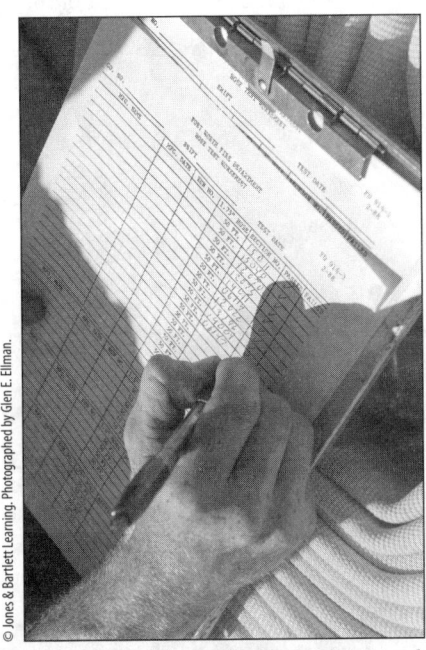

_____ Mark hose that passed. Record the results in the departmental logs.

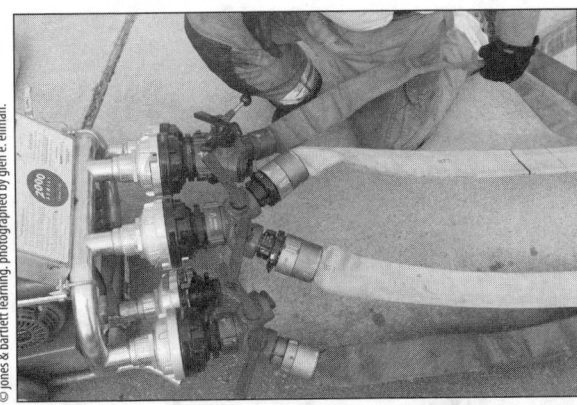

_____ Don turnout gear. Connect up to 300 ft (91 m) of hose to a hose test gate valve on the discharge valve of a fire department pumper or hose tester.

310 Fundamentals of Fire Fighter Skills

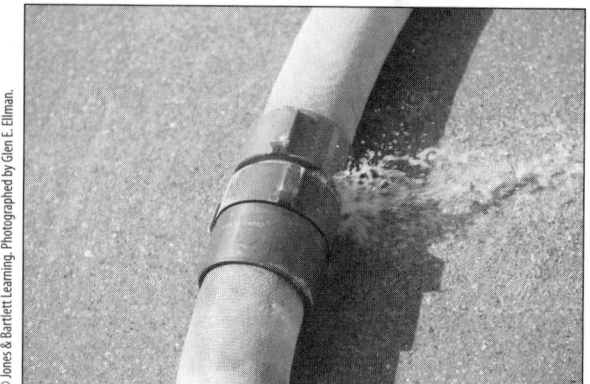

_____ Mark the position of each hose coupling on the hose. This will help determine if slippage occurs during the test (Step 7). Check each coupling for leaks. If leaks are found behind the coupling, remove the hose from service. If the leak is in front of the coupling, tighten the leaking coupling. If the leak continues, replace gaskets if necessary after shutting down the hose line.

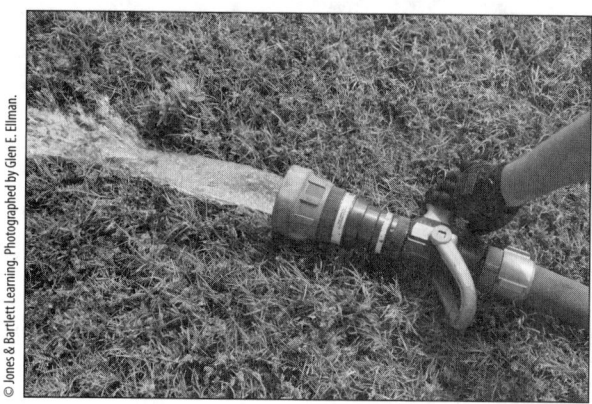

_____ Open the nozzles to purge air from the hose, discharging the water away from the test area. Close the nozzles once the air is purged. Measure and record the length of each section of hose.

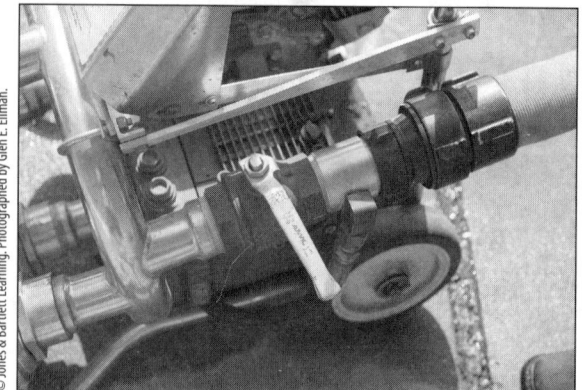

_____ Close each hose test gate valve.

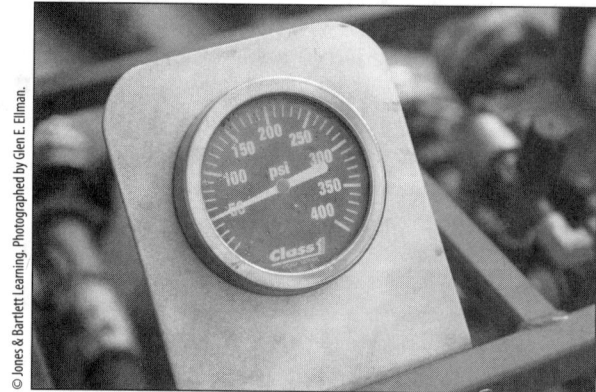

_____ Attach a nozzle to the end of each hose. Slowly fill each hose with water at 50 psi (345 kPa), and remove kinks and twists in the hose.

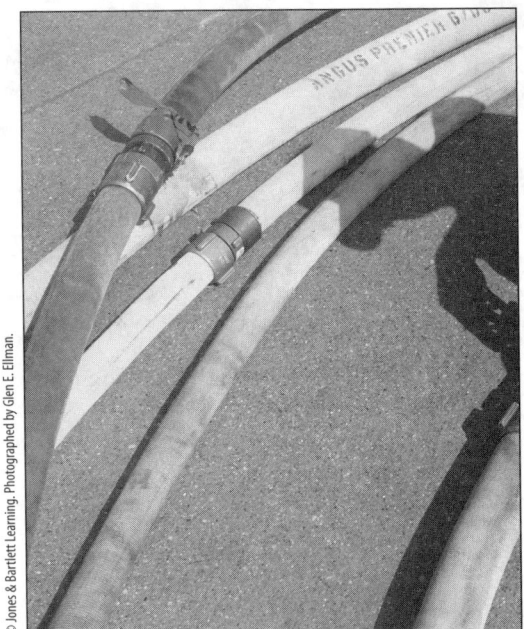

_____ Tag hose that failed.

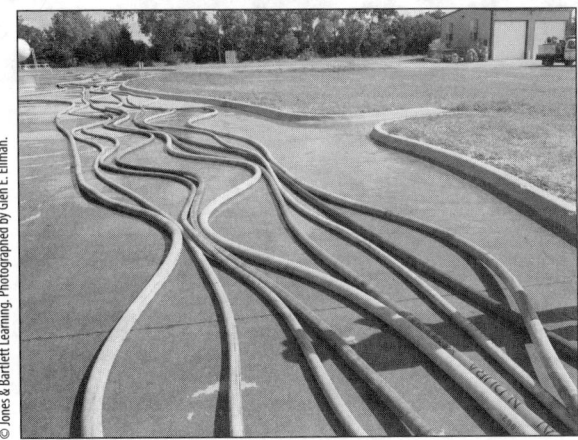

_____ Ensure that all fire fighters are clear of the test area. Increase the pressure on the hose to the pressure required by NFPA 1962, and maintain that pressure for 5 minutes. Monitor the hose and couplings for leaks as the pressure increases during the test. Close the gate valves and open the nozzles to bleed off the pressure. Uncouple and drain the hose.

Vehicle Rescue and Extrication

Workbook Activities

The following activities have been designed to help you. Your instructor may require you to complete some or all of these activities as a regular part of your fire fighter training program. You are encouraged to complete any activity your instructor does not assign you, as a way to enhance your learning in the classroom.

Chapter Review

The following exercises provide an opportunity to refresh your knowledge of this chapter.

Matching

Match each of the terms in the left column to the appropriate definition in the right column.

_____ 1. Conventional vehicles

_____ 2. Rocker panel

_____ 3. Tempered glass

_____ 4. Bulkhead

_____ 5. Rescue-lift air bags

_____ 6. Step chocks

_____ 7. Cribbing

_____ 8. Wedges

_____ 9. Laminated glass

_____ 10. Posts

A. Specialized cribbing assemblies

B. Section of vehicle's frame below the doors, between the front and rear wheels

C. Used to snug loose cribbing under the load or when using lift air bags to fill the void between the crib and the object as it is raised

D. The vertical support members of a vehicle that holds up the roof and forms the upright columns of the occupant cage

E. Glass used to make car windshields

F. Glass used for side and rear car windows

G. A vehicle that uses an internal combustion engine

H. Short lengths of usually hardwood timber used to stabilize vehicles

I. Pneumatic-filled bladders made out of rubber or synthetic material

J. The wall that separates the engine compartment from the passenger compartment

Multiple Choice

Read each item carefully, and then select the best response.

_____ 1. Vehicles that are powered by compressed natural gas are known as
   A. electric-powered vehicles.
   B. hybrid vehicles.
   C. alternative-powered vehicles.
   D. conventional vehicles.

_____ 2. The first step in opening a vehicle door is to
   A. use a pry bar to limit the movement of the door as it is cut.
   B. separate the hinges from the door.
   C. expose the door hinges.
   D. create a purchase point.

_____ 3. What is the first step in displacing the roof of a vehicle?
   A. Remove the "A" posts.
   B. Cut the "C" posts.
   C. Ensure the safety of the rescuers.
   D. Remove the glass.

_____ 4. As soon as you have secured access to the victim, what is your next step as a rescuer?
   A. Remove the excess glass.
   B. Remove the extraneous materials.
   C. Begin to provide emergency medical care.
   D. Begin to communicate with the victims.

_____ 5. When removing a windshield with an axe, one rescuer begins
   A. at the top, in the middle.
   B. at the driver side.
   C. at the passenger side.
   D. at the bottom.

_____ 6. The victim needs to be stabilized and packaged in preparation for removal in the
   A. stabilization phase.
   B. extrication phase.
   C. size-up phase.
   D. rescue phase.

_____ 7. When removing the roof of a vehicle, it is essential to remove the
   A. windshield.
   B. "C" posts.
   C. doors.
   D. bulkhead.

_____ 8. What is the first step of the dash displacement procedure?
   A. Open both front doors.
   B. Remove the bulkhead.
   C. Remove the steering wheel.
   D. Cut the "A" post.

_____ 9. What is the simplest way to displace a seat backward?
   A. Cut the material out of the bottom of the seat.
   B. Remove the backseat.
   C. Tilt the seat backward.
   D. Move the seat backward in its tracks.

_____ 10. The suspension system of most vehicles can be stabilized with
   A. cribbing.
   B. straps.
   C. wedges.
   D. step chocks.

_____ 11. Between the layers of glass that make the vehicle windshield is
   A. an empty space.
   B. a thin layer of flexible plastic.
   C. an epoxy glue.
   D. an invisible wire mesh.

_____ 12. Cribbing, rescue-lift air bags, and step blocks are all types of
   A. stabilization devices.
   B. patient extractors.
   C. bracing tools.
   D. prying tools.

_____ 13. Which posts are located closest to the front of the vehicle?
   A. "A" posts
   B. "B" posts
   C. "C" posts
   D. "D" posts

_____ 14. The rear window of a vehicle is made of
   A. tempered glass.
   B. laminated windshield glass.
   C. block glass.
   D. sheet glass.

_____ 15. Steering wheels can be cut using
   A. a hacksaw.
   B. a bolt cutter.
   C. a hydraulic cutter.
   D. all of the above.

_____ 16. A vehicle windshield is made of
   A. tempered glass.
   B. laminated windshield glass.
   C. block glass.
   D. sheet glass.

_____ 17. Cribbing protects the vehicle from
   A. electrical hazards.
   B. excessive exposure.
   C. rolling.
   D. other transportation.

_____ 18. What are the most efficient and widely used tools for opening jammed doors?
   A. Cutting tools
   B. Manual hydraulic tools
   C. Powered hydraulic tools
   D. Prying tools

_____ 19. When using rescue-lift air bags, use _____ to fill the void between the crib and the vehicle.
   A. step chocks
   B. wedges
   C. posts
   D. bulkheads

_____ 20. What is the most common type of rescue-lift air bag?
   A. Low-pressure lift air bag
   B. Medium-pressure lift air bag
   C. High-pressure lift air bag
   D. Dual-pressure lift air bag

Labeling

Label the following diagram with the correct terms.

1. The anatomy of a vehicle.

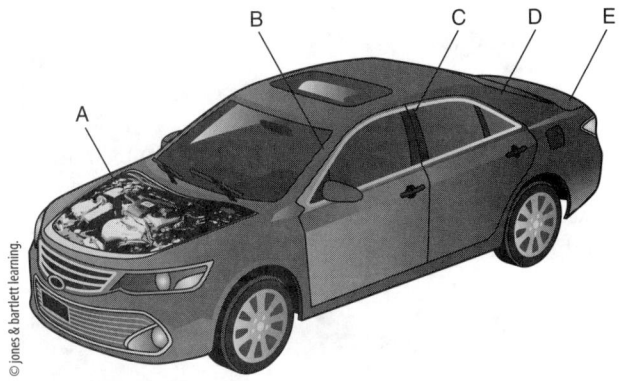

A. _____
B. _____
C. _____
D. _____
E. _____

Vocabulary

Define the following terms using the space provided.

1. Hybrid vehicle:

2. Firewall:

3. Purchase point:

4. Post:

5. Unibody:

Fill-In

Read each item carefully, and then complete the statement by filling in the missing word(s).

1. The simplest way to access a victim of a crash is to open a(n) _____.

2. Vehicles consist of three main compartments; the _____ compartment, the passenger compartment, and the trunk or cargo area.

3. The first step in the extrication process is _____ and _____.

4. If the door cannot be opened or glass removal will not provide access to the victim, the most common technique for gaining access is _____ displacement.

5. After arriving at the scene of a motor vehicle collision, it is important to assess the _____ present and to determine the _____ of the incident.

6. The right side of the vehicle is where the _____ seat is located.

7. One method of displacing the roof is to cut the _____ posts and fold the roof back toward the rear of the vehicle.

8. Traffic hazards are best handled by the appropriate _____ _____ agency.

9. The three types of commonly used pneumatic rescue-lift air bags are low, medium, and high _____.

10. The _____ posts are located between the front and rear doors of a vehicle.

True/False

If you believe the statement to be more true than false, write the letter "T" in the space provided. If you believe the statement to be more false than true, write the letter "F."

1. _____ Unibody construction combines the vehicle body and the frame into a single component.
2. _____ Wedges should be the same width as the cribbing used in stabilization efforts.
3. _____ Rescue-lift air bags are among the best pieces of equipment used to shore a vehicle by themselves.
4. _____ The purpose of disentangling the victim is to remove those parts of the vehicle that are trapping the victim.
5. _____ When it is necessary to force a door to gain access to a victim, choose the door closest to the victim.
6. _____ The steps of scene stabilization consist of reducing, removing, or mitigating the hazards at the incident scene.
7. _____ Downed power lines can create a mechanical hazard.
8. _____ The incident commander will usually perform a size-up of the scene by conducting a 360-degree walk-around the scene.
9. _____ Unstable objects pose a more serious threat to rescuers than do stabilized vehicles.
10. _____ High-pressure rescue-lift air bags are commonly used for recovery operations.

Short Answer

Complete this section with short written answers using the space provided.

1. Identify and provide an example of each of the four general functions of gaining access and disentangling a victim.

_____

_____

_____

_____

2. Identify the five types of alternative-fuel vehicles.

   _____
   _____
   _____
   _____

3. Identify five safety tips for using rescue-lift air bags.

   _____
   _____
   _____
   _____

Fire Alarms

The following real case scenarios will give you an opportunity to explore the concerns associated with vehicle rescue and extrication. Read each scenario, and then answer each question in detail.

1. You have been dispatched to a vehicle accident on the interstate at 1:15 a.m. on a rainy night. Your company is first on the scene, and standard operating procedures (SOPs) state your first actions are to protect the scene from traffic and then do a size-up.

   a. How will you protect the scene from approaching traffic?

   _____
   _____
   _____
   _____
   _____

   b. How will you proceed with your scene size-up?

   _____
   _____
   _____
   _____
   _____
   _____

2. Your company has been dispatched to a motor vehicle accident involving two vehicles with trapped occupants. It is 3:00 p.m. on a bright, clear day; both vehicles are on their wheels. The incident commander (IC) orders your company to stabilize both vehicles.

   a. Which equipment will you use for vehicle stabilization?
   _____
   _____
   _____
   _____
   _____
   _____

   b. How will you stabilize these vehicles?
   _____
   _____
   _____
   _____
   _____
   _____

Skill Drills

Skill Drill 24-1: Disable the Electrical System of an Electric Drive Vehicle Fire Fighter II, NFPA 1001: 5.4.1
Test your knowledge of this skill drill by filling in the correct words in the photo captions.

Immobilize the vehicle by _____ the wheels. Set the parking brake, and place the vehicle in park, if you can access these controls.

Lower all automatic windows, if possible. Disable the low-voltage system by shutting off the vehicle's ignition (power button or conventional key) and disconnecting or cutting the 12-volt battery cables. Cut the _____-_____ negative cable first, and then cut the positive cable. Double cut each cable to remove a short section. This will prevent the cables from accidentally _____. For vehicles equipped with a proximity key, move the key as far away from the vehicle as possible to prevent the possibility of unintentional restart. Because it may take up to 10 minutes for the high-voltage system to discharge, use caution while performing extrication operations.

Skill Drill 24-2: Performing a Scene Size-Up at a Motor Vehicle Accident Fire Fighter II, NFPA 1001:5.4.1

Test your knowledge of this skill drill by placing the photos below in the correct order. Number the first step with a "1," the second step with a "2," and so on.

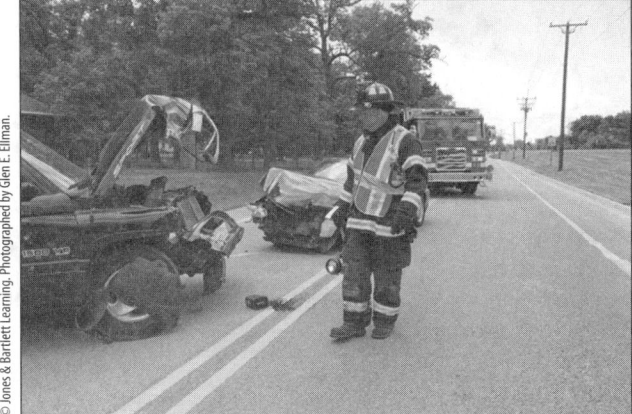

_____ Perform a 360-degree walk-around to identify potential hazards. Look for hazards above and below the vehicle, and determine the stabilization equipment needed to prevent further movement of the vehicle involved in the incident.

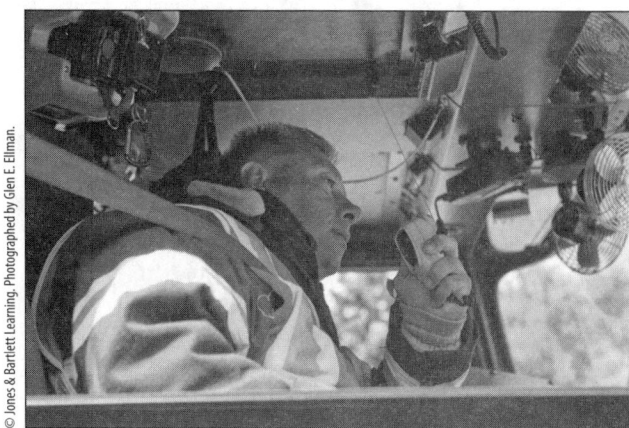

_____ Perform a quick initial assessment as you arrive on the scene, establish command, and give a brief initial radio report. Establish fire suppression protection if fluids are released or if extrication may be required; a minimum of one 1½-in. (38-mm) hose line should be in place.

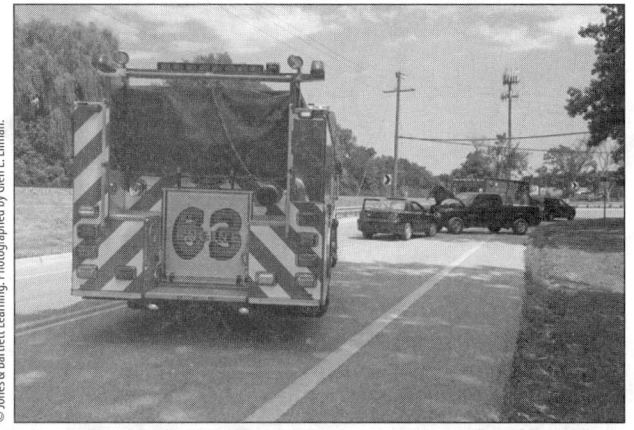

_____ Position emergency vehicles to protect the MVA scene and the rescuers. Take any additional actions needed to prevent further MVAs.

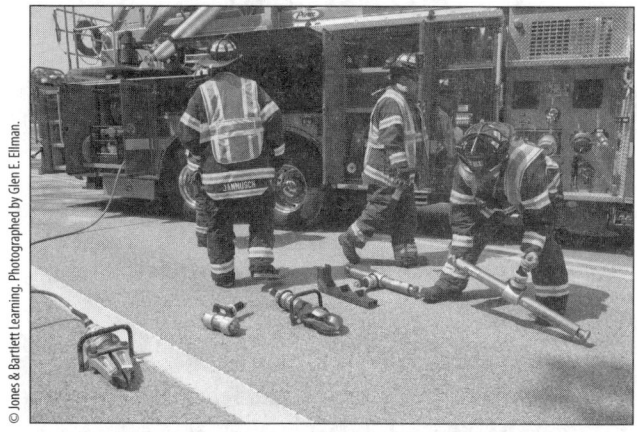

_____ Establish a secure working area and an equipment staging area. Direct personnel to perform initial tasks.

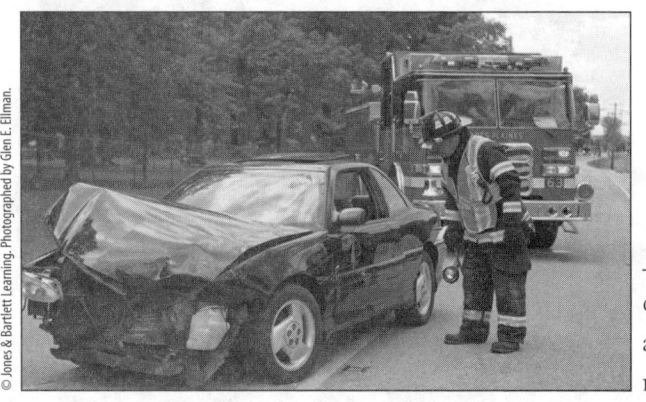

_____ Determine the number of patients, the severity of their injuries, and the amount of entrapment. Give an updated report, and call for additional resources if needed.

Skill Drill 24-3: Mitigating the Hazards at a Motor Vehicle Accident Fire Fighter II, NFPA 1001: 5.4.1

Test your knowledge of this skill drill by placing the photos below in the correct order. Number the first step with a "1," the second step with a "2," and so on.

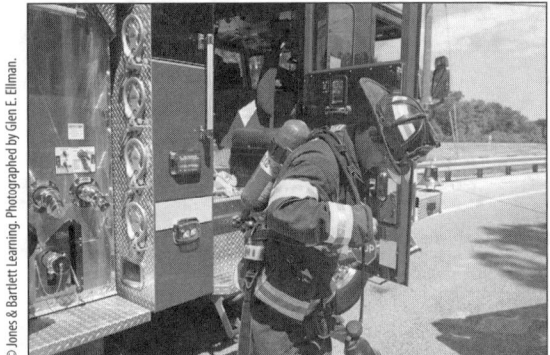

_____ Don PPE, including SCBA. Attach a regulator, if conditions require.

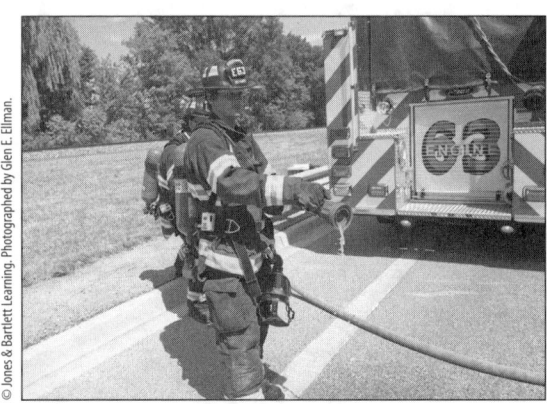

_____ Assess the incident scene for hazards. Communicate with other crews and command. Advance a charged hose line to the proximity of the vehicle. Extinguish any fires.

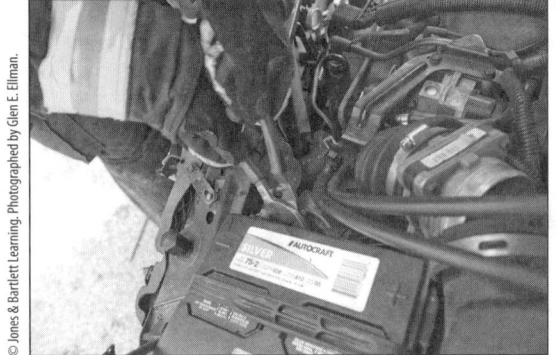

_____ Mitigate electrical sources of ignition by cutting the 12-volt battery cables.

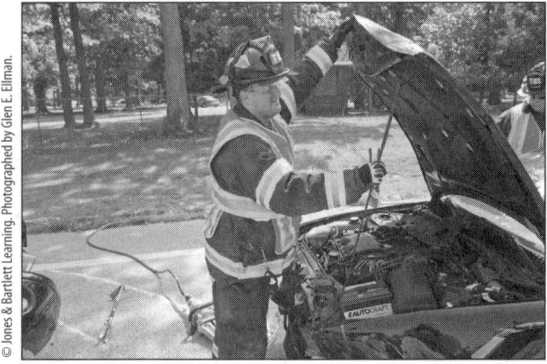

_____ Open the hood of the vehicle.

Skill Drill 24-4: Stabilizing a Vehicle Following a Motor Vehicle Accident Fire Fighter II, NFPA 1001: 5.4.1

Test your knowledge of this skill drill by placing the photos below in the correct order. Number the first step with a "1," the second step with a "2," and so on.

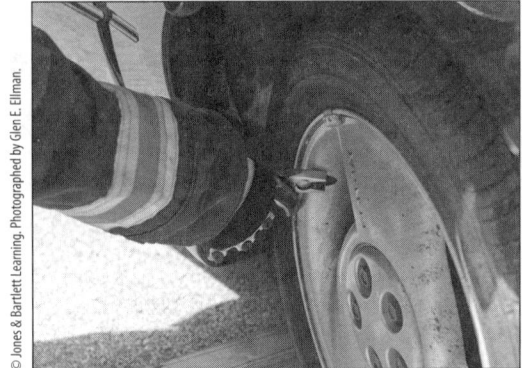

_____ Use additional step chocks and cribbing, as needed. Consider deflating tires for added stability.

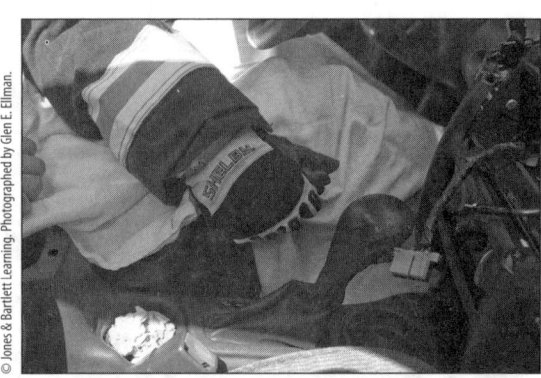

_____ Place the gear shift in park and apply the parking brake, if these controls can be accessed.

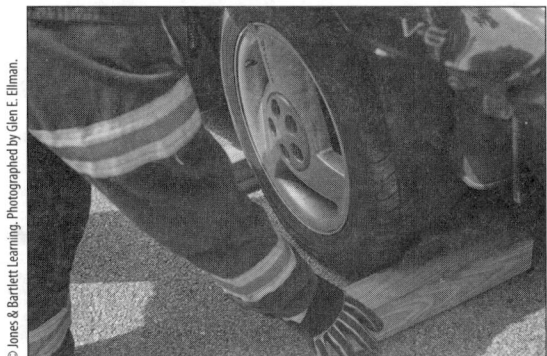

_____ Don PPE, including eye protection. Minimize hazards to rescuers and victims. Chock both sides of one tire to prevent the vehicle from rolling by placing one step chock in front of a wheel and a second step chock in back of the wheel.

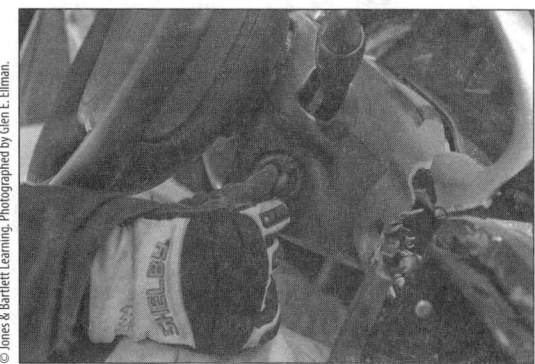

_____ Lower all automatic windows, if possible. Turn off the ignition and remove the key or fob.

Skill Drill 24-5: Breaking Tempered Glass Fire Fighter II, NFPA 1001: 5.4.1
Test your knowledge of this skill drill by filling in the correct words in the photo captions.

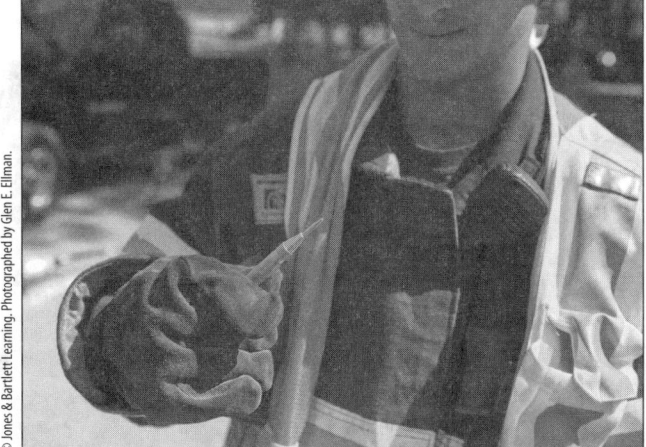

Don PPE, including eye protection. Minimize hazards to rescuers and victims. Ensure stability of the vehicle by using appropriate _____ and _____. Select a tool for breaking tempered glass.

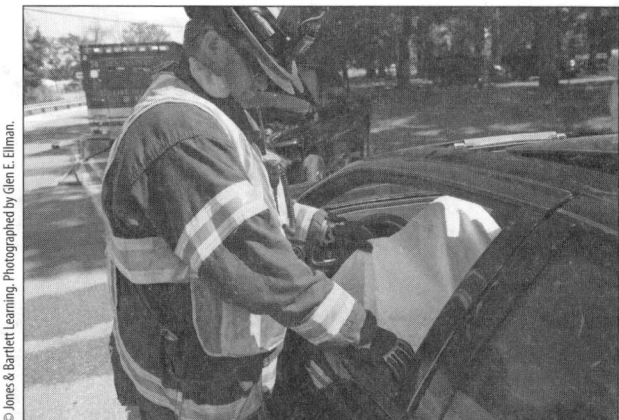

Ensure that the victim and other fire fighters are as _____ as possible.

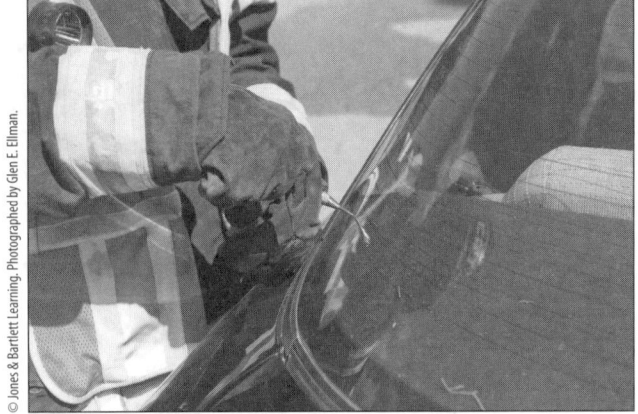

If using a _____-_____ center punch tool, place the tool in the lower corner of the window and sharply apply pressure until the spring is activated. If using a striking tool, strike the lowest corner away from the victim.

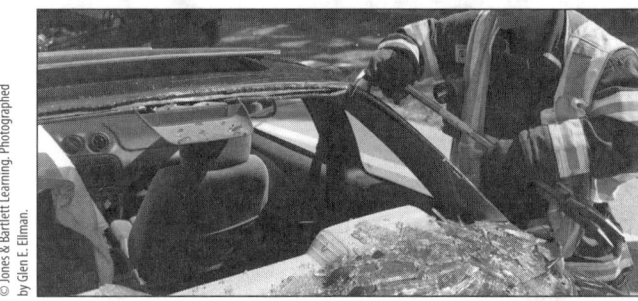

Remove loose _____ around the window opening.

Skill Drill 24-6: Gaining Access to a Vehicle Following a Motor Vehicle Accident Fire Fighter II, NFPA 1001: 5.4.1
Test your knowledge of this skill drill by filling in the correct words in the photo captions.

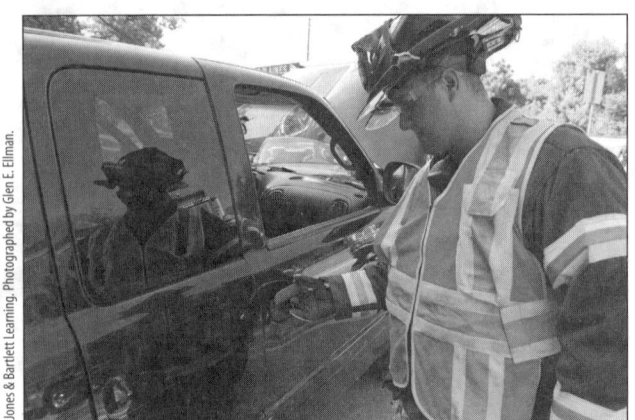

Don PPE, including eye protection. Minimize hazards to rescuers and victims. Ensure stability of the vehicle by using appropriate chocks and cribbing. If you can access the passenger compartment, place the gear shift in _____, apply the parking brake, lower automatic windows, turn off the ignition, and move the _____ key (if applicable) away from the vehicle. Isolate the power by disconnecting or cutting the battery cables. Determine the best access point, and then open a door, break needed glass, or distort metal.

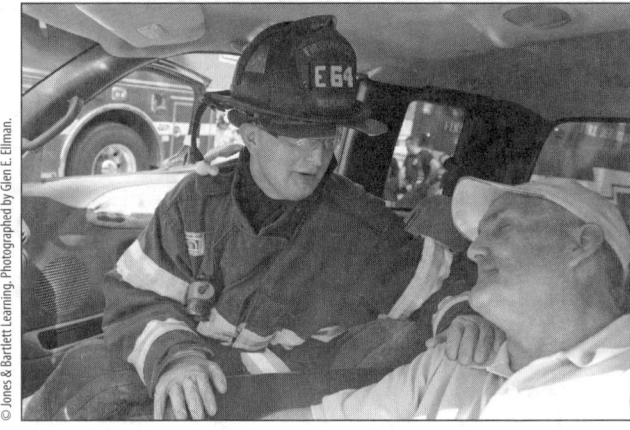

Enter the vehicle, and _____ with the victim.

Skill Drill 24-7: Forcing a Vehicle Door Fire Fighter II, NFPA 1001: 5.4.1

Test your knowledge of this skill drill by placing the photos below in the correct order. Number the first step with a "1," the second step with a "2," and so on.

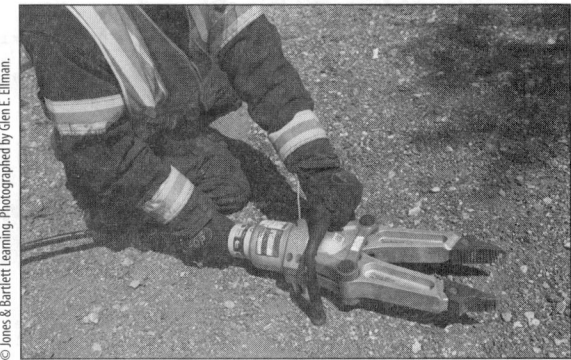

_____ Don PPE, including eye protection. Retrieve and set up the required tools. Check the equipment for readiness. Assess the vehicle for stabilization and hazards, including SRS devices.

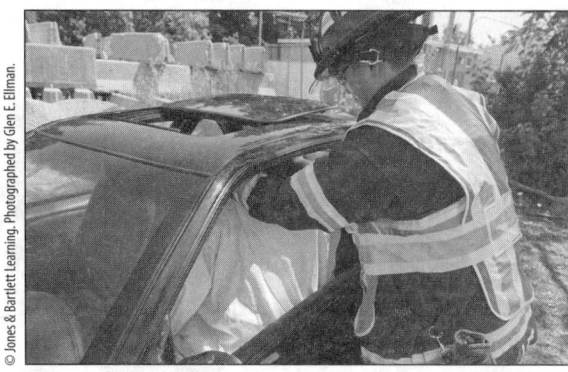

_____ Communicate with the victim; minimize hazards to both the rescuers and the victim.

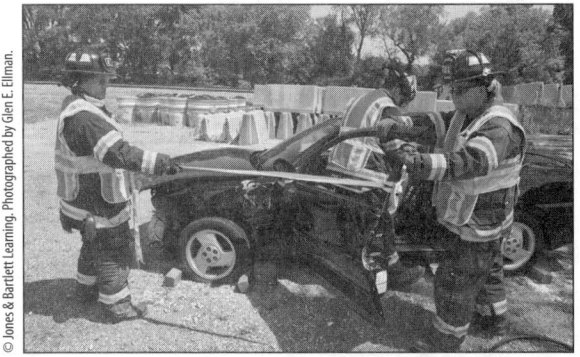

_____ Remove the door, if possible. If rapid extrication is required, secure the door with ropes or cribbing so it does not shift while removing the victim.

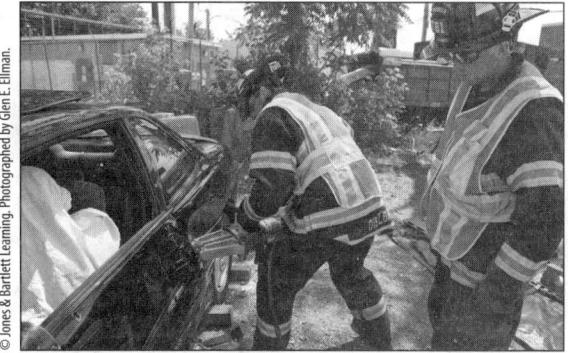

_____ Engage hand tools or a power unit to force the door, using good body mechanics.

Skill Drill 24-9: Performing a Dash Roll Fire Fighter II, NFPA 1001: 5.4.1

Test your knowledge of this skill drill by filling in the correct words in the photo captions.

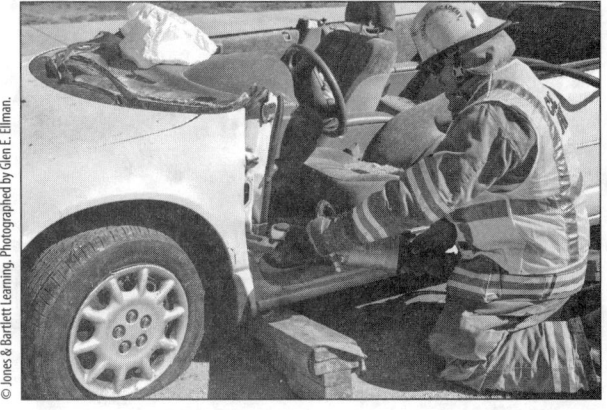

Don PPE, including eye protection. Minimize hazards to rescuers and victims. Prevent the vehicle from rolling by placing a chock in front of one tire and a second chock behind the same tire. Use additional step chocks and cribbing, as needed. Consider _____ tires for added stability. Communicate with the victim, and ensure that both the victim and rescuers are protected from hazards. Make a _____ _____ at the bottom of the A-post.

324 FUNDAMENTALS OF FIRE FIGHTER SKILLS

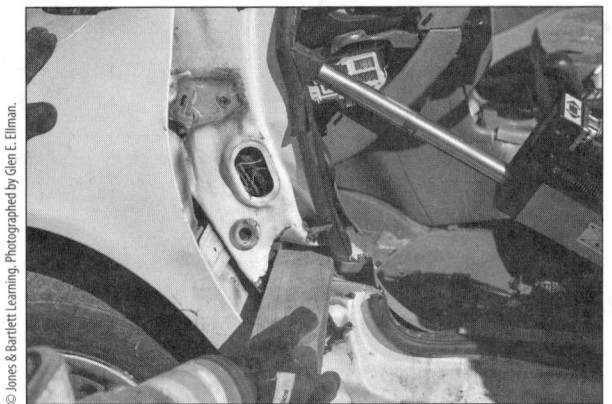

Use a _____ _____ or spreading tool to roll the dash and bulkhead up and away from the victim. Place cribbing under the rocker panel as the dash is being rolled.

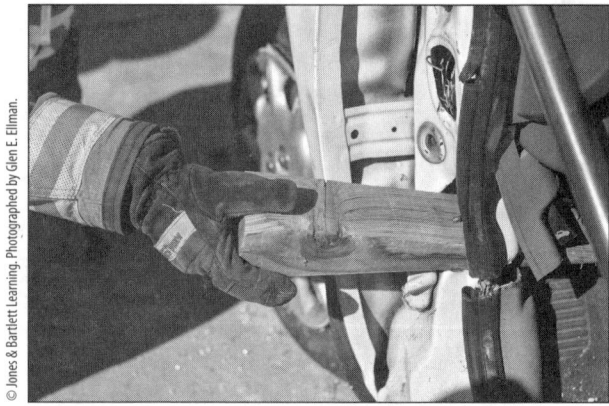

Place a wedge in the _____-_____ cut to prevent the dash from returning to its original position.

Skill Drill 24-10: Performing a Dash Lift Fire Fighter II, NFPA 1001: 5.4.1
Test your knowledge of this skill drill by filling in the correct words in the photo captions.

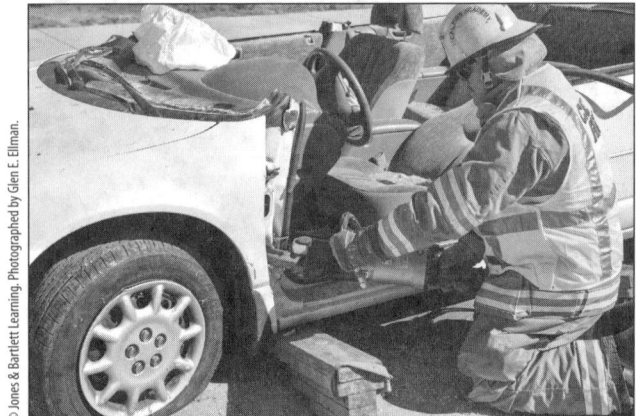

Don PPE, including eye protection. Minimize hazards to rescuers and victims. Prevent the vehicle from rolling by placing a _____ in front of one tire and a second chock behind the same tire. Use additional step chocks and cribbing, as needed. Consider deflating tires for added stability. Communicate with the victim and ensure that both the victim and rescuers are protected from hazards. Make necessary relief cuts in the A-post and other _____ members, as needed.

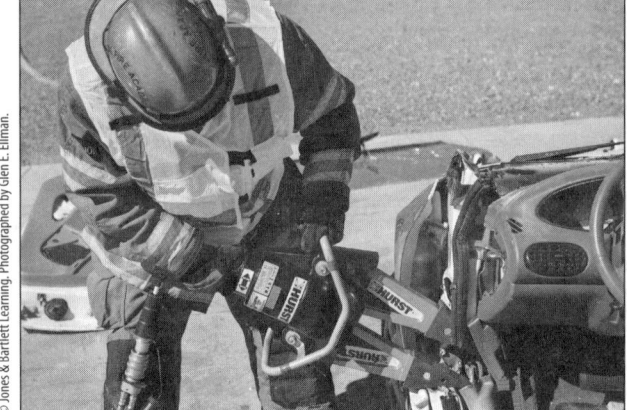

Use a hydraulic spreading tool in the A-post relief cut to lift the dash and bulkhead up and away from the victim. Place _____ under the rocker panel as the dash is being lifted.

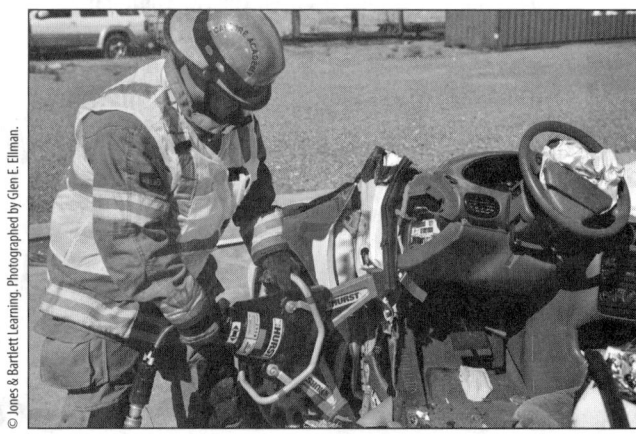

Maintain contact with the hydraulic spreading tool to prevent the tool from _____ while removing the victim.

Skill Drill 24-11: Removing the Roof of a Vehicle Fire Fighter II, NFPA 1001:5.4.1

Test your knowledge of this skill drill by placing the photos below in the correct order. Number the first step with a "1," the second step with a "2," and so on.

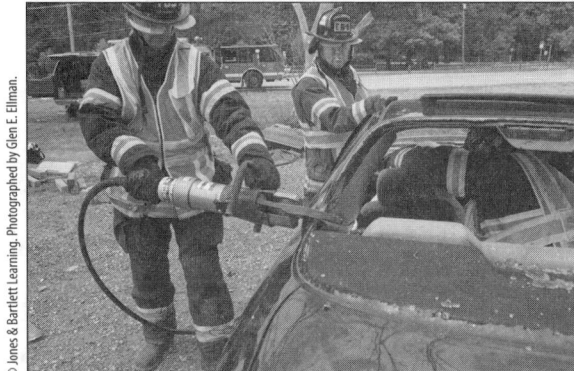

_____ Engage the appropriate tools to remove the roof, while using good body mechanics.

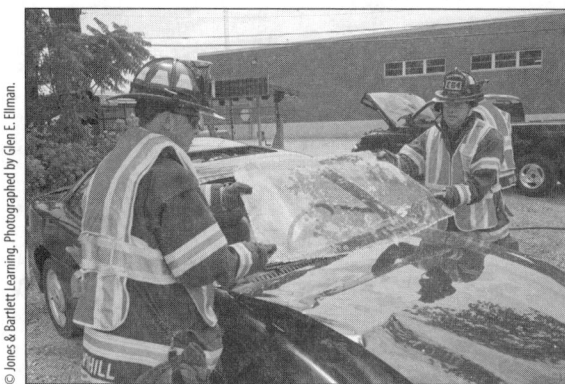

_____ Don PPE, including eye protection. Retrieve and set up the required tools. Check the equipment for readiness. Assess the vehicle for stabilization and hazards. Prior to cutting any materials, be sure to identify the presence and location of any hidden pistons, canisters, electrical wiring, or SRS devices, such as air bags and seat belt pretensioners, and address these hazards accordingly. It may be necessary to remove interior trim around the posts to locate these devices. Communicate with the victim, and minimize hazards to both the rescuers and the victim. Remove any remaining glass.

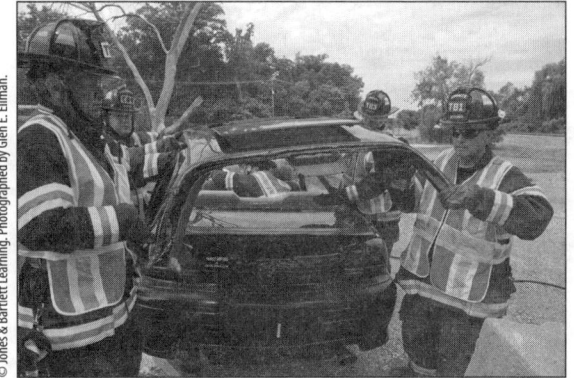

_____ Remove the roof to a safe location. Return the tools to the staging area upon completion of the tasks.

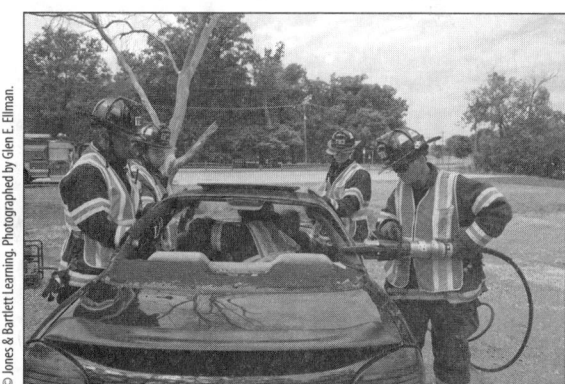

_____ Control the vehicle roof and protect against sharp edges at all times.

Assisting Special Rescue Teams

Workbook Activities

The following activities have been designed to help you. Your instructor may require you to complete some or all of these activities as a regular part of your fire fighter training program. You are encouraged to complete any activity your instructor does not assign you, as a way to enhance your learning in the classroom.

Chapter Review

The following exercises provide an opportunity to refresh your knowledge of this chapter. All questions in this chapter are Fire Fighter II level.

Matching
Match each of the terms in the left column to the appropriate definition in the right column.

_____ 1. High-angle operations
_____ 2. IDLH
_____ 3. Low-angle operations
_____ 4. Supplied air respirator system
_____ 5. PFD
_____ 6. Shoring
_____ 7. Hot zone
_____ 8. Spoil pile
_____ 9. Warm zone
_____ 10. Placards

A. The area immediately surrounding an incident site that is directly dangerous to life and health
B. Allows the body to float in water
C. The slope of the ground is greater than 45 degrees, and fire fighters are dependent on life safety rope for support
D. Signage, required to be placed on all four sides of vehicles, that identifies the hazardous materials contents being transported by the vehicles
E. Flammable, toxic, or oxygen-deficient atmospheres that pose immediate or possible adverse health effects
F. A method of supporting a trench wall to prevent its collapse
G. An emergency breathing system that utilizes an air line running from the rescuers to a fixed air supply located outside of the confined space
H. When fire fighters are dependent on the ground for their primary support, and the rope system is a secondary means of support
I. The area between the hot zone and the cold zone
J. The unstable pile of dirt removed from an evacuation

Multiple Choice
Read each item carefully, and then select the best response.

_____ 1. To ensure the continuity of quality care and proper transfer of responsibility, there must be
   A. a complete team debriefing.
   B. adequate reporting and accurate records.
   C. an incident analysis report.
   D. a critical incident stress management (CISM) intervention.

CHAPTER 25

_____ **2.** A collapse that occurs after an initial collapse is called a
   A. follow-up collapse.
   B. supportive collapse.
   C. shoring collapse.
   D. secondary collapse.

_____ **3.** During elevator and escalator rescue, some activities should be attempted only by
   A. technical rescue team members.
   B. emergency responders.
   C. professionally trained service technicians.
   D. veteran department members.

_____ **4.** A(n) _____ is an enclosed area that is not designed for people to occupy.
   A. vault
   B. confined space
   C. box car
   D. SAR

_____ **5.** In search and rescue, removing a victim from a hostile environment is classified as a
   A. search.
   B. rescue.
   C. recovery.
   D. removal.

_____ **6.** Once the victim has been removed from the hazard area, who transports the victim to an appropriate medical facility?
   A. The technical rescue team
   B. The operations team
   C. EMS
   D. The safety officer

_____ **7.** By using a personnel _____ and working within the ICS, an IC can track the resources at the scene, make appropriate assignments, and ensure that every person at the scene operates safely.
   A. buddy system
   B. tagout system
   C. accountability system
   D. two-in/two-out rule

_____ **8.** What are the most versatile and widely used technical rescue skills?
   A. Disentanglement skills
   B. Medical skills
   C. Rope skills
   D. Hazardous materials knowledge

_____ **9.** Warning _____ are required for most hazardous materials in storage or in transit.
   A. lights
   B. sirens
   C. papers
   D. placards

_____ 10. During a technical rescue incident, whose orders do fire fighters follow?
   A. The company officer's
   B. The incident commander's
   C. The battalion chief's
   D. The rescue captain's

_____ 11. During a rescue incident, emergency medical care should be initiated as soon as
   A. the technical rescue team is clear of the scene.
   B. access is made to the victim.
   C. the medical team arrives on scene.
   D. the incident commander (IC) indicates that medical treatment is required.

_____ 12. The lack of oxygen and the presence of poisonous gases are the greatest hazards associated with a
   A. vehicle or machinery rescue.
   B. high-angle rescue.
   C. hazardous materials rescue.
   D. confined-space rescue.

_____ 13. When responding to a reported technical rescue incident, the _____ should assume command.
   A. first arriving person who has operation-level training
   B. first arriving technical rescue specialist
   C. first arriving Chief officer
   D. first arriving company officer

_____ 14. A technical rescue team will usually respond with a rescue squad,
   A. medic unit, and safety officer.
   B. paramedic, and incident commander.
   C. logistics team, and operational team.
   D. medic unit, engine company, truck company, and chief.

_____ 15. The area used for staging vehicles and equipment is called the
   A. hot zone.
   B. warm zone.
   C. cold zone.
   D. public zone.

_____ 16. In an industrial setting, securing the scene is the responsibility of the
   A. facility supervisor.
   B. incident commander.
   C. emergency response team.
   D. property owner.

_____ 17. Which level of training allows an individual to work in the warm zone and directly assist those conducting the rescue operation?
   A. Awareness level
   B. Operations level
   C. Technician level
   D. Incident commander level

_____ 18. Shutting off the utilities in the area where the rescuers will be working is a responsibility of the
   A. incident commander.
   B. safety officer.
   C. logistics officer.
   D. shift captain.

_____ 19. The overriding objective for each rescue, transfer, and removal is to complete the process as
   A. quickly as possible.
   B. safely and efficiently as possible.
   C. a team.
   D. an integrated team.

_____ 20. In a vehicle accident, disentanglement is the process of
  A. cutting a vehicle away from the victim.
  B. removing the victim from the vehicle.
  C. cutting and removing the doors of the vehicle.
  D. establishing medical control of the victim.

_____ 21. When responding to an industrial facility, the IC should make contact with the
  A. business owner.
  B. property owner.
  C. responsible party.
  D. city office or administration.

_____ 22. The fire fighter should start compiling the facts about an incident from the
  A. captain.
  B. scene size-up.
  C. initial dispatch of the rescue call.
  D. technical rescue team specialists.

_____ 23. NIOSH reports that initial rescuers account for _____ percent of all confined space deaths.
  A. 25
  B. 50
  C. 60
  D. 80

_____ 24. All emergency service personnel at a rescue situation must
  A. constantly assess and reassess the scene.
  B. communicate with the victim(s).
  C. report directly to the incident commander.
  D. be prepared to assist with the technical rescue team.

_____ 25. What is the most common method of establishing the control zones for an emergency incident site?
  A. Barricades
  B. Pylons
  C. Chalk or paint lines
  D. Fire line tape

Vocabulary

Define the following terms using the space provided.

1. Lockout/tagout system:

   _____
   _____
   _____

2. Hazardous materials:

   _____
   _____
   _____

3. Technical rescue incident:

   _____
   _____
   _____

Fundamentals of Fire Fighter Skills

Fill-In

Read each item carefully, and then complete the statement by filling in the missing word(s).

1. Natural gas and liquefied petroleum gas are nontoxic, but are classified as _____ because they displace breathing air.

2. Information gathered _____ to the technical rescue team's arrival will save valuable time during the actual rescue.

3. _____ collapse is the sudden and unplanned collapse of part or all of a structure.

4. Once the rescue is complete, the scene must be _____ by the rescue crew to ensure that no one else becomes injured.

5. If you have the role of assisting a technical rescue team, _____ with the team is probably the most important thing you can do.

6. Scene control activities are sometimes assigned to _____ _____ personnel.

7. To ensure the safety of the rescuers, there must be a(n) _____ _____ _____ in place.

8. The _____ level of training provides an emphasis on recognizing the hazards, securing the scene, and calling for appropriate assistance.

9. It is extremely important that hazardous materials incident victims are _____ prior to transport.

10. To assist in more efficient communication with other rescuers, it is important to know the _____ used in the field.

11. The process of preparing the victim for transport is called _____.

12. A rescue area is an area that surrounds the incident site and whose size is _____ to the hazards that exist.

True/False

If you believe the statement to be more true than false, write the letter "T" in the space provided. If you believe the statement to be more false than true, write the letter "F."

1. _____ Without a solid command structure, it will be difficult to ensure the safety of the rescuers.

2. _____ Rescue efforts often require a small, focused group of individuals to complete the operation.

3. _____ During water rescue incidents, all responders within 10 ft (3 m) of the water must wear an approved personal flotation device.

4. _____ During a rescue, a team member should remain with the victim to direct the rescuers performing disentanglement.

5. _____ Any machine that is involved in a machinery rescue should be considered electrically charged.

6. _____ Wilderness search and rescue incidents are an example of a situation where it is acceptable for searchers to work separately.

7. _____ To assist a victim in remaining calm, you should communicate calmly, at a level that the victim can understand.

8. _____ Tagout procedures are used for personnel accountability.

9. _____ The best way to prepare for the next rescue call is to review the last one.

10. _____ Rescue situations have many hidden hazards.

Short Answer
Complete this section with short written answers using the space provided.

1. List the three types of control zones that should be established at an incident.

2. List the five guidelines that a fire fighter should follow when assisting rescue team members.

3. Identify the paramilitary guidelines for which a fire fighter must have a strong appreciation in order to understand the command and control concept of fire departments.

4. Identify the components of the acronym "FAILURE" used to describe why rescuers fail.

5. Identify five (5) of the types of special rescues encountered by fire fighters.

Fire Alarms

The following real case scenarios will give you an opportunity to explore the concerns associated with assisting special rescue teams. Read each scenario, and then answer each question in detail.

1. Your company is dispatched to a trench collapse where a worker is trapped. How should you make a safe approach to the collapse zone?

   _____
   _____
   _____
   _____
   _____
   _____

2. Your company has been dispatched to a call of wires down, with an individual who is conscious and inside a vehicle that has come in contact with the downed wires. There are several citizens in the immediate area. Your company officer has ordered you to secure the scene and establish a barrier. How should you accomplish these orders?

   _____
   _____
   _____
   _____
   _____
   _____
   _____
   _____

Skill Drills

Skill Drill 25-1: Establishing a Barrier Fire Fighter II, NFPA 1001: 5.4.2
Test your knowledge of this skill drill by filling in the correct words in the photo captions.

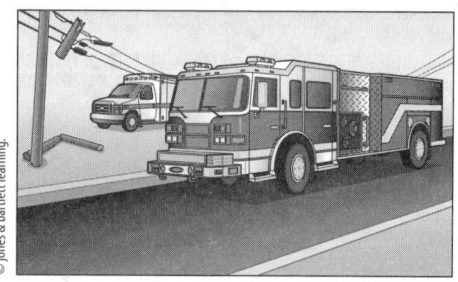

Respond safely to the emergency scene. Place the emergency vehicle in a _____ position that protects the scene. Don the appropriate PPE.

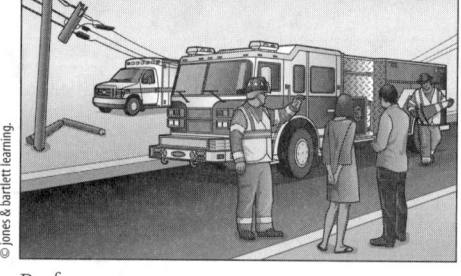

Perform a _____-_____ to assess for hazards. Secure the scene.

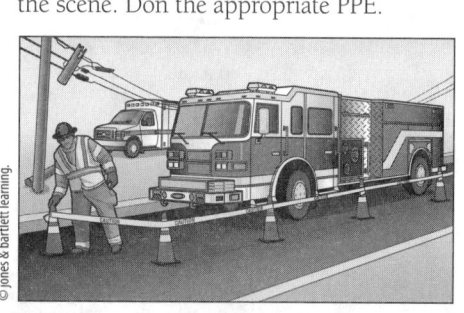

Call for needed assistance. Use appropriate devices to establish a _____, following the orders of the IC.

Skill Drill 25-3: Conducting a Weekly/Monthly Generator Test Fire Fighter II, NFPA 1001:5.5.4

Test your knowledge of this skill drill by placing the photos below in the correct order. Number the first step with a "1," the second step with a "2," and so on.

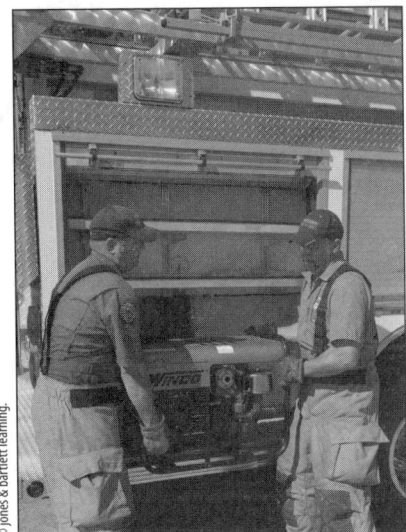

_____ Remove the generator from the apparatus compartment, or open all doors as needed for ventilation. Install the grounding rod, if needed.

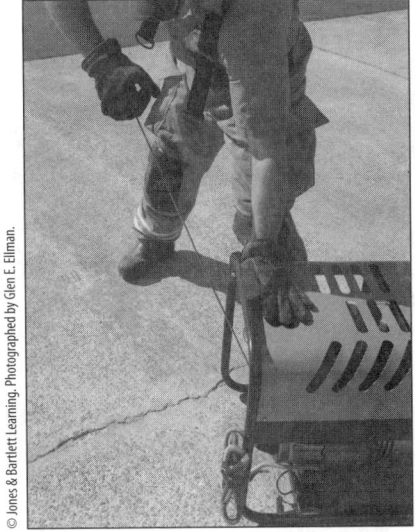

_____ Run the generator under load for 15 to 30 minutes. Turn off the load, and listen as the generator slows down to idle speed. Allow the generator to idle for approximately 2 minutes before turning it off. Disconnect all power cords and junction boxes; clean all power cords, plugs, adaptors, GFCIs, and tools; and replace them in proper storage areas. Allow the generator to cool for 5 minutes. Refill the generator with fuel and oil, as needed, and return the generator to its compartment. Fill out the appropriate paperwork.

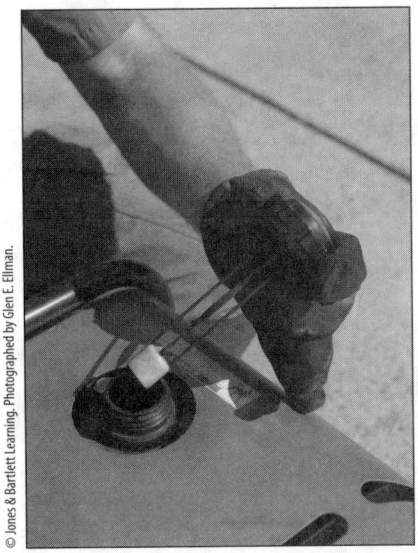

_____ Check the oil and fuel levels, and start the generator. Connect the power cord or junction box to the generator, connect a load such as a fan or lights, and make sure the generator attains the proper speed. Check the voltage and amperage gauges to confirm efficient operation.

Fire Detection, Suppression, and Smoke Control Systems

Workbook Activities

The following activities have been designed to help you. Your instructor may require you to complete some or all of these activities as a regular part of your fire fighter training program. You are encouraged to complete any activity your instructor does not assign you, as a way to enhance your learning in the classroom.

Chapter Review

The following exercises provide an opportunity to refresh your knowledge of this chapter. All questions in this chapter are Fire Fighter II level.

Matching

Match each of the terms in the left column to the appropriate definition in the right column.

_____ 1. Cross-zoned system   **A.** The valve assembly on a dry sprinkler system that prevents water from entering the system until the air pressure is released

_____ 2. False alarm   **B.** A sprinkler head usually marked SSU

_____ 3. Early suppression fast response sprinkler head   **C.** A sprinkler system in which the pipes are normally filled with water

_____ 4. OS&Y valve   **D.** A sprinkler head designed to react quickly and suppress a fire in its early stages

_____ 5. Dry-pipe valve   **E.** A device that increases the removal of the air from a dry-pipe or preaction sprinkler system

_____ 6. Upright sprinkler head   **F.** A sprinkler control valve with a valve stem that moves in and out as the valve is opened or closed

_____ 7. Gas detector   **G.** The activation of a fire alarm system when there is no fire or emergency condition

_____ 8. Accelerator   **H.** A fire alarm system that requires activation of two separate detection devices before initiating an alarm

_____ 9. Nuisance alarm   **I.** A device that measures the concentration of dangerous gases

_____ 10. Wet sprinkler system   **J.** A device within a piping system that allows water to flow in only one direction

_____ 11. Line detector   **K.** A standard fire alarm audible signal for alerting occupants of a building

_____ 12. Clapper mechanism   **L.** Wire or tubing that can be strung along the ceiling of large open areas to detect an increase in heat

_____ 13. Temporal-3 pattern   **M.** A fire alarm signal caused by malfunction or improper operation of a fire alarm system or component

_____ 14. Deluge head   **N.** A sprinkler head that has no release mechanism

CHAPTER 26

Multiple Choice

Read each item carefully, and then select the best response.

_____ 1. Which of the following is the name for a special extinguishing system that operates by discharging a gaseous agent into the atmosphere at a concentration that will extinguish a fire?
   A. Wet chemical extinguishing system
   B. Clean agent extinguishing system
   C. Dry chemical extinguishing system
   D. Carbon dioxide extinguishing system

_____ 2. Which type of sprinkler head has a glass bulb filled with glycerin to hold the cap in place?
   A. Fusible-link sprinkler head
   B. Chemical-pellet sprinkler head
   C. Deluge head
   D. Frangible-bulb sprinkler head

_____ 3. The network of pipes and outlets for fire hoses built into a structure and designed for use by the building occupants is designated
   A. Class I.
   B. Class II.
   C. Class III.
   D. Class IV.

_____ 4. The most current codes require new homes to have a smoke alarm
   A. on every floor.
   B. in every room.
   C. in every bedroom and on every floor level.
   D. in every bedroom, hallway, and floor level.

_____ 5. To allow the fire department's engine to pump water into the sprinkler system, each sprinkler system should also have a
   A. primary feeder.
   B. secondary feeder.
   C. pumper outlet.
   D. fire department connection.

_____ 6. A network of pipes and outlets for fire hoses built into a structure to provide water for firefighting purposes is called a
   A. residential pipe system.
   B. grid system.
   C. standpipe system.
   D. closed flow system.

_____ 7. Fire alarm systems are activated by the
   A. remote annunciator.
   B. ESFR device.
   C. alarm initiation device.
   D. line detector.

_____ 8. Which type of valve is mounted on the outside wall of a building?
   A. PIV
   B. OS&Y valve
   C. WPIV
   D. Support control valve

_____ 9. In most cases, the entire sprinkler system can be shut down by
   A. closing the main control valve.
   B. using the remote annunciator panel.
   C. deactivating the alarm.
   D. using a sprinkler wedge.

_____ 10. Which type of detectors are triggered by the invisible products of combustion?
   A. Ionization smoke detectors
   B. Photoelectric smoke detectors
   C. Heat detectors
   D. Spot detectors

_____ 11. Which type of detectors detect the electromagnetic light waves produced by a flame?
   A. Beam detectors
   B. Line detectors
   C. Air sampling detectors
   D. Flame detectors

_____ 12. Most modern sprinkler systems are connected to the building's fire alarm system to alert the occupants by a pressure switch or a
   A. tamper switch.
   B. flow switch.
   C. clapper switch.
   D. trigger switch.

_____ 13. Which type of sprinkler head is triggered by the melting of a metal alloy at a specific temperature?
   A. Fusible-link sprinkler head
   B. Frangible-bulb sprinkler head
   C. ESFR sprinkler head
   D. Pendant sprinkler head

_____ 14. Which type of fire alarm requires two steps before the alarm will activate?
   A. Single-action pull-station
   B. Double-action pull-station
   C. Protected pull-station
   D. Tamper alarm

_____ 15. The temporal-3 pattern is a(n)
   A. verification system.
   B. standardized audio pattern.
   C. alarm activation system.
   D. photoelectric detector system.

_____ 16. A smoke detector is designed to sense the presence of
   A. smoke.
   B. heat.
   C. fire.
   D. toxic gases.

_____ 17. The activation of a single smoke detector plus the activation of a second smoke detector is characteristic of a
   A. double-pull alarm system.
   B. verification system.
   C. cross-zoned system.
   D. nuisance system.

_____ 18. Which type of detectors are calibrated to detect the presence of a specific gas that is created by combustion?
   A. Gas detectors
   B. Combustion detectors
   C. Beam detectors
   D. Rate-of-calibration detectors

_____ 19. Which type of detectors use wire or tubing strung along the ceiling of large open areas to detect an increase in heat?
   A. Spot detectors
   B. Heat detectors
   C. Beam detectors
   D. Line detectors

_____ 20. Many buildings have an additional fire alarm control display panel in the front of the building called a
   A. remote alarm station.
   B. remote control panel.
   C. remote annunciator.
   D. remote visual board.

Labeling

Label each photo with the correct term.

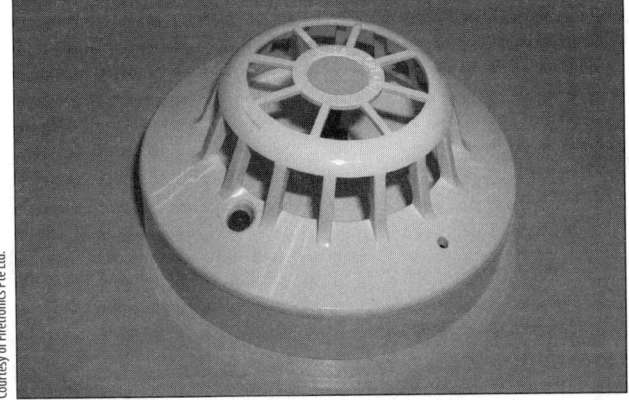

1. _____   2. _____

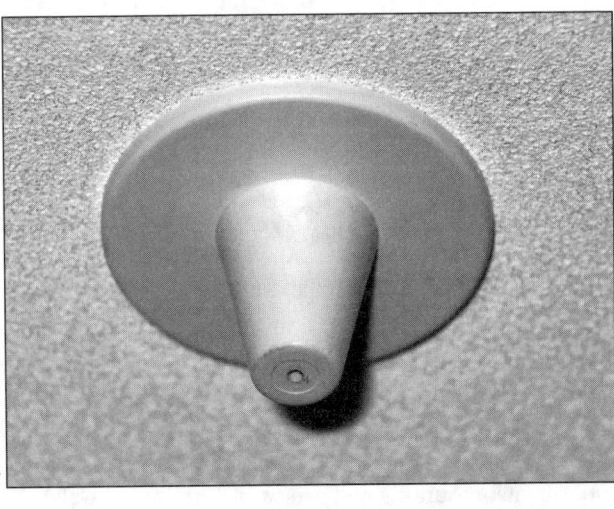

3. _____   4. _____

Fundamentals of Fire Fighter Skills

Vocabulary

Define the following terms using the space provided.

1. Zoned system:

   _____
   _____
   _____

2. Deluge sprinkler system:

   _____
   _____
   _____

3. Smoke control system:

   _____
   _____
   _____

4. Clean agent extinguishing system:

   _____
   _____
   _____

5. Fire department connection:

   _____
   _____
   _____

Fill-In

Read each item carefully, and then complete the statement by filling in the missing word(s).

1. A(n) _____ suppression system is often installed in areas where computers or sensitive electronic equipment is used.

2. The Class _____ standpipe is designed for use by fire department personnel only.

3. A(n) _____ detector is a type of photoelectric smoke detector used to protect large open areas.

4. The network of pipes that delivers water through the sprinkler system is the sprinkler _____.

5. A(n) _____ _____ system sends a signal directly to the fire department or to a monitoring location via telephone or radio signal.

6. _____ sprinkler heads are designed for horizontal mounting and projecting out from a wall.

7. Sprinkler heads are rated according to their _____ temperature.

8. _____ _____ _____ heat detectors will be activated if the temperature of the surrounding air rises more than a set amount in a given time period.

9. The fire alarm control panel should monitor the entire alarm system to detect any_____.

10. _____ smoke control uses building features such as fire-rated walls and draft curtains to limit the spread of smoke.

True/False

If you believe the statement to be more true than false, write the letter "T" in the space provided. If you believe the statement to be more false than true, write the letter "F."

1. _____ An activated alarm sounds throughout a building.
2. _____ Smoke alarms can be either hard-wired to a 110-volt electrical system or battery operated.
3. _____ All sprinkler systems should be equipped with a method for sounding an alarm whenever there is water flowing in the pipes.
4. _____ Fire alarm systems can control doors and elevators.
5. _____ An activated sprinkler head in an automatic sprinkler system triggers the water-motor gong.
6. _____ A photoelectric detector has a small amount of radioactive material inside a chamber.
7. _____ A central station is operated by the fire department.
8. _____ Bimetallic strips are made to respond to a rapid increase in temperature.
9. _____ Heat detectors provide reliable life-safety protection.
10. _____ Nuisance alarms are caused by individuals who deliberately activate fire alarms when there is no fire.

Short Answer

Complete this section with short written answers using the space provided.

1. List the five fire department notification systems.

   _____
   _____
   _____
   _____

2. Identify the three fire suppression systems.

   _____
   _____
   _____
   _____

3. Identify the four categories of sprinkler systems and provide a brief description of each category.

4. Identify the three categories of standpipes, with a description of their intended use.

5. List the variations that are different in a residential sprinkler system compared to a commercial system.

Fire Alarms

The following real case scenarios will give you an opportunity to explore the concerns associated with fire protection, suppression, and detection systems. Read each scenario, and then answer each question in detail.

1. It is 10:00 on a Wednesday morning when your engine is dispatched to deal with an alarm activation at an office building. You and the crew check the annunciator panel. The annunciator indicates that the carbon dioxide extinguishing system has been activated in the computer server room. One of the managers of the company meets you at the door and reports that light smoke was seen in the server room. What are the special hazards of a carbon dioxide extinguishing system?

2. It is Sunday morning and you have completed checking the apparatus. Your Lieutenant calls the crew together for a practice drill. She tells you that the drill will familiarize you with the fire suppression system at the new city courthouse. The fire suppression system at the courthouse has a supplied wet sprinkler system with fire department connections. Why is it important for fire fighters to have a basic understanding of fire suppression systems?

_____
_____
_____
_____
_____

Fire and Life Safety Initiatives

Workbook Activities

The following activities have been designed to help you. Your instructor may require you to complete some or all of these activities as a regular part of your fire fighter training program. You are encouraged to complete any activity your instructor does not assign you, as a way to enhance your learning in the classroom.

Chapter Review

The following exercises provide an opportunity to refresh your knowledge of this chapter. All questions in this chapter are Fire Fighter II level.

Matching

Match each of the terms in the left column to the appropriate definition in the right column.

_____ 1. Public education
_____ 2. Target hazard
_____ 3. EDITH
_____ 4. Static water supply
_____ 5. Stop, Drop, and Roll program
_____ 6. Horizontal evacuation
_____ 7. Fire prevention
_____ 8. Defend-in-place
_____ 9. Fire codes
_____ 10. Preincident planning

A. Instructs people on what to do if their clothing catches fire
B. A strategy of moving occupants from a dangerous area to a safe area
C. Teaches techniques to reduce fire deaths and injuries
D. Properties that pose an increased risk to fire fighters
E. A strategy in which victims are protected from the fire without relocation
F. Teaches residents how to get out of their homes safely during a fire or other emergency
G. The process of obtaining information about a building and storing the information in a system where it can be quickly retrieved
H. Regulations adopted to ensure a minimum level of fire safety
I. Examples include a lake or stream
J. Activities intended to prevent the outbreak of fires

Multiple Choice

Read each item carefully, and then select the best response.

_____ 1. Activities that are intended to help prevent the outbreak of fires or to limit the damage if a fire does occur are referred to as
   A. fire prevention.
   B. fire codes.
   C. fire regulations.
   D. public awareness.

CHAPTER 27

_____ 2. The preincident survey should be conducted in
   A. a systematic, uniform format.
   B. normal duty uniform.
   C. scheduled annual visits.
   D. teams of four.

_____ 3. Kitchen fires are responsible for _____ percent of all residential fires.
   A. 8
   B. 22
   C. 47
   D. 62

_____ 4. The most challenging problem during an emergency incident at a healthcare facility is
   A. the limited access to patients.
   B. the limitations of the floor plans.
   C. protecting nonambulatory patients.
   D. negotiating traffic en route to the facility.

_____ 5. The main objectives of fire prevention activities are to limit life loss, to prevent injuries, and to
   A. provide education.
   B. minimize property damage.
   C. provide an emergency response.
   D. avoid regulation infractions.

_____ 6. Lightweight construction
   A. can be found only in newer buildings.
   B. utilizes trusses as structural support.
   C. is the sturdiest of the newer construction types.
   D. is the most cost-effective type of construction.

_____ 7. Regulations that have been legally adopted by a government body with the authority to pass laws and enforce safety regulations are called
   A. fire bylaws.
   B. jurisdictional laws.
   C. jurisdictional regulations.
   D. fire codes.

_____ 8. The classifications of buildings by major use group include
   A. lightweight, tested development, heavyweight, open.
   B. public assembly, institutional, commercial, industrial.
   C. renovated private, renovated public, commercial development, industrial.
   D. public assembly, institutional, commercial.

_____ 9. Accumulated trash and a visible house number should be checked during the
   A. walk-by assessment.
   B. interior survey.
   C. exterior survey.
   D. home escape plan.

_____ 10. Facility security and personnel safety are both major concerns at
   A. schools and daycare.
   B. hospitals and nursing homes.
   C. residential occupancies.
   D. detention and correctional facilities.

_____ 11. Which of the following is a set of documents from the National Fire Protection Association that is intended to address a wide range of issues relating to fire and safety?
   A. National Fire Codes
   B. National Training Standards
   C. Jurisdictional Regulations
   D. Recommended Building Safety Codes

_____ 12. Drafting sites should be included in a preincident plan because they identify
   A. which adjoining structures are most susceptible to fire spread.
   B. open areas that can trap fire fighters.
   C. the best routes for ventilation.
   D. locations where an engine can draft water directly from a static source.

_____ 13. A voluntary inspection of a private dwelling is called a
   A. fire department visitation.
   B. public fire safety inspection.
   C. legal requirement.
   D. home fire safety survey.

_____ 14. A preincident plan should include information about
   A. a building's floor plan.
   B. entrance and exit locations.
   C. hazardous materials stored in the building.
   D. all of the above.

_____ 15. A comprehensive all-hazard approach to community programs to prevent the loss of life or property is known as
   A. All Hazard Planning.
   B. Community Risk Reduction.
   C. Community Prevention Planning.
   D. Master Risk Reduction.

_____ 16. The primary role of a fire alarm system is to
   A. alert the occupants of a building when an incident occurs.
   B. alert the fire department of an incident.
   C. meet safety standards of the building code.
   D. all of the above.

_____ 17. Helping people to understand how to prevent fires from occurring and teaching them how to react if a fire does occur are the goals of
   A. local governments.
   B. fire departments.
   C. public fire safety education.
   D. teachers.

_____ 18. The five types of building construction, in descending order of fire resistance, are
   A. fire resistive, noncombustible, ordinary, heavy timber, wood frame.
   B. ordinary, noncombustible, fire resistive, wood frame, heavy timber.
   C. fire resistive, noncombustible, ordinary, wood timber, heavy frame.
   D. ordinary, fire resistive, noncombustible, wood frame, heavy timber.

_____ 19. The primary causes of fires in living rooms include electrical equipment and
   A. smoking.
   B. children playing with matches.
   C. storage of combustible or flammable materials.
   D. unattended cooking food.

_____ 20. Horizontal ventilation can be accessed through
   A. windows and doors.
   B. windows and chimneys.
   C. ceiling and pressure fans.
   D. windows and skylights.

Vocabulary

Define the following terms using the space provided.

1. Community risk reduction (CRR):

   _____

   _____

   _____

2. Fire codes:

   _____

   _____

   _____

3. Exit Drills In The Home (E.D.I.T.H.):

   _____

   _____

   _____

4. Fire safety survey:

   _____

   _____

   _____

5. Conflagration:

   _____

   _____

   _____

6. Preincident plan:

   _____

   _____

   _____

346 FUNDAMENTALS OF FIRE FIGHTER SKILLS

7. Ordinary construction:

8. Exposure:

9. Defend-in-place:

10. Nonambulatory patient:

Fill-In
Read each item carefully, and then complete the statement by filling in the missing word(s).

1. Teach students to use the back of a(n) _____ to sense the temperature of a door.

2. _____ are installed in high-rise buildings to eliminate the need to extend hose lines from a pumper at the street level up to the fire level.

3. Your highest priority as a fire fighter should always be to _____ fires.

4. Moving patients from a dangerous area to a safer area on the same floor is known as _____ evacuation.

5. Home fire safety surveys should be conducted in a(n) _____ fashion for both the inside and outside of the home.

6. Schools and hospitals are in the _____ major use classification.

7. Fire fighters should stress the importance of keeping _____ in working order.

8. The preincident survey should consider both _____ and _____ access problems.

9. Citizens have a(n) _____ obligation to comply with the fire codes.

10. Wood-frame buildings are classified as Type _____.

True/False

If you believe the statement to be more true than false, write the letter "T" in the space provided. If you believe the statement to be more false than true, write the letter "F."

1. _____ Every kitchen should be equipped with an approved ABC-rated fire extinguisher.
2. _____ All properties have the potential to create a conflagration.
3. _____ Smoke alarms should be tested once a year using the test button.
4. _____ Wood-frame building construction has floors and walls made of combustible wood material.
5. _____ An EDITH presentation should include stressing the importance of sleeping with bedroom doors open.
6. _____ A target hazard is any property large enough to catch fire.
7. _____ Having working smoke alarms on each level of a home reduces the risk of death from fire by 80 percent.
8. _____ Potential natural barriers should be included in the preincident plan.
9. _____ Good housekeeping is one of the most important issues when addressing fire safety in garages and basements.
10. _____ Buildings with unprotected steel beams are considered Type I: Fire Resistive, according to NFPA220, *Standard on Types of Building Construction*.

Short Answer

Complete this section with short written answers using the space provided.

1. Identify five recommendations for kitchen safety.

   _____
   _____
   _____
   _____
   _____

2. List typical target hazard properties that may be found in the community.

   _____
   _____
   _____
   _____
   _____

3. Provide six examples of public fire safety education programs.

   _____
   _____
   _____
   _____
   _____

4. Describe the two Firefighter Life Safety Initiatives that relate specifically to public education and fire prevention.

___

5. List four of the issues that should be considered during preincident planning for water supply where no fire hydrants are available.

___

Fire Alarms

The following real case scenarios will give you an opportunity to explore the concerns associated with vehicle rescue and extrication. Read each scenario, and then answer each question in detail.

1. Your company has been assigned a list of buildings that must have a preincident survey conducted. As the rookie, you have been assigned the task of developing a plan for conducting each survey. Which steps should be used for conducting a good preincident survey?

___

2. You are in the middle of a home fire safety survey of a private home. So far, the survey is going well. You enter the basement and notice that the occupant is storing five full gasoline cans next to the gas water heater. How should you proceed?

_____
_____
_____
_____
_____
_____

Fire Origin and Cause

Workbook Activities

The following activities have been designed to help you. Your instructor may require you to complete some or all of these activities as a regular part of your fire fighter training program. You are encouraged to complete any activity your instructor does not assign you, as a way to enhance your learning in the classroom.

Chapter Review

The following exercises provide an opportunity to refresh your knowledge of this chapter.

Matching

Match each of the terms in the left column to the appropriate definition in the right column.

_____ 1. Ignitable liquid   A. Intentionally set fires

_____ 2. Undetermined   B. Fire cause classification that includes fires for which the cause has not been or cannot be proven

_____ 3. Contaminated   C. Evidence that is reported first-hand

_____ 4. Incendiary fires   D. Person who sets three or more fires near the same location in a limited period

_____ 5. Mass arsonist   E. Items that can be examined in a laboratory and presented in court to prove or demonstrate a point

_____ 6. Arsonist   F. Classification for liquid fuels including both flammable and combustible liquids

_____ 7. Circumstantial evidence G. A term used to describe evidence that may have been altered from its original state

_____ 8. Demonstrative evidence   H. A person who deliberately sets a fire to destroy property with criminal intent

_____ 9. Direct evidence   I. The means by which alleged facts are proven by deduction or inference from other facts that were observed first hand

_____ 10. Physical evidence   J. Evidence that can be used to validate a theory

Multiple Choice

Read each item carefully, and then select the best response.

_____ 1. The NFPA standard that establishes the guidelines for fire and explosion investigations, is NFPA
   A. 921.
   B. 1403.
   C. 1500.
   D. 1671.

CHAPTER 28

_____ 2. If a fire intensifies in a short period of time, it may indicate
   A. poor dispatch information.
   B. the use of an accelerant.
   C. extreme weather conditions.
   D. multiple points of origin.

_____ 3. What might charring on the underside of a low horizontal surface, such as a tabletop, indicate?
   A. The fire's point of origin was on top of the surface.
   B. The fire was accidental.
   C. There was a pool of a flammable liquid.
   D. The fire started from a cigarette butt.

_____ 4. An ignition source that has enough energy and is capable of transferring that energy to the first fuel long enough to heat the fuel to its ignition temperature is known as a
   A. definitive ignition source.
   B. competent ignition source.
   C. circumstantial ignition source.
   D. primary ignition source.

_____ 5. An accelerant may have been used if the fire _____ when water is applied.
   A. spreads
   B. decreases
   C. is extinguished
   D. rekindles

_____ 6. The cause of a fire can be classified as either incendiary or
   A. malicious intent.
   B. criminal intent.
   C. undetermined.
   D. accidental.

_____ 7. Which of the following terms is used to describe a device or mechanism that is used to start a fire?
   A. Arsonist device
   B. Incendiary device
   C. Accelerant
   D. Trailer

_____ 8. In most jurisdictions, the _____ determines the cause of a fire.
   A. law enforcement agency
   B. chief of the fire department
   C. property owner
   D. fire investigator

_____ 9. A charred V-pattern on a wall indicates that fire spread
   A. along the floor before reaching the wall.
   B. up and out from an unknown material at the base of the V.
   C. along the ceiling before reaching the wall.
   D. slowly.

_____ 10. "Chain of custody" is a legal term that describes the process of maintaining continuous possession and control of evidence from
   A. the time it is discovered until it is presented in court.
   B. investigator to incident commander.
   C. investigator to law enforcement agency.
   D. discovery to isolation.

_____ 11. One of the first steps in a fire investigation is identifying the
   A. fuel supply.
   B. accelerants.
   C. point of origin.
   D. evidence.

_____ 12. An arson investigation must determine not only who was responsible for starting the fire but also
   A. why the person started the fire.
   B. when the person started the fire.
   C. the property damage caused by the fire.
   D. the cause and origin of the fire.

_____ 13. Child firesetters are children from the age of _____.
   A. 1 to 12
   B. 1 to 10
   C. 2 to 6
   D. 2 to 18

_____ 14. The process of carefully looking for evidence within the debris is referred to as
   A. layering.
   B. overhaul.
   C. evidence recovery.
   D. digging out.

_____ 15. An arsonist who sets three or more fires at separate locations with no emotional cooling-off period between fires is called a
   A. spree arsonist.
   B. serial arsonist.
   C. mass arsonist.
   D. motivated arsonist.

_____ 16. An arsonist who sets three or more fires, with a cooling-off period between fires, is called a
   A. spree arsonist.
   B. serial arsonist.
   C. mass arsonist.
   D. motivated arsonist.

_____ 17. Which category of youth firesetters frequently targets buildings such as churches, schools, or vacant homes?
   A. Serial
   B. Child
   C. Adolescent
   D. Juvenile

_____ 18. The fire department's authority over an incident ends when
   A. the property is formally released to the property owner.
   B. the property is under the investigator's supervision.
   C. any criminal or malicious intent regarding the fire's origin is ruled out.
   D. the property is secured and no hazards to public safety exist.

_____ 19. Which type of evidence can be used to prove a theory?
   A. Demonstrative evidence
   B. Trace evidence
   C. Circumstantial evidence
   D. Physical evidence

_____ 20. An arsonist who sets three or more fires at the same site or location during a limited period of time is called a
   A. spree arsonist.
   B. serial arsonist.
   C. mass arsonist.
   D. motivated arsonist.

Vocabulary
Define the following terms using the space provided.

1. Competent ignition source:
   _____
   _____
   _____

2. Chain of custody:
   _____
   _____
   _____

3. Trailers:
   _____
   _____
   _____

4. Depth of char:
   _____
   _____
   _____

Fill-In
Read each item carefully, and then complete the statement by filling in the missing word(s).

1. An arsonist may place _____ to hinder the efforts of fire fighters.

2. _____ removed from any victim should be preserved as evidence.

3. The _____ of any victims found in the building should be noted.

4. Smoke residue and _____ patterns can be helpful in identifying the point of origin.

5. Evidence should not be _____ or altered from its original state in any way.

6. What a fire fighter _____ during an incident could be significant in an investigation of an incident.

7. At the point of origin, an ignition source comes into contact with a(n) _____ _____.

8. Until the fire is under control, fire fighters must concentrate on fighting the fire and not investigating the _____.

9. The fire investigation process usually begins with an examination of the building's _____.

10. Anything that can be used to validate a theory is _____ evidence.

11. Insurance companies often investigate fires to determine the _____ of a claim.

12. A type of unwanted fire caused by earthquakes or tornadoes is known as _____ fires.

True/False

If you believe the statement to be more true than false, write the letter "T" in the space provided. If you believe the statement to be more false than true, write the letter "F."

1. _____ The appearance and behavior of people at the scene of a fire can provide valuable clues.
2. _____ A cause-and-origin investigation determines where, why, and how a fire originated.
3. _____ Evidence is most often found during the size-up phase of a fire.
4. _____ When a fire is determined to be accidental, the company officer is responsible for filing the necessary reports.
5. _____ Arsonists often open the shades and windows of structures they burn.
6. _____ Charring is usually deepest on the edges of the object.
7. _____ The color of the smoke often indicates what is burning.
8. _____ A fire can be caused by an act or by an omission.
9. _____ To avoid contaminating evidence, fire investigators always wash their tools between taking samples.
10. _____ Only one person should be responsible for collecting and taking custody of all evidence at a fire scene.

Short Answer

Complete this section with short written answers using the space provided.

1. List the three categories of youth firesetters, including the age range of each.

   _____
   _____
   _____
   _____

2. List the six common arson motives listed in NFPA 921, *Guide to Fire and Explosion Investigations*.

   _____
   _____
   _____
   _____

3. Identify the four classifications of fire cause.

   _____
   _____
   _____
   _____

4. Describe the six types of fire evidence.

_____
_____
_____
_____

Fire Alarms

The following real case scenarios will give you an opportunity to explore the concerns associated with fire cause determination. Read each scenario, and then answer each question in detail.

1. Your engine has responded to a structure fire in a church. A serial arsonist has been setting fire to churches in your community. This fire has some of the same characteristics as the other church fires. You and your partner confined the fire to the basement of the church. Now you and your partner have been assigned to help the fire investigator overhaul the fire scene. How should you proceed?

    _____
    _____
    _____
    _____
    _____
    _____

2. You are on the scene of a suspected arson at a waterfront restaurant. You are assigned to work with one of the arson investigators in your department to help collect and process possible evidence. How do you proceed?

    _____
    _____
    _____
    _____
    _____
    _____